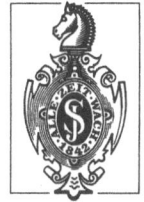

Susanne Klein-Vogelbach

Therapeutic Exercises in Functional Kinetics

Analysis and Instruction of Individually Adaptable Exercises

Foreword by W. M. Zinn

With 111 Figures
in 275 Separate Illustrations

Springer-Verlag
Berlin Heidelberg New York
London Paris Tokyo
Hong Kong Barcelona
Budapest

Dr. med. h. c. Susanne Klein-Vogelbach
Felixhäglistraße 12
CH-4103 Bottmingen, Switzerland

Translator:
Linda Sloan-Ecker
Sternwaldstraße 6
W-7800 Freiburg, FRG

Translation of the 2nd German edition:
Therapeutische Übungen zur funktionellen Bewegungslehre
© Springer-Verlag Berlin Heidelberg 1978, 1986

ISBN-13:978-3-540-52731-2   e-ISBN-13:978-3-642-75794-5
DOI: 10.1007/978-3-642-75794-5

21/3145-543210 – Printed on acid-free paper

Foreword

In these analyses and instructions for economical movement therapy, Dr. Klein-Vogelbach, for many years head of the Physiotherapy School of the Kantonsspital in Basel, presents the second part of her published work on the school of functional kinetics which is her creation. This is a system of physiotherapy that has grown out of creative observation and consistent, independent development, one that, in its manner of observing and interpreting human movement, I have long regarded as a fundamental contribution to physio- and ergotherapy.

Although no explicit references are cited, this work accords with the findings of modern neurophysiology and biomechanics in every field. Here I will mention only the preventive and therapeutic value of economical posture and movement, the conception of the human being as an organism constantly reacting to gravity and other external stimuli, the therapeutic use that is made of postural reflexes, and a multitude of other facilitation techniques.

Repetition of an exercise or any other performance of the central nervous system results not only in a reduction of resistance at the synapses of the feedback control through which the stimulation potentials pass – this is the physiological basis of all learning, without which there could be no development – but also, in addition to the specific targeted increase in strength and performance, in an additional, generalized global facilitation. Perception training, self-experience and other types of body image training are highly important elements of any therapy aimed at alleviating pain and normalizing disturbances in the human support and movement apparatus. Thus, functional kinetics and the exercises developed from it constitute a method which is likely to pass with flying colours the test of comparative studies with control groups of differently treated or even untreated patients which will be necessary before it can achieve universal recognition.

This book contains a series of exercise instructions for physiotherapists, and I can only recommend most urgently that referring doctors should read them too. Once again, the author's decades of study and work with her material have resulted in a concise but extremely dense, closely packed text which will require concentrated reading. The thoroughness of presentation gives therapists immediate access to meaningful, practical work and will allow them later to develop independently an unlimited and eminently individualizable exercise repertoire of their own. Special mention should be given here to the possibilities for physiotherapy in disorders of the spine and the shoulder and pelvic girdles, and the first logically constructed attempt to treat aerophagia: all methods whose value I can confirm after employing them for years in treating numerous patients in Bad Ragaz and Valens.

We rheumatologists too have been awaiting this book with impatience, and express our thanks to the author not merely for her important contribution to physio- and ergotherapy, but also for the great work she has taken on in addition in publishing her life's work in the service of our patients. A mastery of functional kinetics will allow therapists to understand the needs of sick and handicapped patients and to confine themselves to essentials. This will form a basis from which they can extend their knowledge of different specialties, such as proprioceptive neuromuscular facilitation, the treatment of rheumatic fever, psychosomatic disturbances or central and peripheral neurological symptoms, to name but a few. In this way, they will be helped to avoid the great temptation to one-sidedness by employing a variety of therapeutic methods, and to fulfil the requirements of the highest standards in their invaluable work.

Bad Ragaz, February 1978   W. M. Zinn

Preface to the English Edition

The best way to understand functional kinetics is by using it to treat patients. Practice was where it started; the theoretical underpinning followed later, when functional kinetics became a subject taught at training colleges. That, at any rate, is what happened in the German-speaking countries: in the English-speaking world it has yet to make its way.

The exercises presented here are models or norms: in practice, they need to be adapted to each individual patient, but without the goal of the exercise being lost. To overcome deficits in the patient's movement behaviour, it is not the patient who must adapt to the exercise, but the exercise which must be adapted to the patient. This is a challenge to the therapist that is demanding, but also stimulating. I hope that these therapeutic exercises will succeed in fascinating physiotherapists in the English-speaking world.

My thanks are due to all those mentioned in the prefaces to the German editions. For the English edition, special thanks go to: the translator, Linda Sloan-Ecker; Kersti Wagstaff, who edited the translation with me; and Elisabeth M. Bürge and Irene Gantert, who helped me in reading the English translation. At Springer-Verlag I have been cared for as sympathetically and patiently as always, and for this my warmest thanks go to Bernhard Lewerich, Marga Botsch (Medical Editorial I) and Heidrun Rieble (Book Production III).

Basel 1991   Susanne Klein-Vogelbach

Preface to the Second German Edition

Functional kinetics has made pleasing progress in the past few years. The number of people interested in further training in functional kinetics, the need to train instructors, and the recent appearance of functional kinetics on the basic training curriculum at many schools of physiotherapy mean that a clear presentation of this method is now needed that will help students towards observation and a treatment-oriented understanding of movement. To this end, the basic textbook, *Funtional Kinetics,* essential to an understanding of *Therapeutic Exercises,* was reissued in 1984 in a third, fully revised edition.

The analytical concept "actio-reactio, conditio-limitatio" has continued to prove its worth in *Ball Gymnastics in Functional Kinetics* (second edition 1985) and is beginning to become generally accepted. The movement analyses in this new edition of *Therapeutic Exercises* have therefore been revised in accordance with this concept. New exercises have been added: in particular, the treatment of posture-related syndromes of the vertebral column has been expanded and completed with a detailed and systematic presentation of the techniques of lift-free/reduced lift mobilization of the joints, especially those of the vertebral column, and mobilizing massage of the lumbar, thoracic and cervical areas.

The reward for all this work is that it is possible, using these movement analyses, to adapt every exercise and technique individually to each patient. Because the point of reference is always the normal movement behaviour of a healthy person, exercise programmes geared to particular pathologies become superfluous, and the danger of schematic treatment of a person, turned by the circumstance of illness into a patient, is avoided. The complexity of these movement analyses, on the other hand, is unavoidable – for normal movement is extremely subtle and finely differentiated.

This book is intended as the basic textbook for introducing functional kinetics into physiotherapeutic practice. For this reason an extensive reference list seemed unnecessary.

My warmest thanks are owed to Springer-Verlag for sympathetic guidance and collaboration, especially from Bernhard Lewerich and Ilse Wittig of Medical Editorial and J. Sydor of Book Production. Sincere thanks go also to Katrin Eicke-Wieser, who read through the whole manuscript with great care; her constructive criticism corrected many oversights and improved the clarity of the text in many places.

In addition, I should like to thank the models, Vreny Lüscher, Beatrix Lütof-Keller, Margrit Meier-Waldstein and Isabelle Gloor-Marconi, the photographer, Dietmar Hund (Kantonsspital Basel), Foto Fetzer (Bad Ragaz), Foto Zimmer, Cécile Zimmer (Basel), and the graphics artist, Holger Hammerich (Basel).

Basel, June 1986   Susanne Klein-Vogelbach

Preface to the First German Edition

A normal child learns during the early years of its life how to walk, talk and use its hands. For this it needs no other teacher than its environment, which allows the child to develop according to its own natural tendencies and the stimuli around it, and, through endless repetition, to organize the messages it receives. If the child wants to acquire particular skills, however, such as playing a musical instrument, hard work and endurance are needed, and, if possible, a competent teacher. But these alone are not enough to achieve the exceptional. The potential contained in the child's innate gifts also defines the child's limits and possibilities. There are many ways of fostering talent, but none of creating it.

A patient doing a Therapeutic Exercise for medical reasons finds himself in the position of wanting to acquire a physical skill for which he has no talent. In other words, even the ideal, most cooperative, best motivated patient, no matter how hard and determinedly he works, will be able to achieve no better than a "good average" with his Therapeutic Exercise. In therapy he will have to come to terms, perhaps for the first time consciously, with a painful discovery: that things that one finds difficult because one has no talent for them, and which one – for whatever reason – tries hard at, never earn much praise from comparative criticism, while things that one finds easy, having a gift for them, earn admiration and are often praised even when one puts no particular effort into them.

Being confronted in therapy with his own difficulties in movement, the patient finds that he has to learn by self-experience to recognize and demand his own best, within the range of his own possibilities. Comparisons with "the others", whom he perhaps admires and envies, are something he has to accept and cope with.

The therapist, on the other hand, should be able to give a just evaluation of the patient's achievement. She knows how much continuous effort and patience he has to put into reducing the gap between his motor behaviour and the "good average". That hard work deserves praise and confirmation, and the therapist is the person of reference who should provide both. Pleasure in the confirmation he has earned and honest assessment of his motor behaviour will help the patient to both learn and perceive more quickly. When he perceives and understands his motor behaviour, he will find it easier to accept his handicap with equanimity. If this self-motivation succeeds in firing the patient to work constantly at his motor behaviour, he will also find the way to plan and shape his own reality economically and to live it with his own particular vitality.

Basel, February 1978   Susanne Klein-Vogelbach

Contents

Note on Pronouns

For clarity and brevity, "she" has been assigned to the physiotherapist throughout, and "he" to the patient.

Definition

Therapeutic Exercises are carefully targeted and planned sequences of movement or of changes in activity designed to demarcate and isolate a defined functional deficit in motor behaviour in such a way that avoidance mechanisms are ruled out and the desired function necessarily arises in response to a clear stimulus.

Note

- A Therapeutic Exercise is useful if, through being performed with precision, it achieves its goal.
- All Therapeutic Exercises need to be made automatic by frequent repetition.
- Regular repetition of a Therapeutic Exercise once automated reduces the functional deficit.
- The self-monitoring required of the patient in Therapeutic Exercises, by conscious awareness and perception of movements and activities, is quite high.
- Therapeutic Exercises are uncomfortable because they emphasize the weaknesses in motor behaviour.
- A badly performed Therapeutic Exercise is useless and may even be harmful.
- It is characteristic of Therapeutic Exercises that they can rarely be performed spontaneously.

General Introduction

The goal of this book is to enable the therapist to set up instructions for model Therapeutic Exercises that solve a defined movement problem and can in addition be varied in adaptation to the patient's constitution and condition.

The path towards this goal starts with definition of the movement problem, by determining the patient's "functional status". If the damage to the motor behaviour is reversible, the therapist aims at regaining normal motor behaviour. If the damage is irreversible, she aims at the best compromise possible. The next step is to choose as a model a Therapeutic Exercise suitable for resolution of the defined functional problem.

Functional movement therapy can also take the form of *manipulation*. There are many kinds of manual techniques. A physiotherapist should have as many of these as possible at her command, so that she can choose one specifically for each patient or combine several techniques. Manual techniques are used to try to elicit particular functional reactions from the patient. Sensitive manipulation gives the patient training in kinaesthetic and tactile perception, through which he experiences – i. e. feels – new movement situations. The success of these techniques depends chiefly on the professionalism and craftmanship of the therapist. Therapy should start to show success before the end of the treatment period.

Manipulation has various forms, for example:
- Manual working of tissues
- Resistance offered by the therapist, allowing the patient to hang from her
- Support offered by the therapist, allowing the patient to use her as a support area
- Manipulation by the therapist of a change in the position of the patient's axes of movement in relation to gravity.

Functional movement therapy can also take the form of *verbal instruction*. The therapist must have an understanding of how to teach by verbal instruction. Whether she has this or not will be shown by whether she succeeds in eliciting the movement she wants and – what is more important – in winning the patient's co-operation in doing so.

Training the patient's perceptive capacities is essential for his self-experience of his own body in movement and at rest. This is the key to motivation of the patient and thus also essential for precisely targeted movement therapy. The less a patient realizes his movement deficit, and the less pain he has, the more difficult it is to motivate him in therapy.

Obviously, the manipulative and verbal methods of movement training are inseparable and often overlap. As long as the therapist continues to work with the patient, she will always be using both.

Principles of Movement Training

- A person's motor behaviour reflects both his physical and his psychological condition.
- Normal motor behaviour is beyond the conscious control of the individual.
- The attempt to consciously control or direct motor behaviour results in hyperactivity and may easily lead to tenseness of posture and movement.
- Posture is affected by many things. It is on the one hand an expression of personality, but it also constitutes a complex reaction to a multitude of influences from the environment.
- Sequences of movement can be practised. Obviously, a person is always practising movement as long as he goes on moving. All the therapist has to do, therefore, is to direct this constant practice into the right channels.
- Posture is a physiological and psychological phenomenon. All normal people have a natural talent for posture and movement. This talent is best trained by specific, finely differentiated processes of perception. The patient therefore has to be motivated to self-education through self-experience in motor behaviour. What will win him over is discovering, first, that he has a talent for movement, secondly, that practising movement can be fun – even fascinating – and, thirdly, that he feels better for it.

Teaching the patient to enjoy practising posture and movement is a top priority for the therapist. Playing is fun, so she has to awaken the patient's sense of play.

The changes regarded as necessary in the patient's motor behaviour should be practised until the patient can reproduce them automatically. During the learning process, however, the control of the movements must be made conscious through appropriate perceptual signals. It is important for the instruction to appeal to movement reactions that are already tendentially present and can therefore be "called upon". How far this is successful depends on the therapist's ability to engage the patient's perceptual capacity, imagination and feel for melody and rhythm.

- The patient will recognize successful normalization of his motor behaviour as a kind of "anti-stress condition". This condition can only be called "relaxed" if that word is used to mean "*as much* or *as little* activity *as is necessary* for a particular posture or movement". This is the condition of economical activity.
- Having felt the condition of wellbeing which we have just defined as economical activity, and having acquired the ability to call up this condition, the patient feels a need to reproduce it when its loss forces itself upon his awareness through tension, pain, lack of strength or unexplained tiredness. The surest way to motivate a patient to self-education in motor behaviour is by helping him, via his potential for kinaesthetic and tactile perception, to experience economical activity in posture and movement.

Therapeutic Exercises

The first essential for successful therapeutic exercising is to choose a suitable Exercise as a model for the solution of the functional problem in hand and to adapt this model to the patient's *condition, constitution, postural statics* and *mobility*.

A functionally trained therapist will always know or be able to invent suitable models for Therapeutic Exercises once she has identified the existing functional problem.

A patient's somatic and psychological *condition* will alter during the course of treatment. For this reason, one must always be prepared to readapt the exercise. Functional therapy of patients who have recently undergone surgery or are suffering acute pain or are in a state of depression will be different to the therapy given at a later point when the patient's condition has changed. A major change in weight, growth in a child or adolescent, or the ageing process can all have a considerable effect on movement sequences.

The patient's *constitution* is a constant, requiring, if any, a basic, once-for-all adaptation of the exercise to the patient.

The way in which the patient's *postural statics* deviate from the norm show the "deficit" in his motor behaviour. This "deficit" is the visible functional problem to be treated.

Mobility has constitutional and conditional elements which must be registered separately. *Constitution* governs the patient's general mobility, while *conditional* elements include the many possible pathological changes in motor behaviour. *Conditional and constitutional mobility* together determine the best variant of adaptation of the model of a Therapeutic Exercise. *Condition, postural statics* and *condition-determined mobility* – or restrictions of mobility – define the rate at which an exercise is taught and learnt: how big each step in learning is and how long is spent on one step before passing to the next. The therapist chooses her verbal and manipulative cues according to these considerations.

Setting Up a Therapeutic Exercise

This book shows you how to:
– Define Therapeutic Exercises by functional analysis
– Set out instructions for Therapeutic Exercises that can be followed by anyone interested in doing so.

■ Goal of the Exercise

Resolution or partial resolution of the defined functional problem and incorporation of the individually adapted Exercise into the patient's motor behaviour.

▶ Functional Analysis in Therapist Language

● Conception of the Exercise

● Position and Activation in the Starting Position

Position in space of the critical axes
Points of contact between the body and the environment
Components of movement in relation to the neutral position of the joints

Movement tolerances at the critical joints in relation to the intended primary movement

Distribution of body weight on a base support or suspension device, against a supportive device, or over a support area, and the resulting activity states of the musculature

Intensity of muscle activity required with economical activity; respiration

Potential accelerating and braking weights in relation to the intended primary movement

● Actio–Reactio of the Movement Sequence

Actio: The primary movement
Reactio: Activated passive buttressing
Reactio: Change in the support area

Actio: Accelerating weights
Reactio: Braking weights

● Conditio–Limitatio of the Movement Sequence

Conditio: Constant distances between body distance points
Limitatio: Active buttressing and stabilization

Conditio of absolute and/or relative fixed spatial points
Limitatio through limiting the primary movement, activated passive buttressing and/or change in the support area

Conditio of movement speed
Limitatio of economical activity by finding the optimal speed

● Position and Activation of the End Position and Return to the Starting Position

▶ Instruction in Patient Language

● **Instruction Appealing to the Patient's Perception**

● **Verbal Instruction**

● **Instruction by Manipulation**

▶ Adapting the Exercise to the Patient's Constitution and Condition

● **Adaptation to Constitution: Role of Lengths, Widths, Depths and Distribution of Weights**

● **Adaptation to Condition**

Poor physical fitness or wish to increase performance

Pain arising during the exercise a contraindication

Muscular weakness or depressed reactivity; adaptation of lifting strain and/or extent and/or speed of movement

Restricted movement or hypermobility

Movement disorders originating in the central nervous system

1 The Frogs: Functional Training of the Abdominal Muscles

Functional training of the abdominal muscles activates the abdominal muscles as for their normal physiological function.

Note

Functional training of the abdominal muscles is not training for strength through the employment of drastic increases in load (e.g., lifting the extended legs from supine), but a method of training in fine skill through the economical employment of strength at the right moment.

The goal is for the abdominal muscles to contract according to the following functional principles:

- When the upper abdominals contract, the epigastric angle should narrow but the distance from distance point (DP) navel to DP xiphoid process remains the same. The *upper abdomen becomes narrow*. The activity of the oblique abdominal muscles pulls the ribs down. This necessitates active buttressing by extensional stabilization of the thoracic spine in the neutral position.
- When the lower abdominals contract, the distance from DP navel to DP symphysis becomes shorter. The *lower abdomen becomes short.* The activity of the rectus abdominis muscle causes the lumbar spine to flex, enhancing the motive components of these muscles.

Functional training of the abdominal muscles requires the involvement of all the numerous switchpoints of movement affected by the activity of these muscles.

Function of the Abdominal Muscles

The abdominal muscles regulate pressure inside the abdomen:
- They should be able to react to different abdominal contents, e. g., the fetus during pregnancy, adipose tissue in cases of obesity, or food during digestion.
- They should be able to compensate for constitutional variations of the shape of the pelvis and lumbar spine and for postural variations of the position of the pelvis in the hip joints.

The abdominal muscles are involved in respiration :
- During inspiration, the increased tone in the abdominal wall acts as a buttress against the diaphragm as it flattens out by contraction in the subphrenic space.

– In prolonged expiration, the abdominal muscles are activated in concentric-isotonic work, which is coordinated with the buttressing extensional stabilization of the thoracic spine.

The abdominal muscles help to stabilize the long axis of the body during equilibrium reactions, particularly by rotational movement components in the spinal column.

The abdominal muscles participate in equilibrium movements of the pelvis in the hip joints by extensional, flexional and lateroflexional movement components in the lumbar spine.

The abdominal muscles are also involved in all movements of the extremities, coordinating the effects of these movements on body segments (BSs) thorax and pelvis. They are particularly involved in lifting of the legs by flexion at the hips.

Position in Space of the Long Axis of the Body During Training of the Abdominal Muscles

When the long axis of the body is roughly vertical, the spinal column is subjected to compressive load. Compressive loading is normal and physiological for the spinal column.

Distally arising movements of the extremities are to be coordinated by the abdominal muscles, automatically and with fine adjustment.

Caudally arising activation: When the hip flexes to lift the leg, the leg hangs ventrally from the pelvis and the pelvis ventrally from the thorax. In order to keep the long axis of the body vertical, the extensional stabilization of the thoracic spine, as active buttressing of the ventrally attached weight of the leg, will automatically increase. This increases the compressive load on the spinal column. Depending on the weight of the hanging leg, the long axis of the body may also lean somewhat backwards.

Cranially arising activation: Flexional arm movements and extensional head movements prompt actively buttressing coordinating activity in the abdominal muscles. Extensional arm movements and flexional head movements trigger continuing coordinating activity in the abdominal muscles.

Automatic activity of the abdominal muscles arises during equilibrium movements of the pelvis in the hip joints and in the joints of the lumbar spine, and in association with breathing.

It is often required in therapy that the abdominal muscles be exercised with the long axis of the body horizontal and the patient supine. However, a body which is lying down is only minimally activated and not prepared for sudden physical stress except that arising from the need to roll over or get up.

When the long axis of the body is roughly horizontal, the spinal column is subjected to torsional and shearing stress. Any weights suspended from the ventral muscles in this starting position will only help to train these muscles if the inherently mobile spinal column is stabilized at the right moment. If the weights are too heavy or suspended too suddenly, the passive holding structures of the spinal column are subjected to shearing stress. This faulty stress affects the vertebral joints and vertebral-intervertebral disc articulations, and may cause herniation in the groin, in the rectus abdominis muscle, and at surgical scar sites.

If such stress arises *caudally,* from lifting the legs, and if the lumbar spine is stabilized too late, the lumbar spine will extend, which has a deleterious effect on the motive components of the caudal rectus abdominis muscle.

If the stress arises *cranially,* from lifting the head, the shoulder girdle with the arms, and the thorax, and if the thoracic spine is not stabilized extensionally, the overheavy lever arm will shorten by translating the head ventrally and further flexing the thoracic spine. An undesired contraction of the upper abdomen will occur.

1.1 The Classic Frog (Figs. 1–3)

The "Classic Frog" is an invented name. The end position of the exercise reminds one of a frog on its back.

■ Goal of the Exercise

The goal is for the patient to learn to functionally contract his abdominal muscles, i.e.
- Narrow his upper abdomen by narrowing the epigastric angle
- Contract his lower abdomen by moving his symphysis towards his navel and use his abdominal muscles powerfully and skilfully.

▶ Functional Analysis in Therapist Language

The Classic Frog is a suitable exercise for functional training of the abdominal muscles in persons with a normal spinal column or a variant of the norm. Moderate lumbar lordosis and thoracic kyphosis with a relatively large frontosagittal diameter of the thorax are pathological deviations from the norm which can also be improved by practising the Classic Frog.

● Conception of the Exercise

We want to bring about physiological contraction of the abdominal muscles by employing movements which flow from distal to proximal. To this end, we choose a starting position which stretches the abdominal muscles so that the upper abdomen becomes wide and the lower abdomen long. The best position for this is supine with the arms flexed at the shoulder joints and resting on the floor alongside the head. Activation out of this starting position, with the five extremities head, arms and legs pulling away from the body's centrepoint, intensifies the functional stretching of the abdominal muscles. ·

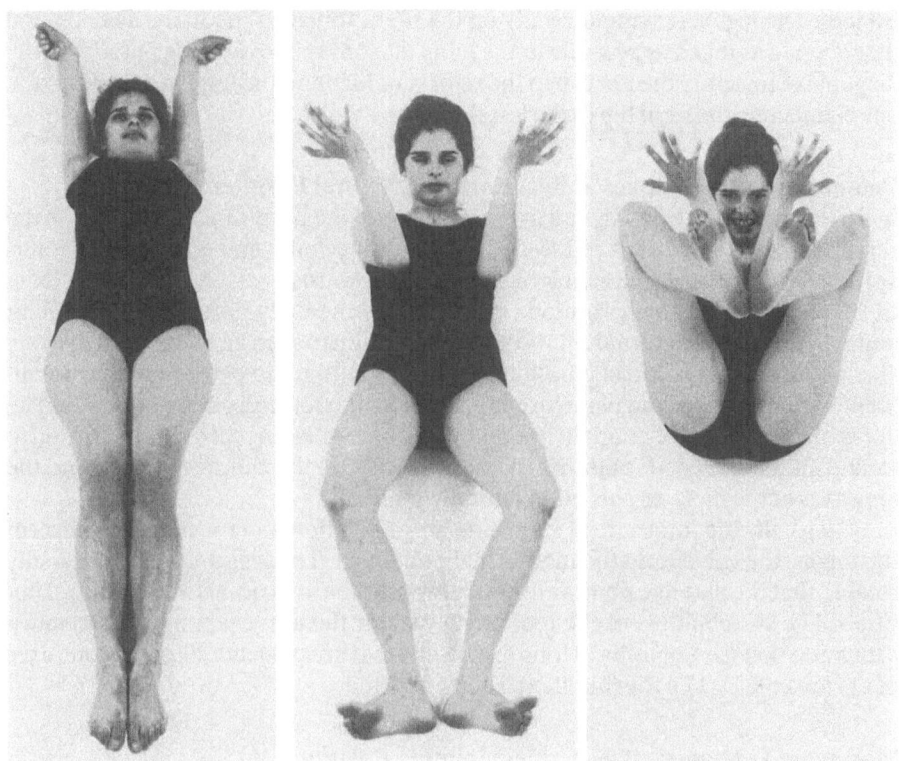

a, b   c

Fig. 1 a–c. The Classic Frog. **a** Starting postion, **b** middle of the movement sequence, **c** end position

An exhalation at the beginning of the movement sequence initiates the functional contraction of the muscles. In addition, BS arms should bring about a narrowing of the upper abdomen and BS legs a contraction of the lower abdomen, both by a continuing movement. BS head has the task of checking the movement initiated by the legs and also of preventing the upper abdomen from contracting.

The supine position in this exercise promotes strength and skill in the abdominals. This is because, owing to the way they are arranged in space, the weights of the extremities have to be lifted and moved at the same time.

● **Position and Activation in the Starting Position**

Position in Space of the Critical Axes
Points of Contact Between the Body and the Environment
In supine, the flexion/extension axes of the spinal column and of the proximal joints of the extremities are horizontal.

BS head is aligned in the horizontal long axis of the body.

BS arms: The arms rest symmetrically on the floor, almost parallel to the cranial projection of the long axis of the body.

9

BS legs: The legs rest symmetrically on the floor, touching medially. The legs are thus aligned as much as possible in the body diagonals, the right leg parallel to the diagonal connecting the left hip to the right shoulder and the left leg parallel to the one connecting the right hip to the left shoulder.

Components of Movement in Relation to the Neutral Position of the Joints
In BS head, DP vertex is aligned in the long axis of the body and the lordosis in the cervical spine is somewhat reduced. The atlanto-occipital and atlanto-axial joints are flexed such that the patient looks ventrally/upwards.
In BS arms (Fig. 2), the acromions face cranially/medially/dorsally; the shoulder joints are in flexion, internal rotation, and abduction to such an extent that the long axes of the arms are almost parallel; the elbow joints are in extension; the switch-points of the forearm and hands are in pronation, flexion and ulnar abduction. The dorsa of the wrists face cranially/medially. The interphalangeal joints are flexed to form a closed fist (PNF pattern fist; see Knott 1969) the thumbs oppose and the long axes of the metacarpals point laterally/cranially.
In BS legs, the hip joints are in extension and adduction and the medial aspects of the thighs, the calves and the medial malleoli touch. The legs are so far internally rotated that the patellae point ventrally/upwards; the knee joints are in neutral position. The switchpoints of the feet are in plantar flexion, eversion, and so much pronation that the anatomical long axes of the feet are projections of the long axes of the lower legs. The toes are flexed and adducted.

**Movement Tolerances at the Critical Joints in Relation
to the Intended Primary Movement**
BSs arms and legs have the largest tolerance for movement on their way into the antagonistic, end-stopped final position. The vertebral joints have movement tolerance for all components of movement; the flexional components are under maximum lifting strain.
The horizontal components of the primary movements cancel each other out, because the legs move cranially/laterally, the arms caudally/medially, and the head slightly caudally. The upwardly directed vertical components ensure positive lifting strain on the abdominal muscles.

**Distribution of Body Weight on a Base Support or Suspension Device,
Against a Supportive Device, or over a Support Area,
and the Resulting Activity States of the Musculature**
In the starting position, the floor is the body's base support. BSs pelvis, thorax, head, legs and arms are all parked on the floor. As the extremities stretch away from the body's centrepoint, the body segments become linked by stretching, supported leaning, and bridging activities. A support area is formed: the smallest area encompassing the body's points of contact with the base support. The centrifugal pull of the extremities away from the centrepoint causes the support area to become slightly larger.
The critical distance points for the stretching away from the body's centrepoint are:

- In BS head, the vertex, stretching cranially.
- In BS arms, the dorsa of the right and left wrists, stretching cranially and somewhat laterally.
- In BS legs, the toes, stretching caudally.

This activation, which we have described emphasizing direction, brings about the following continuing movements:
- From BS head: the thoracic spine extends and the upper abdomen becomes moderately longer.
- From BS arms: the ribs lift, the epigastric angle opens and the upper abdomen widens markedly.
- From BS legs: the pelvis flexes in the hip joints, the lumbar spine extends, causing the lower abdomen to lengthen. The extensional bridging activity in the lumbar area activates particularly the lumbosacral articulation, extensionally and with reduced lift.

Intensity of Muscle Activity Required with Economical Activity
Respiration
The stretch is performed slowly with a corresponding increase in the intensity of economical activity. The patient breathes in until the yawn reflex is triggered; this is the signal for the movement sequence to start.

● **Actio – Reactio of the Movement Sequence**

The Classic Frog is a constant-location exercise in which the support area becomes concentrically smaller as the patient nears the end position and becomes eccentrically larger as he moves back into the activated starting position.
In the starting position, the long axis of the body is horizontal. The primary movements that flow from distal to proximal have not only vertical but also horizontal components, which are directed in towards the body centrepoint. These horizontal components are capable of triggering unwanted equilibrium reactions, subjecting the spinal column to uneconomical torsional stress (see Klein-Vogelbach 1990, hereafter cited as *Functional Kinetics*), and this would in fact happen if the horizontal components were to run only footwards or only headwards (orientation within the body). For this reason we choose five primary movements for the Classic Frog – the movements of the arms, legs and head – whose horizontal components cancel each other out, because some of them run footwards, some headwards, and they are symmetrical. The resultant of these movements is now vertical and directed upwards. Because the effects of the horizontal components of the primary movements are neutralized in this way, no predominant reactio occurs.

Actio: The Primary Movement
The five coordinated primary movements of BSs arms, legs and head bring these body sections into free play. The movements of the arms and legs are antagonistic to their starting positions and continue on into the abdominal muscles, causing the upper abdomen to narrow and the lower abdomen to contract. The weight of the five extremities imposes an appropriate amount of lifting strain on the abdominal muscles.

11

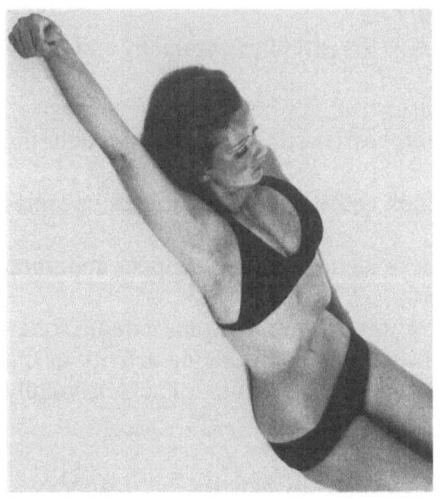

Fig. 2. Arm position at the start of the Classic Frog

In BS arms, DPs right and left olecranons move ventrally/upwards/caudally/medially towards the plane of symmetry, roughly above the navel. Fulcrum displacement brings the elbow joints into 90° flexion and the forearms into supination. The switchpoints of the hands form opened hands (PNF; see Knott 1969) with the thumbs abducted. The palms have rotated first medially then dorsally. At the end of the movement sequence they face cranially and the long axes of the hand point ventrally/upwards. The shoulder joints move into extension/adduction/external rotation; the acromions have migrated caudally/laterally/ventrally. The continuing movement has now pulled the ribs down and the oblique abdominal muscles have narrowed the upper abdomen (critical fulcrum; Figs. 2, 3).

In BS legs, DPs right and left heels first move cranially along the floor in the plane of symmetry. When they leave the floor they continue cranially/ventrally/upwards, coming to rest approximately over the navel. In doing so, the talocrural joint moves into dorsiflexion, the subtalar and talocalcaneonavicular joints into inversion, and the toes into extension and abduction. This displacement of the heels has brought the knee joints into flexion and external rotation and the hip joints into flexion (abduction) external rotation. By continuing movement the lumbar spine flexes, the caudal end of the sacrum leaves the floor and the lower abdomen contracts (critical fulcrum).

In BS head, flexion in the atlanto-occipital and atlanto-axial joints causes the critical distance point of the fifth primary movement, DP vertex, to move slightly ventrally/upwards/caudally.

Reactio: Activated Passive Buttressing

As the movement sequence nears completion, the caudal portion of the pelvis lifts off the floor. The weight of the pelvis plus that of the legs suspended from it now place such severe strain on the straight abdominal muscles that the head, in activated passive buttressing, is reactively lifted up off the floor as a counterweight by the ventral cervical muscles, with flexion in the atlanto-occipital and atlanto-axial joints, and becomes suspended from the rectus abdominis muscle.

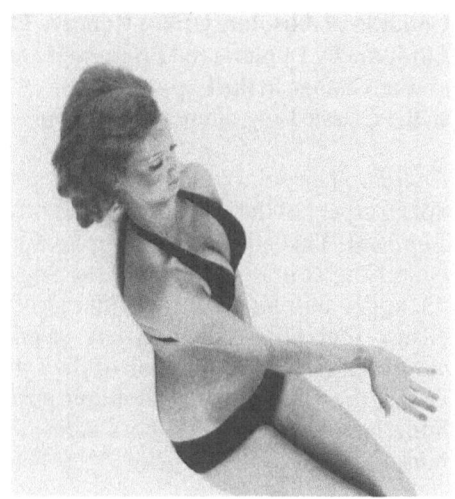

Fig. 3. Arm position at the end of the Classic Frog

Reactio: Change in the Support Area
The continuing primary movements that bring the arms, legs and head into free play are centripetal and reduce the support area.

● Conditio – Limitatio of the Movement Sequence

Conditio: Constant Distances Between Body Distance Points
Limitatio: Active Buttressing and Stabilization
In the Classic Frog, we see the following:

Conditio: The distance from DP navel to DP xiphoid process remains constant.
Limitatio: This distance remains constant if the external rotation components of the humeroscapular joints counteract the direction of the primary movement by adducting and counterstabilizing the scapulae against the thoracic spine, thus stimulating the latter in extensional activity. Now we have extensional stabilization of the thoracic spine in neutral position, which in functional terms constitutes active buttressing against the tendency of the thoracic spine to flex in response to the activity in the straight abdominal muscles (which are activated by continuing movement from the primary movements of the arms and head). The narrowing of the upper abdomen by lowering the ribs – part of the goal of the exercise – is possible only if this active buttressing takes place.

Conditio: The distance from DP left heel to DP right heel does not change once the heels have touched each other.
Limitatio: The heel-to-heel contact will remain throughout the movement sequence if it is maintained by buttressing pressure activity of the heels against each other and the legs move symmetrically. The opposing pressure of the heels activates the external rotators of the hips. The transverse abduction in the hip joints, by which the bending knees move apart, also facilitates the flexion at the hips.

Conditio of Absolute and/or Relative Fixed Spatial Points
Limitatio by Limiting the Primary Movement, Activated Passive Buttressing
and/or Change in the Support Area
In the Classic Frog, there are absolute and relative fixed spatial points.

Conditio: The point of contact dorsal aspect of BS thorax/floor remains, even if the dorsal aspect of the shoulder girdle rises up off the floor.
Limitatio: This absolute fixed spatial point stops the primary movement of the head from continuing and checks any potential cranially-arising contraction of the upper abdomen. The shoulder girdle rises off the floor at the right moment to ensure that DPs right and left olecranons are able to keep the ventral/upward/caudal/medial direction of their movement precisely. In anticipation of this lifting, the weight of the shoulder girdle together with that of the arms is first hung onto the thorax on both sides, thereby activating the oblique abdominal muscles.

Conditio: DPs right and left heels always move in the plane of symmetry. They do not lose contact with the floor until the separate weights of the two legs have been united by the pressure of the heels against each other.
Limitatio: This relative fixed spatial point brings about a symmetrical movement of the legs with flexion in the knee joints. The hip flexors suspend the united weight of the legs from the pelvis, which in turn is suspended from the thorax at the xiphoid process. This symmetrical distribution of weight ensures that the spinal column is not only stabilized against rotation and lateral flexion, but is also able to maintain equilibrium. Since the heels may not leave the floor until they have actively joined together, they must first be dragged cranially along the floor until the amount of flexion and transverse abduction in the hip joints and the flexion in the knee joints permits adequate purchase of the heels against each other. The lever of BS legs has now been sufficiently shortened that the strain on the abdominal muscles of lifting the legs from the floor is within their capacity. This prevents unwanted shearing stress to the lumbar area.

Conditio: In the contraction of the lower abdomen, DP navel is a fixed spatial point towards which DP symphysis moves.
Limitatio: For DP navel to remain an absolute fixed spatial point, the pelvis must, in co-rotational continuation of the primary movement of the legs, lift its caudal part from the floor by flexion in the lumbar spine. This causes DP symphysis to move ventrally/upwards/cranially.

Conditio of Movement Speed
Limitatio of Economical Activity by Finding the Optimal Speed
Conditio: The movement sequence is initiated by triggering the yawn reflex. The patient then breathes out continuously until he reaches the final position.
Limitatio: In order for the primary movements of the arms and legs to start smoothly and simultaneously with the yawn, the first phase of the movement sequence consists of slow relaxation of the stretch in the activated starting position. This involves eccentric isotonic muscle work. However, before this let-

up of tension allows the arms and legs, under the influence of gravity, to go into the activity state called parking function, the concentric isotonic lifting work of the coordinated primary movements serving the goal of the exercise is begun, with an increase in the speed of movement and in the intensity of economical activity.

During the eccentric isotonic movement phase, the elasticity of the lung enhances the expiration and lowering of the ribs; during the concentric isotonic movement phase, prolonging the exhalation increases the strength of the abdominal muscles and promotes their physiological contraction.

Conditio: The legs and arms perform their primary movements simultaneously while the head continues to pull away from the body centrepoint until the pressure of its weight on the floor begins to diminish. This is the signal for DP chin to move towards DP jugular notch.

Limitatio: The reactive lifting of the head from the floor can be seen and palpated in the activation of the sternocleidomastoid. It occurs at the precise moment when, during the concentric positive lift phase of the coordinated primary arm and leg movements, the caudal part of the pelvis is lifted off the floor. The weight of the head responds with activated passive buttressing. Through flexion at the atlanto-occipital and atlanto-axial joints, BS head enters the movement sequence from cranially as the fifth primary movement and checks the entire movement of the Classic Frog.

● **Position and Activation in the End Position
and Return to the Starting Position**

The end position is reached when the five primary movements have fulfilled the goal of the exercise and the functional contraction of the abdominal muscles under appropriate stress (i.e. stress which does not overtax them) has taken place. The end position is held for a few seconds. During this time, the patient can either breathe shallowly through the nose with double panting or breathe through the mouth, whistling during both inspiration and expiration (see pp. 151–152).

The movement sequence from the end position back into the starting position begins with another eccentric isotonic release of tension. The patient's breathing is also coordinated to this activity, in that inhalation is initiated by the relaxation of expiratory activity combined with the natural elasticity of the lung. The concentric isotonic activity begins distally in the hands and feet. The critical distance points in BS arms on the way back the starting position are DPs fingers of the right and left hand. The activity in the extremities does not increase until the weights of the pelvis and the extremities, no longer suspended eccentrically from the abdominal muscles, have reached the floor again and increased the support area. In BS arms, this happens when the shoulder girdle touches the floor; in BS legs, it occurs when the heels are once again supported by the floor, and in BS pelvis, it occurs when the pelvis has dorsal contact with the floor. The heels must touch the floor before the harmful avoidance mechanism of eccentric isotonic extension in the lumbar spine can take place due to overstrain on the abdominal muscles. BS head ensures that the straight abdominal muscles remain activated until the weight of the pelvis is no longer suspended from the xiphoid process. Once the pelvis is on the floor, the weight of the head is no longer needed as an activated passive buttress. When all five extremities have touched the floor and the arms and legs have moved concentric-isotonically back into the starting position, activation of the starting position can begin again.

▶ Instruction in Patient Language

● Instruction Appealing to the Patient's Perception

The easiest way for the patient to learn the arm movement is for him lie on his back with his eyes closed, the therapist to manipulate one of his arms through the precise primary movement, and the patient simultaneously to copy this movement with his other arm. From the outset, the breathing should be coordinated with the movement.

● Verbal Instruction

● Instruction by Manipulation

Position and Activation in the Starting Position

"Lie comfortably on your back with your arms resting alongside your head. Make yourself as tall as you can – make your stomach long, your neck, your legs, your arms. As your stomach stretches, your back forms a bridge, wrinkling the small of your back. As you stretch the back of your neck, your throat grows shorter. Your eyes can wander; the top of your head is pulling away from your navel. Your hands are fisted and can wave outwards. The skin on the back of your wrists is tight. Your legs are long and the insides are touching; your knees face upwards. Try to touch your anklebones together. Your toes try to ball into a fist, but otherwise your feet are pointed like a ballet dancer's, so the soles of your feet now face the floor. Your stomach is nice and long and is wide at the top. You keep on stretching and stretching until you start to yawn."

For *BS arms:* The therapist asks the patient not to resist the manipulation. She then carefully and precisely manipulates one arm into the starting position. The dorsum of the hand is stretched away from the navel, ensuring that the arm activation will continue down into BSs thorax and pelvis. Now the patient copies the movement of the manipulated arm with his free arm.

Since the patient is intended to feel *BS legs,* touching medially, to be a single unit, the therapist manipulates both legs together, allowing the patient to coordinate his arms as she moves his legs.

BS head is manipulated by fine, directed compression along the long axis of the body, applied at the vertex. The five extremities are repeatedly activated. At various intervals, the patient is asked to either turn over or to get up and then, with a progressively improving kinaesthetic sense, to resume the starting position.

Correct activation of the extremities brings *BSs pelvis and thorax* into the desired position. Manipulation is the best way of demonstrating how we want the distance between two distance points (e. g. symphysis pubis to navel) to be changed.

Actio, Conditio and Limitatio of the Movement Sequence

"As you yawn, the fists of your hands and feet slowly open and start to look like powerful, wide, flat fans. Each hand becomes a fan, with the little finger turning inwards. The feet, connected at the heels, together make one large erect fan. Have you noticed how your breath is flowing away after your yawn? Make sure to keep it flowing away, and then you'll clearly feel your waist becoming narrow and your lower abdomen becoming short. That's the signal for you to pull your elbows towards the middle of your body, as quick as a flash, over your navel. As you do this, your fan-like hands turn so that your thumbs point out and the wrinkled backs of your hands face your feet. At the same time, your knees start to spread apart, to make room for the fan formed by your feet. This fan begins to lift off from the floor; your heels, firmly pressed together, move in a shallow arc through the air until they are just about over your navel. Now you're nearly there: your bottom is up in the air and now, as if by magic, your head begins to float too. Now bend your neck even farther forwards so that you can look through the hole between your legs, as if it were a window. You can see that the fan of the feet is spread wide and floating high in the air. The fans of the hands are erect and open upwards."

Teaching the patient the movement sequence by manipulation is similar to teaching him the starting position. Because the patient is now learning a movement and not a position, we must prevent any deviation from the precise path we want him to trace through space by skilful contact stimulus and verbal cues. When the time comes for significant weight to be lifted from the support area and become suspended from the body, the therapist must physically assume as much of this weight as necessary so that the movement sequence' flows smoothly and without deviating in direction. With progress, the patient should be able to manage without the therapist's help.

Position and Activation in the End Position

"Now the Frog is finished. You'll enjoy breathing most if you quietly whistle a little tune through your teeth. When you run out of air, just keep on whistling inwards as you breathe in. Your stomach is now working hard. That's good. That's exactly how it should be."

Like the starting position, the end position can also be reached by manipulation in several stages, and the patient then be told to hold it, with verbal cues: "Stay there!" "Don't move!" Manipulating an arm into the end position allows the patient to feel the activity of the oblique abdominal muscles distinctly, while manipulating BS legs activates the straight muscles. The compressive resistance applied at the vertex and directed along the long axis of the body emphasizes the active buttressing and stabilizing components in the thoracic spine. In the final position, the stress on the abdominal wall can be increased by applying resistance to, for instance, the heels (for the rectus abdominis muscle) or the elbows (for the oblique abdominal muscles). Applying resistance also helps to imprint the position in the patient's awareness.

Return to the Starting Position

"Now, remember how nice the beginning was with the stretching and yawning. When you think about them you forget all about the whistling and the hard work. The fans gently close. Your hands fall in on themselves like withered leaves. The feet-fan closes too, ends its flight, and lands carefully on the floor. Now that the stomach doesn't have to work so hard, you can turn all your thoughts to your nice long legs, long arms and long stomach. Your fists turn to wave outwards again and your feet are again those of a ballet dancer. Your long neck helps you pull all five body segments away from your navel. Now you feel like yawning, and everything can start all over again from the beginning."

During this phase of the exercise, the therapist must make sure, through manipulation, that the transfer onto the support area of the weight previously suspended from the body is properly coordinated with the activity states of the body segments involved.

► Adapting the Exercise to the Patient's Constitution and Condition

● Adaptation to Constitution: Role of Lengths, Widths, Depths and Distribution of Weights

If the patient has any lengths, widths, depths or weights that are significantly greater than the norm, the strain on the moving levers may increase disproportionately. By the same token, if any lengths, widths, depths or weights are significantly less than the norm, an imbalance in the moving levers may occur and interfere with the coordination of the five primary movements.

● Adaptation to Condition: Common "Faults" Requiring Adaptation of the Exercise

- Insufficiency of the abdominal muscles, so that even the low strain of the Classic Frog cannot be managed without an avoidance mechanism
- Paretic abdominal or back muscles
- Conditional overweight such as overlarge (trained) muscles in the extremities, which can overload the levers, or excessive accumulations of fat, which can restrict movement excursions, especially in the hip and shoulder joints
- Limited joint mobility, particularly limited flexion in the hips, knees and elbows, which may disturb the movement sequence or cause deviations of direction
- Pain occurring during the exercise

● Abnormalities of Postural Statics Requiring Adaptation of the Exercise

- Severe pathological spinal curvatures, such as severe scoliosis, for which this type of abdominal training would appear inadvisable
- Severe, pathological abnormalities of the thorax – such as severe funnel chest – or of the hip joints which so impede the continuing and buttressing movements that the goal of the exercise is unattainable.

For such cases, the exercise Short and Sharp (p. 354) is recommended.

Adaptation of the Classic Frog
If it appears that the continuing effect of the primary movements of the arms and legs is better transmitted to the abdominal musculature (the goal of the exercise) *without* buttressing movement components in the proximal joints of the extremities, the movement components of the primary movements of the arms and legs are adapted accordingly. These adaptations are called the **Primitive** and the **Diagonal Frog**.
If the pelvis, the arms and the head are too heavy for the abdominal muscles when the long axis of the body is horizontal, the adaptation can be made by **changing the position in space of this axis**.

1.2 Adaptation: The Primitive Frog (Figs. 4–6)

The "Primitive Frog" is an invented name. The "primitive" refers to the more basic, developmentally more primitive arm and leg movements employed in this exercise.

■ Goal of the Exercise

The goal of the exercise is for the patient with a flat back, especially a flat thoracic spine with large frontotransverse diameter of the thorax, and/or with marked lumbar hyperlordosis, and/or a small distance between the greater trochanters, to learn to functionally contract the abdominal muscles.

▶ Functional Analysis in Therapist Language

The Primitive Frog for functional training of the abdominal muscles is suitable for patients with a flat back or with lumbar hyperlordosis, two conditions often associated with excessive widths, especially of the thorax.

● Conception of the Exercise

As in the Classic Frog, the goal is to effect physiological contraction of the abdominal mucles by employing distal-to-proximal continuing movements of the extremities. Supine is the chosen starting position. Because patients with flat backs have insufficient physiological spinal curvature, the divergence between the long axes of the arms and legs is increased in this adaptation in order to have a stabilizing rather than a mobilizing effect upon the spine on activation in the starting position. In selecting the movement components for the proximal joints of the extremities in the movement sequence, all counterstabilization must be avoided, so that the movements of the arms and legs can continue on unimpeded into the abdominal muscles. With the exception of the adaptations described below, the Primitive Frog is performed the same way as the Classic Frog.

● Position and Activation in the Starting Position

Position in Space of the Critical Axes
Points of Contact Between the Body and the Environment
In supine, the long axis of the body, the long axes of the arms and legs, and the flexion/extension axes of the spinal column are horizontal. In this position in space, if the abdominal muscles have to work, they perform positive lifting.
BS head is positioned in the horizontal long axis of the body.
In BS arms, the arms lie symmetrically on the floor, perfectly aligned in the imaginary extensions of the body diagonals: the right arm extends the diagonal connect-

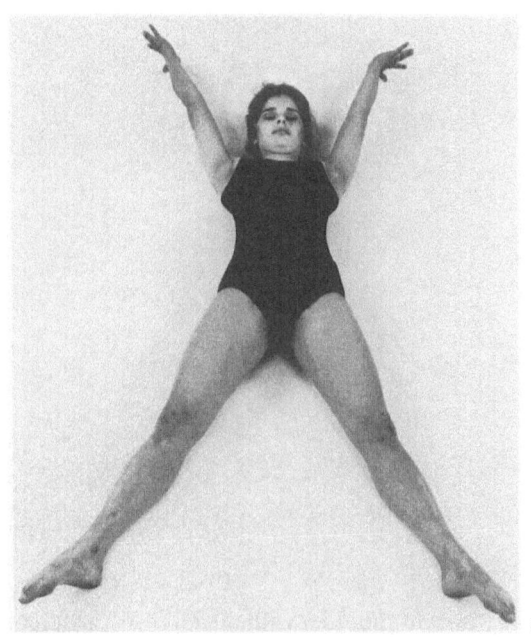

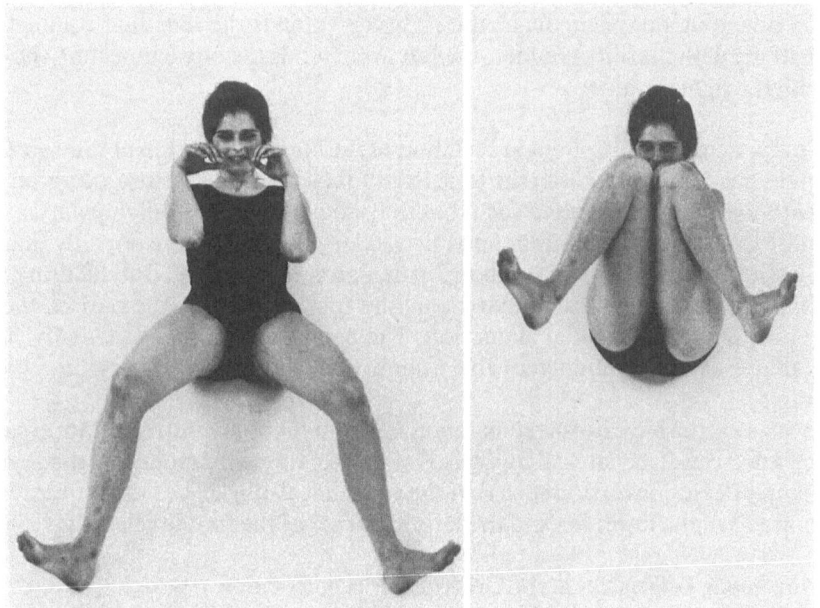

Fig. 4 a–c. The Primitive Frog: symmetrical arm and leg pattern. **a** Starting position, **b** middle of the movement sequence, **c** end position

21

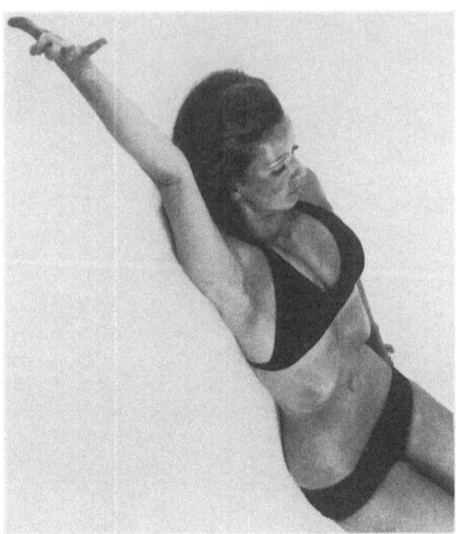

Fig. 5. Arm position at the start of the Primitive Frog

ing the right shoulder with the left hip, the left arm extends the one connecting the left shoulder with the right hip.

In BS legs, the legs lie symmetrically on the floor. They are clearly positioned in the diverging body diagonals: the right leg extends the diagonal connecting the right hip with the left shoulder, the left leg extends the one connecting the left hip with the right shoulder.

Components of Movement in Relation to the Neutral Position of the Joints

In BS head, DP vertex is in the long axis of the body. The atlanto-occipital and atlanto-axial joints are flexed such that the patient looks ventrally/upwards.

In BS arms, the acromions are positioned less cranially, more dorsally than in the Classic Frog; the shoulder joints are in flexion and pronounced abduction/external rotation; the elbows are in extension; the forearms are in supination, the wrists in dorsiflexion and radial abduction. The palms face cranially/medially. The fingers are extended/abducted; the thumb is retroposed, its tip against the floor (Fig. 5).

In BS legs, the hips are in extension/marked abduction/external rotation such that the knee caps face laterally/upwards (Fig. 4a); the switchpoints of the feet are in plantar flexion/inversion such that the anatomical long axis of the foot extends the long axis of the lower leg and the lateral border of the foot touches the floor.

Movement Tolerances at the Critical Joints in Relation to the Intended Primary Movement

BSs arms and legs have the greatest movement tolerance on their way into the antagonistic end position. The vertebral joints have tolerance for movement in all movement components; the flexional components are under maximum lifting stress. The horizontal components of the primary intended movements of the five extremities cancel each other out: the legs move cranially/medially, the arms caudally/medially, the head slightly caudally. The upward vertical components ensure positive lifting stress on the abdominal muscles.

Distribution of Body Weight on a Base Support or Suspension Device,
Against a Supportive Device, or Over a Support Area,
and the Resulting Activity States of the Musculature

In the starting position, the floor is the body's base support. BSs pelvis, thorax, head, arms and legs are parked on the floor. As the extremities pull away from the body centrepoint, the muscular activity links the body segments together and a support area is formed: the smallest area encompassing all points of contact of the activated body with the base support.

Activation in the starting position of the Primitive Frog is fundamentally different from that in the Classic Frog. In the Classic Frog, the flexion/extension axes of the hip and knee joints and the metatarsophalangeal joints of the big toes are horizontal and parallel. The critical distance points of the legs for the activation in the starting position, DPs toes of the right and left foot, lie ventral to and above the flexion/extension axes of the hips. To bring about the horizontal component of direction caudally away from the body centrepoint, the proximal lever of the hip joints, the pelvis, effects a flexional movement at the hip joints, causing extensional distortion of the lumbar spine, which thus goes into bridging activity. If we wished to prevent this continuing effect of the activation in the starting position, we would have to change the distance points in BS legs to DPs right and left heels, which lie dorsal to and below the flexion/extension axes of the hips. Then, to bring about the horizontal caudal component of direction, the proximal lever of the hip joints, the pelvis, would effect an extensional movement at the hips, and the distortion of the lumbar spine would be flexional. This adaptation suffices for patients experiencing moderate pain in the lumbar spine; more severe pain requires a switch to the Primitive Frog.

In BS legs in the starting position of the Primitive Frog, the internal rotational component is replaced by external rotation, and the adduction component by abduction. The long axes of the legs of the Primitive Frog diverge markedly from the long axis of the body. In the activation of the starting position, the critical distance points of the primary leg movement have horizontal but, within the horizontal, divergent direction components: critical DP right toes stretches caudally/outwards to the right, while critical DP left toes stretches caudally/outwards to the left. Since external rotation has been added to the abduction component at the hips, the activation in the starting position stabilizes the hips extensionally, because there is a discreet extension of the hip joints by upwards/ventral displacement of the fulcra. The lumbar spine stabilizes with the hips, in discreet flexion. The diverging activities of the primary movements of the legs meet the vertebral column at the rotation level of the lower thoracic spine, which they stabilize by buttressing. Thus the activated primary movements of the legs in the starting position of the Primitive Frog are designed entirely with a view to neutralizing hyperlordosis and/or lesions of the lumbar spine.

In the starting position of the Classic Frog, the long axes of the arms are almost parallel and the shoulders internally rotated. In the activation of the arms in the starting position, to bring about the horizontal direction component of critical DPs right and left wrists cranially, away from the body centrepoint, the distal levers of the sternoclavicular joints, the clavicles, effect movement at the joints to end-stop, with DPs right and left acromions moving cranially/medially, the shoulder girdle pulling away from the thorax and the pincer jaws closing on both sides. The neck disappears between the right and left pincer jaws.

In the starting position of the Primitive Frog, the component of internal rotation in BS arms is replaced by external rotation and the previously nearly parallel long axes of the arms diverge in marked abduction from the long axis of the body. There is also an "open hand" (PNF). In activation in the starting position, the critical distance points of the arms possess horizontal but, within the horizontal, divergent direction components: critical DP right middle fingertip stretches away cranially/outwards to the right while critical DP left middle fingertip stretches away cranially/outwards to the left. Since external rotation has been added to the divergent components at the shoulder joints, activation in the starting position has a counterstabilizing effect on the shoulder girdle, opening the pincer jaws and adducting the scapulae against the thoracic spine. The neck appears long and the thoracic spine becomes stabilized in slight extension. These diverging primary movements of the arms meet the spinal column at the rotation level of the lower thoracic spine, stabilizing it by buttressing.

● **Actio – Reactio of the Movement Sequence**

The Primitive Frog is a constant-location movement sequence with centripetal reduction of the support area on the way to the end position and centrifugal enlargement of the support area on the way back to the starting position.

For the Primitive Frog we choose five primary movements – those of the arms, legs and head – whose horizontal components cancel each other out, because some of them run towards the feet, others towards the head, and they are symmetrical. Because the horizontal components cancel each other out in this way, there is no predominant reactio in this exercise.

Actio: The Primary Movement
Reactio: Activated Passive Buttressing
Reactio: Change in the Support Area
The five coordinated primary movements of BSs arms, legs and head bring these body sections into free play. These primary movements of the arms and legs are antagonistic to their activation in the starting position and continue on into the abdominal musculature of patients with flat back and/or unstable spinal columns, causing the muscles to contract. The weight of the five extremities imposes an appropriate amount of lifting stress on the abdominal musculature; this must occur at the right moment, and thus the abdominal muscles are trained for not only strength but skill as well.

Actio: In BS arms, critical DPs right and left olecranons move ventrally/upwards/caudally/medially in the direction of the plane of symmetry, approximately above the navel. Fulcrum displacement brings the elbows into roughly 135° flexion and the forearms into pronation. The switchpoints of the hands form

24

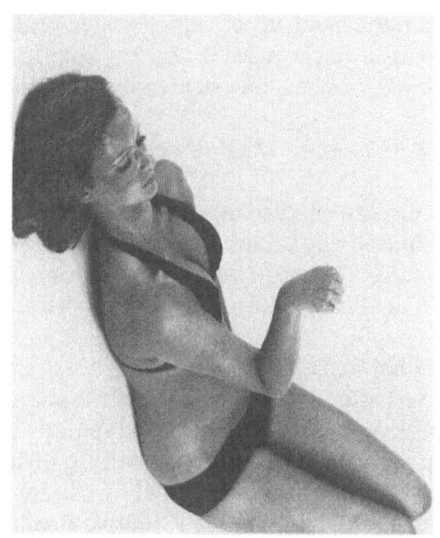

Fig. 6. Arm position at the end of the Primitive Frog

closed fists with opposing thumbs and ulnar abduction by fulcrum displacement. The long axes of the forearms cross and the fists face ventrally/upwards. The shoulders are in extension, internal rotation and adduction such that the elbows almost touch medially. By continuing movement, DPs right and left acromions have moved caudally/quite a bit ventrally/medially. Because the counterstabilizing components (see p. 13) in the shoulder girdle have been left out, the movement now continues smoothly into the thorax. The ribs drop and the thoracic spine undergoes slight cranial-to-caudal flexion – both desirable effects in patients with thoracic flat blacks. The upper abdomen has narrowed and contracted slightly (Fig. 6).

In BS legs, fulcrum displacement in the knees moves critical DPs right and left knees ventrally in flexion upwards/cranially/medially towards the plane of symmetry and over the navel. The talocrural joints dorsiflex, the subtalar and talocalcaneonavicular joints evert, the toes extend and abduct. The long axis of each lower leg is now in the vertical plane of the body diagonal belonging to it. The thighs flex/transversely adduct/internally rotate at the hip joints. In a co-rotational continuing movement the lumbar spine goes into flexion and the caudal end of the sacrum leaves the floor. The lower abdomen has contracted markedly and the weight of the pelvis is now suspended from the straight abdominal muscles.

In BS head, the critical distance point of the fifth primary movement, DP vertex, moves ventrally/upwards/caudally by flexion in the atlanto-occipital and atlanto-axial joints and in the cervical spine,

Reactio: The five distal-to-proximal continuing primary movements bring about a centripetal reduction in the support area because BS arms and legs lose contact with the floor and go into free play. When, towards the end of the movement, the caudal part of the pelvis leaves the floor, the weight of the pelvis with the legs suspended from it constitute such an intense stress on the straight abdominal muscles that the head, in activated passive buttressing, is also lifted up off the floor by the ventral neck muscles and by flexion in the atlanto-occipital and atlanto-axial joints, and becomes suspended from the rectus abdominis muscle.

- **Conditio – Limitatio of the Movement Sequence**

Conditio of Absolute and/or Relative Fixed Spatial Points
Limitatio by Limiting the Primary Movement, Activated Passive Buttressing and/or Change in the Support Area
In the Primitive Frog, there are both absolute and relative fixed spatial points.

Conditio: Point of contact dorsum of BS thorax from T7 to L1/ floor remains fixed even after the dorsal aspect of the shoulder girdle leaves the floor.
Limitatio: This absolute fixed spatial point checks the continuation of the primary arm and head movements, thereby ensuring that the upper abdomen, despite contracting slightly in a cranial-to-caudal direction, can also become markedly narrower. Because, in the Primitive Frog, the movement of the shoulder girdle continues so effortlessly on to the thorax, this limitation is important.

Conditio: DPs right and left heels move in the vertical plane of their respective body diagonals.
Limitatio: The movement of these relative fixed spatial points within the vertical planes of their body diagonals either limits or increases the internal rotation component of the primary leg movements in the hip joints, depending on whether the antetorsion angle of the femoral neck is large or small. This makes it easier to lift the pelvis off the base support. If the angle of antetorsion is large, the internal rotation in the hip joints must be limited; if it is small, the internal rotation must be increased.

Conditio: The critical distance points of the primary arm and leg movements, DPs right and left olecranons and DPs right and left knees respectively, should meet in the plane of symmetry, which functions as a relative fixed spatial point.
Limitatio: With the touching of the elbows and knees in the plane of symmetry, we have the extreme adduction in the proximal extremities needed to effectively train the abdominal muscles in patients with flat backs and hyperlordosis.

Conditio: The joined elbows should reach the vertical transverse plane of the navel.
Limitatio: This relative fixed spatial point guarantees optimal continuation of the primary arm movements into the oblique abdominal muscles.

Conditio: The joined knees should at least reach if not cross the vertical transverse plane of the navel.
Limitatio: This relative fixed spatial point makes it possible to lift the caudal part of the pelvis from the floor and thus to contract the lower abdomen. If the knees go beyond the navel, they are higher than the elbows.

Conditio of Movement Speed
Limitatio of Economical Activity by Finding the Optimal Speed
See pp. 14–15, movement analysis of the Classic Frog.

● **Position and Activation of the End Position**
   and Return to the Starting Position

See p. 15, movement analysis of the Classic Frog.

▶ **Instruction in Patient Language**

● **Verbal Instruction**   ● **Instruction by Manipulation**

Position and Activation in the Starting Position

"You are lying on your back, stretching your arms and legs. You are being broken on a comfortable wheel. Your right leg is being pulled out towards the right, your left arm in the opposite direction out towards the left. Your left leg is being pulled out towards the left, your right arm out towards the right. Your toes are pointed, making your feet long, the soles of your feet face in. Your hands are open fans. They rest on the tips of their thumbs on the floor. Stretch again, your head, too; the back of your neck becomes long. Stretch until you have to yawn. That's the signal that the Primitive Frog is about to begin."

If the patient does not succeed in assuming the starting position exactly (it is important that it is exact), the therapist manipulates one arm and one leg into the correct position, allowing the patient to imitate the position with the other arm and leg with his eyes closed. This procedure is repeated until the motor image becomes imprinted in the patient's memory. The patient can then turn over on the floor, then come back to supine and see if he has retained the kinaesthetic image correctly by trying to take up the starting position. The therapist corrects any minor positional errors by manipulating one side.

Actio and Conditio of the Movement Sequence

"While your hand-fans close during the relaxation of yawning, your elbows take over the initiative. They try to meet up with each other above your navel. As they move, your fists close up and cross over each other. Each fist moves to the opposite shoulder, but continues to face forward. Don't forget your breathing.
Now we'll look for the way back. This return route ends exactly at the mo-

Carefully manipulating the movement of one arm is the most efficient way to teach this unfamiliar hand and arm movement. The therapist must be especially careful that, when the shoulder girdle leaves the floor, the shoulder joints move not only medially but also well caudally, so that the thoracic spine flexes slightly when the abdominal muscles are activated. If each elbow follows its path through space correctly

27

ment when the open hand-fans rest on the floor with their thumb tips. These movements to and fro are quiet. But you can't rest at the end, because your arms go on trying to stretch further in the same direction, even through the movement is over.

The arms can rest. You turn your attention to your legs. When you yawned, your toes stopped trying to stretch away. Your knees try to come together above your navel. For a little while your heels slide along the floor and your feet form fans facing outwards. When your knees touch each other, your feet have to keep apart. Your bottom has now come up a little bit from the floor and you can feel how your stomach has to work. That's good.

On the way back to the starting position, your heels find the floor again, far apart from each other but still pretty close to your bottom. Now it's up to your toes to find the shortest way away from your navel back to the starting position. As they go, your knees face outwards and the soles of your feet inwards. The movement is quiet and the stretching away further in the same direction is kept up after the end of the movement, just as with the arms.

Now you are ready to move your arms and legs together, and at the end your head also joins in, lifting off the floor a little bit later than your bottom does. Actually, it *is* lifted – you can feel it happening. All you have to do is pull in your chin.

The Primitive Frog is over now. You can feel this in your abdomen, and you keep breathing. The best thing is to pant very lightly through your nose".

and its movement is coordinated in time with the closing of the fist, while the hand, with internal rotation in the shoulder joint, moves towards the opposite shoulder, we will obtain the relatively large flexion we require in the elbow joints. If the therapist makes sure, right from the beginning, that as the hand closes it turns ventrally/upwards by pronation in the forearm, the patient will experience the movement as simple and in a straight line. The desired continuing effect on the abdominal muscles is optimal.

In the primary leg movements the therapist makes sure, as the tension of the stretch subsides, that, although the knees turn medially with internal rotation in the hip joints, the feet do not move towards each other by adduction in the hip joints. When the critical distance points of the primary movements of the legs, DPs right and left knees, move ventrally/upwards/cranially/medially, the heels should slide cranially/slightly medially along the floor in order to shorten the lever of the legs. They should not leave the floor until the pelvis will not make even the slightest avoidance mechanism in the form of flexion at the hips, deforming the lumbar spine into extension.

The greatest difficulty for the patient will be in maintaining the distance between the heels without overdoing the internal rotation at the hips.

1.3 Adaptation: The Diagonal Frog (Fig. 7)

The "Diagonal Frog" is an invented name. The modifier "diagonal" applied to the familiar "frog" refers to the fact that only one arm and its opposite leg ever become "frog's legs" at a time, while the other two "legs" (extremities) remain in the starting position.

■ Goal of the Exercise

The goal of the exercise is for patients with a hypermobile and/or unstable spinal column to learn to functionally contract the abdominal muscles and to use these muscles with skill and strength.

▶ Functional Analysis in Therapist Language

● Conception of the Exercise

We have both a Diagonal Classic Frog and a Diagonal Primitive Frog. The purpose of these two Diagonal Frogs is to provide vigorous functional training of the abdominal muscles in individuals with either a hypermobile and/or an unstable spinal column without sacrificing the principles of all the Frog exercises: to activate the abdominal muscles, contract them, and bring them into play with strength at the moment they are needed, using continuing movements that flow from distal to proximal from the extremities.

While one arm and the opposite leg move correctly through the primary movement, the other arm and leg remain in the activated starting position, thereby acting as active buttressing to the primary movement. The head can reinforce either the primary movement of the one arm or the activated starting position of the other. The rotation level in the thoracic spine can be used either from cranially or from caudally, but a rotational buttressing movement between the pelvis and the thorax always takes place. In the lumbar and thoracic spine, there is only a little movement tolerance for flexion, just enough for a slight flexional deformation to occur; owing to the extensional active buttressing, large flexional movements cannot arise. As long as these opposing forces remain balanced, the development of even strong force and counterforce carries no risk for the hypermobile and/or unstable spine column.

The following analysis of the Diagonal Classic Frog and the Diagonal Primitive Frog will focus only on the minor changes necessary to the exercises described above.

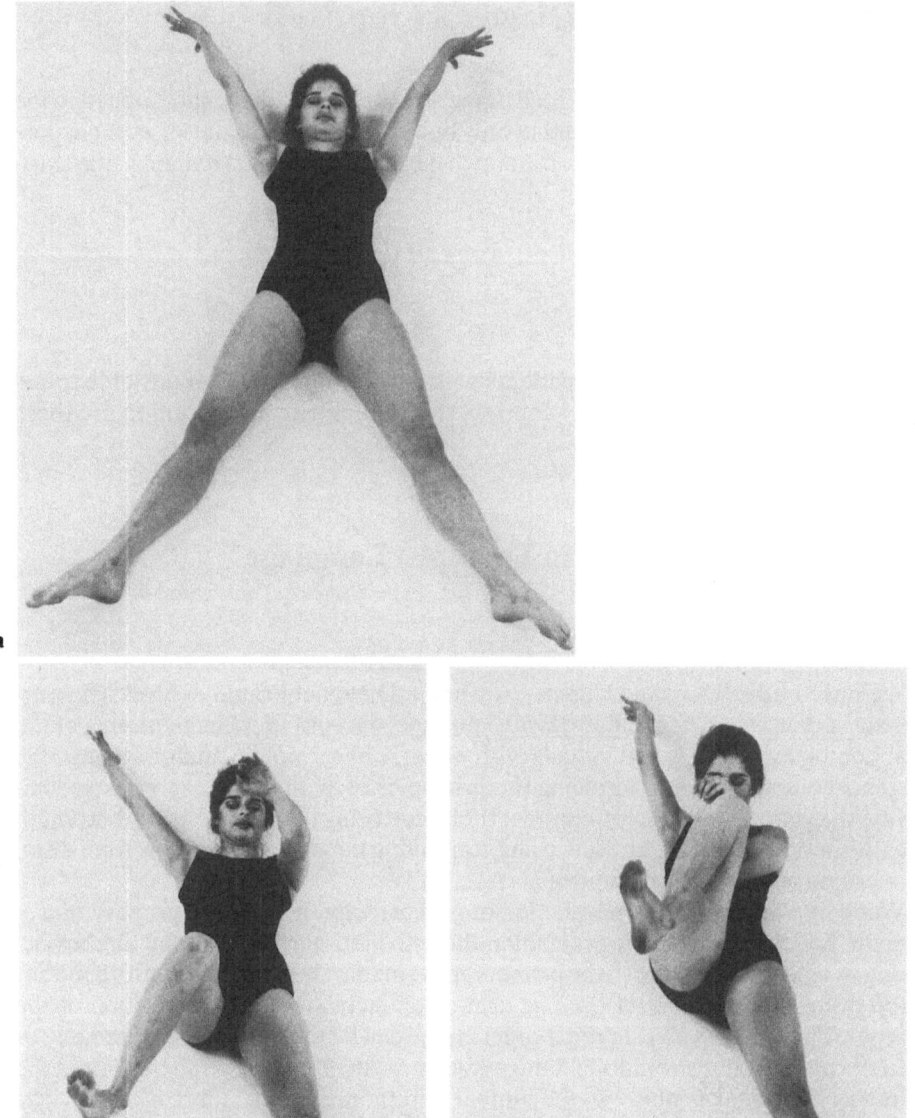

Fig. 7 a–c. The Diagonal Frog (Primitive Frog). **a** Starting position, **b** middle of the movement sequence, **c** end position

● **Position and Activation in the Starting Position**

Position in Space of the Critical Axes
Points of Contact Between the Body and the Environment
Components of Movement in Relation to the Neutral Position of the Joints
Change to the Primitive Frog: In BS legs, one leg can approach the other by adduction in the hip joint, until their medial aspects touch. This means that the leg lying in the original position is able to execute its primary movement alone without difficulty, because the change in the support area is limited.

● **Actio – Reactio of the Movement Sequence**

The Diagonal Frog is a constant-location movement sequence in which the support area becomes smaller during movement into the end position and becomes larger again during movement back into the activated starting position.
We choose three primary movements for the Diagonal Frog: of one arm, of the contralateral leg and of the head. The horizontal components of these movements cancel each other out because some of them flow footwards, some headwards, and in regard to the plane of symmetry they flow towards each other. We will analyse the primary movements of the right arm and the left leg.

Actio: The Primary Movement
Reactio: Activated Passive Buttressing
Reactio: Change in the Support Area
The three coordinated primary movements of the Diagonal Frog bring one arm, the leg opposite to it and the head into free play. The arm and the leg perform movements that are antagonistic to the starting position and which continue into the abdominal muscles. The weight of the three extremities imposes a not excessive, smooth lifting stress on the abdominal muscles, causing especially the oblique muscles to contract at the right time and thus training them for strength and skill.

Actio: In the right arm, the critical distance point of the primary movement, DP right olecranon, moves ventrally/upwards/caudally/medially.
The arm movement of the Classic Frog has already been described in detail (p. 12). The continuing movement causes the ribs on the right side to drop; the pull of the oblique abdominal muscles from cranial/right to caudal/left has narrowed the right upper abdomen and negatively rotated the thorax at movement level lower thoracic spine.
The arm movement of the Primitive Frog has been described in detail on pp. 24–25. The continuing movement causes the ribs on the right side to drop; the pull of the oblique abdominal muscles from cranial/right to caudal/left has narrowed the right upper abdomen and negatively rotated the thorax at movement level lower thoracic spine. However, there is also a slight contraction of the upper abdomen, arising cranially as the thoracic spine flexes.
In the left leg, the critical distance point of the primary movement, DP left knee, moves ventrally/upwards/cranially/medially and crosses the plane of symmetry at about the level of the navel; fulcrum displacement causes the knee to flex.

In the Diagonal Classic Frog, the thigh does not move in the left hip into flexion/external rotation/abduction but rather into flexion/external rotation/adduction. By continuing movement, the pelvis moves to cause extension and internal rotation in the right hip. This movement of the pelvis continues into the spinal column, bringing about caudally arising flexion in the lumbar spine and pelvis-positive rotation in the lower thoracic spine. At the same time, the lower abdomen contracts. The emphasis is on the contraction of the oblique abdominal muscles from caudal/left to cranial/right.

The leg movement of the Primitive Frog is described on pp. 22 and 25. The continuing effect of the pelvic movement in the right hip has an adduction component in addition to extension and internal rotation components. Of the oblique abdominal muscles, those inserting in the area of the left iliac spine contract particularly markedly.

In BS head, the critical distance point DP tip of the nose moves ventrally/upwards/caudally with flexion and rotation in the atlanto-occipital and atlanto-axial joints and in the cervical spine.

Reactio: Because in the Diagonal Frog the horizontal components of the primary movements cancel each other out and the head reinforces the primary arm movement, there is no reactio in the form of activated passive buttressing.

The support area becomes smaller by the lifting of the three primarily moving body parts – left leg, right arm and BS head – off the base support. The support area in the end position is the smallest area encompassing the points of contact between the right leg, left arm, BSs pelvis and thorax and the floor.

● **Conditio – Limitatio of the Movement Sequence**

Conditio: Constant Distances Between Body Distance Points
Limitatio: Active Buttressing and Stabilization
Conditio: The distance from DP left acromion to DP left wrist remains constant.
Limitatio: If the distance from DP acromion to DP wrist in the stationary arm is to remain constant, the humeroscapular, elbow and forearm joints must be stabilized in their starting position by active buttressing in order to withstand an undesired continuing effect of the primary movements. In the Diagonal Classic Frog, this active buttressing is flexional and internal rotational in the shoulder joint, extensional in the elbow and pronational in the forearm joint. In the Diagonal Primitive Frog it is flexional/abductional/external rotational in the shoulder, extensional in the elbow and supinational in the forearm joints.

Conditio: The distance from DP right greater trochanter to DP right lateral malleolus remains constant.
Limitatio: If the distance from the greater trochanter to the lateral malleolus in the stationary leg is to remain constant, the knee must be stabilized in its starting position by active buttressing in order to withstand an undesired continuing effect of the primary movements. The active buttressing in the knee is extensional.

Conditio of Absolute and/or Relative Fixed Spatial Points
Limitatio by Limiting the Primary Movement, Activated Passive Buttressing
and/or Change in the Support Area
Conditio: In the Diagonal Classic Frog, points of contact right heel/floor and ulnar border of the left wrist/floor represent absolute fixed spatial points during the pressure activity in the activated starting position.

Limitatio: The undiminished pressure activity guarantees extensional stabilization of the lumbar and thoracic spines, actively buttressing them against their tendency to flex in a continuation of the primary movement. This active buttressing is the effect of the pressure activities at the points of contact between the left arm and right leg and the floor. The active buttressing brings the proximal extremity joints into bridging activity which, as a continuing movement, causes extensional buttressing stabilization of the lumbar and thoracic spines.

Conditio: In the Diagonal Primitive Frog, the points of contact lateral border of the right heel/floor and tip of the left thumb/floor are absolute fixed spatial points during the pressure activity in the starting position.
Limitatio: The same as in the Diagonal Classic Frog.

Conditio: In the Diagonal Classic Frog, the upward-facing right patella is an absolute fixed spatial point.
Limitatio: This checks the continuing primary movement of the pelvis, internal rotation at the right hip. Moreover, a shift of the support area to the right, onto the lateral aspect of the right leg, is checked, maintaining the positive lifting stress on the abdominal muscles.

Conditio: In the Diagonal Primitive Frog, the upward-/right-facing right patella is an absolute fixed spatial point.
Limitatio: This fixed point checks the continuing primary movement of the pelvis, internal rotation at the right hip, by internal rotational active buttressing of the right leg at the right hip. Although the tolerance for internal rotation of the pelvis is greater than it is in the Diagonal Classic Frog, because of the external rotation of the right leg in the right hip in the starting position, the positive lifting stress on the abdominal muscles is still maintained because the support area cannot be displaced any further to the right.

Conditio of Movement Speed
Limitatio of Economical Activity by Finding the Optimal Speed
See pp. 14–15, analysis of the Classic Frog.

● **Position and Activation in the End Position**
  and Return to the Starting Position

See pp. 15–16, analysis of the Classic Frog.
Note: The diagonals in the Diagonal Classic Frog can be alternated without any change to the starting position. Ultimately, we can go on to diagonal countermove-

ments in which the abdominal muscles contract concentric-isotonically along one diagonal, performing positive lift, while along the other diagonal they contract eccentric-isotonically, performing negative lift.

Possible Combinations of the Classic Frog, Primitive Frog and Diagonal Frog

- Primary arm and leg movements of the Classic Frog
- Primary arm and leg movements of the Primitive Frog
- Primary arm movements of the Classic Frog, primary leg movements of the Primitive Frog
- Primary arm movements of the Primitive Frog, primary leg movements of the Classic Frog
- Diagonal Classic Frog
- Diagonal Primitive Frog
- Diagonal Frog: primary arm movement of the Classic Frog, primary leg movement of the Primitive Frog
- Diagonal Frog: primary arm movement of the Primitive Frog, primary leg movement of the Classic Frog with hip adduction.

Possible Combinations of Movement Directions "Into the End Position" and "Into the Starting Position"

- Symmetrical primary arm and leg movements from the starting position into the end position.
- Symmetrical primary arm movements from the starting position into the end position with simultaneous symmetrical primary leg movements from the end position into the starting position, or symmetrical primary arm movements from the end position into the starting position with simultaneous symmetrical primary leg movements from the starting position into the end position.
- Primary movements of the right arm and right leg from the starting position into the end position and back into the starting position, or primary movements of the left arm and left leg from the starting position into the end position and back into the starting position. The leg of the Classic Frog is adducted at the hip in the end position. The leg of the Primitive Frog begins from the adapted starting position of the Diagonal Frog (see p. 31).
- Primary movement of the right arm from the starting position into the end position and back into the starting position with simultaneous primary movement of the left leg from the end position into the starting position and back into the end position, or primary movement of the left arm from the starting position into the end position and back into the starting position with simultaneous primary movement of the right leg from the end position into the starting position and back into the end position.

Application of the Frog Exercises to Common Postural Deviations from the Hypothetical Norm

– Hollow back with + flexion of pelvis at the hips/ + LS/ + TS/ + CS[1]: use primary arm movements of the Classic Frog, primary leg movements of the Primitive Frog.
– Flat back with + flexion of pelvis at the hips/ + LS/ – TS/ – CS: use Primitive Frog and Diagonal Primitive Frog.
– Flat back with + extension of pelvis at the hips/ – LS/ – TS/ – CS: use standard or diagonal primary arm movements of the Primitive Frog, standard or diagonal primary leg movements of the Classic Frog with adduction at the hips
– Thoracic round back with + extension of the pelvis at the hips/ – LS/ + TS/ + CS: use primary arm and leg movements of the Classic Frog and of the Diagonal Classic Frog
– Complete round back with + flexion of the knees/ + flexion of the thighs at the hips/ – LS/ + TS/ + CS: use the Diagonal Classic Frog.

1.4 Adaptation of the Frogs by Altering the Position in Space of the Long Axis of the Body (Figs. 8-14)

If for any reason the possible combinations of the Classic Frog and the adaptations of the Primitive Frog and the Diagonal Frog, in which the long axis of the body is always horizontal, do not permit functional training of the abdominal muscles without imposing uneconomical stress on the spinal column, a further possibility of adapting the Frogs exists: we keep the primary arm and leg movements of the Classic, Primitive and Diagonal Frogs, but change the position in space of the long axis of the body. In so doing, we are able to neutralize the effect of relative overweight in individual body segments.

Adaptation for + LS/Weak, Atonic Abdominal Muscles/ + Weight in the Legs, Especially in the Thighs/ + Weight Around the Pelvis (Fig. 8)

● **Position and Activation in the Starting Position**

Using a pillow or folded towel, BS pelvis is raised as high above BS thorax as is necessary to bring the critical lumbar section of the spine into neutral or slight flexion. By flexing the thighs at the hips, the weight of the legs is brought to rest in such a position over the upper body and in space that the abdominal muscles need not perform any fall-preventing activity. The knees are flexed so far that the "ischiocrural brake" is ready to lift the weight of the pelvis up off the

---
[1] For notation, see *Functional Kinetics*, pp. 213 ff.

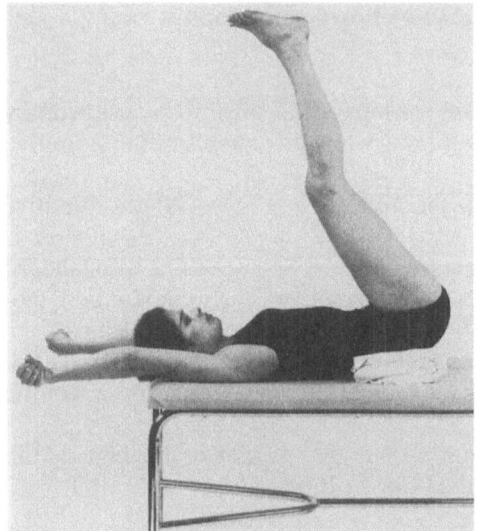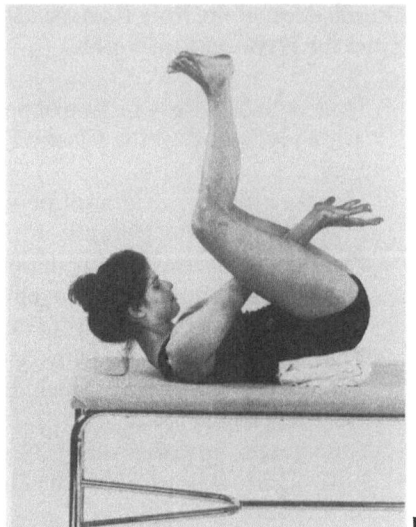

Fig. 8 a, b. Adaptation of the Classic Frog. **a** Starting position, **b** end position

base support. This enhances the caudal-to-cranial motive components of the straight abdominal muscles. BS arms is in the starting position of the Classic Frog.

● Actio and Conditio of the Movement Sequence

The critical distance point of the primary leg movement, DP right and left heels joined, moves dorsally/downwards/cranially. As it does so, flexion is effected in the lumbar spine by the caudal lever and DP symphysis pubis moves towards the navel, contracting the lower abdomen.

The critical distance point of the primary head movement, DP vertex, moves ventrally/upwards/caudally, activating the straight abdominal muscles in a cranial-to-caudal continuing movement. Because of the body's position in space in this exercise, the thoracic spine is not lifted up from the base support, and contact point dorsal aspect of BS thorax/floor is an absolute fixed spatial point that checks the contraction of the upper abdomen. If the abdominal muscles are very weak and the arms are short in proportion to the length of the upper body, the primary arm movements can be adapted by moving the critical distance point of BS arms from the olecranons to the hands and keeping the conditio that the distance from DP shoulder joint to DP wrist remains constant throughout the movement sequence. The elbows then stabilize in extension, the lever constituted by the arms becomes longer and, in relation to the flexion/extension axes of the vertebrae, more weight is now brought caudally. The external rotation component in the shoulder joints ensures that the upper abdomen will narrow in a continuing movement.

36

Adaptation for + Length and + Weight of BS Thorax/ + Length and + Weight of BS Head/ + Weight of BS arms, Particularly in the Shoulder Girdle (Fig. 9)

● **Position and Activation in the Starting Position**

The patient sits on his ischial tuberosities on a relatively high treatment bench. In BS legs touch the floor the soles of the feet. The knee joints are in the neutral position and the talocrural joints are plantarflexed accordingly. The legs are in parking function. BSs pelvis, thorax and head, their joints in neutral, are aligned in the long axis of the body, which is vertical. BS arms assumes the starting position of the Classic Frog. The long axes of the arms incline forwards slightly. The way the weight of the arms is arranged stimulates dynamic extensional stabilization of the thoracic spine in the neutral position. The arms are in free play.

● **Actio and Conditio of the Movement Sequence**

From this starting position, the patient finds the position from which, using the primary arm and leg movements, he can manage to perform the Classic Frog.
When the long axis of the body inclines backwards by extension of the proximal lever in the hip joints, held by eccentric isotonic braking activity of the flexors, the

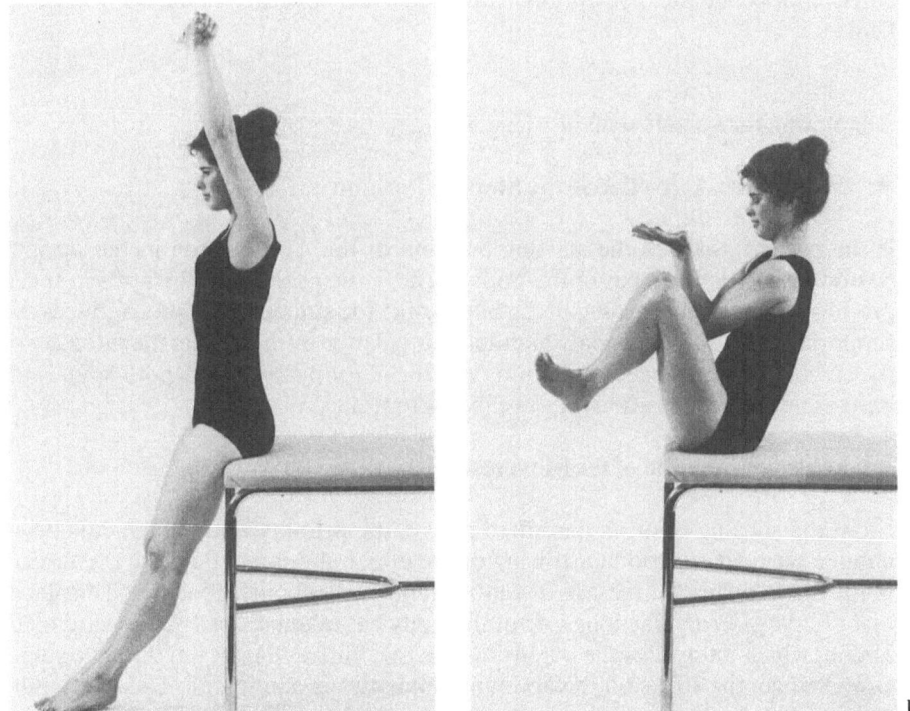

a   b

Fig. 9 a, b. Adaptation of the Classic Frog. **a** Starting position, **b** end position

pelvis extends at the hip joints by high intensity economical activity of the extensors working isotonic-concentrically, and there is flexion at the lumbosacral articulation. At the same time, the feet are dragged backwards along the floor slightly, such that first the heels then the forefeet leave the floor. The legs become the activated passive buttress of the backwards-leaning long axis of the body weighted with BSs pelvis, thorax, head and arms. They have to balance each other, like a set of beam scales: the point on which the beam pivots is the edge of the treatment bench. Although the abdominal muscles, already contracted in the lower abdomen and stretched in the upper abdomen, have a strong motive component, what is most required of them is maximum intensity fall-preventing activity. If the primary weight is too great, the exercise can be adapted by altering the position of the arms: their long axes can be inclined forwards more or less by extension in the shoulder joints.

From this "ready-to-go position", the arms and legs perform the primary movements of the Classic Frog. These primary movements are coordinated in time and space such that the long axis of the body is kept as a virtual axis of the body (see p. 46 and Glossary), inclining backwards enough to balance the legs – which are the counterweight – even when the arms have reached their end position.

This adaptation of the Classic Frog is an exercise in autodidactic training with the patient's own body weights; there can therefore be no prescribed angle for the backward inclination of the long axis of the body. However, the conditio that BSs pelvis, thorax and head be optimally aligned in the long axis of the body must be kept.

Adaptation for Spinal Instability (Fig. 10)

● **Position and Activation in the Starting Position**

If the patient assumes the starting position of the Classic Frog in the upright position with the long axis of the body vertical, the position of the arms in space produces an overlengthening of the body while the standing on tiptoe reduces the support area. He can then only maintain his balance by increasing the intensity of the stabilizing muscle activity. This is beneficial for patients with poor spinal stability. The starting position thus also helps to train skill.

● **Actio and Conditio of the Movement Sequence**

From the starting position described above, the primary arm movements bring about a particularly good narrowing of the upper abdomen. Because the flexion of the hip joint has, for reasons of equilibrium, come about by backward displacement of the fulcrum, the long axis of the body has taken on a slight forward inclination, which intensifies the extensional active buttressing in the thoracic spine. In exchange, the stress on the abdominal muscles is eliminated. The continuing activity of the oblique abdominal muscles which narrows the upper abdomen must be maintained by the constant directional pull caudally/downwards/me-

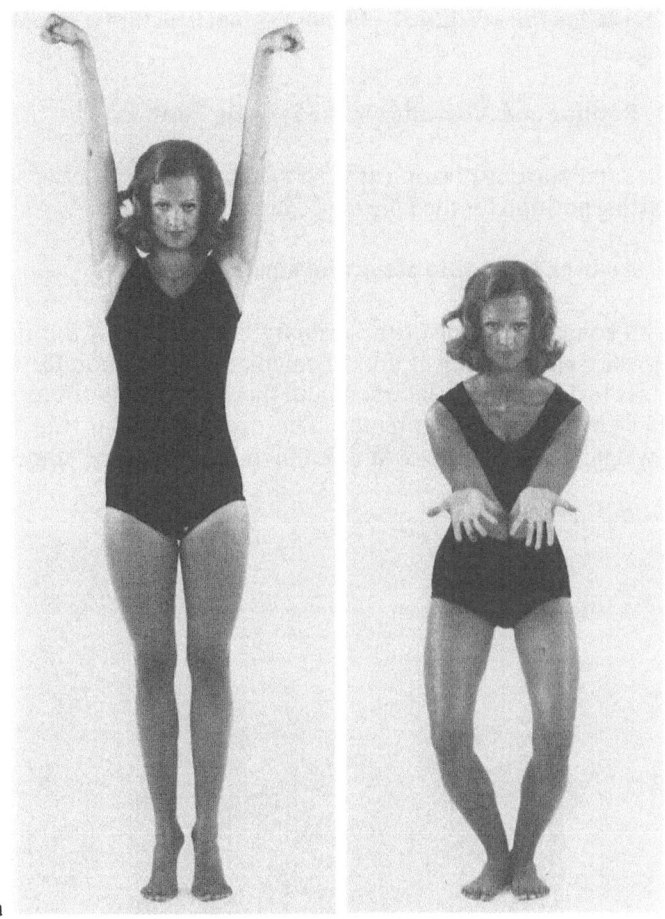

Fig. 10 a, b. Adaptation of the Classic Frog. **a** Starting position, **b** end position

dially/backwards of the critical distance points of the primary movements of the arms, DPs right and left olecranons. Because the legs are now in supporting function, their primary movement is completely altered. With the backward/downward displacement of the flexion/extension axes of the hips in flexion, and with dorsiflexion in the talocrural joints by dorsal/downward displacment of the fulcrum, the heels bring about full sole contact with the floor, thus expanding the support area backwards. As reactio, the flexion/extension axes of the knees automatically move forwards/downwards, bringing about the necessary horizontal compensation of equilibrium. The flexion in the hip joints gives the pelvis, as proximal lever, enough movement tolerance for extension so that, to perfect the end position, extension of the pelvis at the hip joints can bring about caudally arising flexion in the lumbar spine and, with it, contraction of the lower abdomen.

Adaptation for + Widths/ − Depths/Spinal Instability/Spinal Hypermobility
(Fig. 11)

● **Position and Activation in the Starting Position**

The same starting position as described for the previous adaptation is used as the starting position for the Diagonal Classic Frog.

● **Actio and Conditio of the Movement Sequence**

With commencement of the primary movements of the right arm and the left leg, the right heel moves dorsally/medially to the floor, the talocrural joint dorsiflexes by fulcrum displacement and there is external rotation at the left hip joint effected by the distal pointer. The displacement of the heel medially makes a weight shift to the right for the right-leg stance unnecessary because the

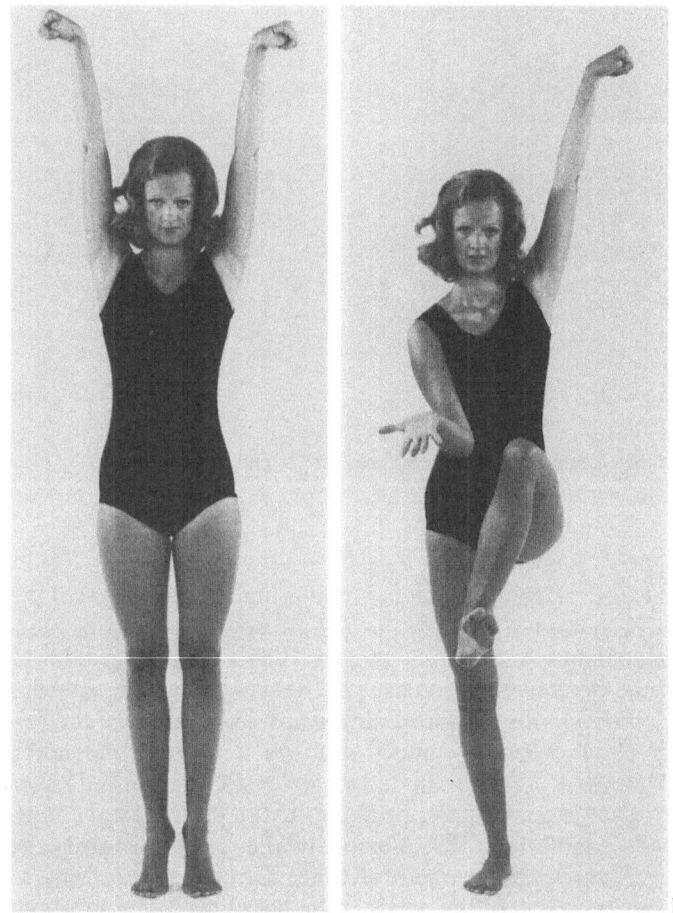

a   b

Fig. 11 a, b. Adaptation of the Diagonal Frog, diagonal, standing. **a** Starting position, **b** end position

40

heel has shifted underneath the centre of gravity and the primary moving extremities bring their weight towards the plane of symmetry and forwards. Because of the conditio that the long axis of the body, a fixed spatial point, remains vertical, the weight of the left leg forces the abdominal muscles to engage in lifting work, while the right arm finds in the extensionally stabilized spinal column an active buttress resisting the contraction of the oblique abdominal muscles from the right/above to the left/below. This extensional active buttressing is reinforced by the tendency of BS head to translate dorsally, keeping the upper abdomen long. The left arm also helps to sustain the extensional stabilization of the spine. The primary movement of the left leg brings the pelvis as the last lever into the continuing movement which, as it flows, extends the right hip, flexes the lumbar spine caudal-to-cranially, and shortens the lower abdomen. The abductional movement component of the pelvis at the right hip is neutralized by the external rotation occurring in the left hip effected by the distal pointer.

Adaptation for Flatback and Spinal Instability (Figs. 12 and 13)

● **Position and Activation of the Starting Position**

The arms move in the Original Frog and in the Diagonal Original Frog, while one leg moves through the Diagonal Classic Frog sequence.
The starting position has the larger support area. For the Diagonal Frog, the right heel just drops backwards/medially and assumes the weight for one-legged standing.

● **Actio and Conditio of the Movement Sequence** (see pp. 12 and 24)

**Adaptation for + Length and + Weight in BSs Thorax and Head
and/or When Coming to Sit from Supine Without Avoidance Mechanisms
or Incorrect Stressing of the Spinal Column Is Desired** (Fig. 14)

● **Position and Activation in the Starting Position**

The patient's BSs thorax and head, being constitutionally longer or heavier than the norm, make it impossible for him to sit up from supine without the use of weights accelerating footwards. So as not to injure the spine, and to maintain the integrity of the long axis of the body, this acceleration will be assigned to the arms and legs.
As a good starting position for the arms and legs we take that of the Classic Frog. BSs pelvis, thorax and head are aligned in the long axis of the body, which is horizontal, and their dorsal aspects form the contact with the base support.
BS arms is in the starting position of the Classic Frog, but the elbows are in flexion effected by the distal lever.
BS legs is almost in the end position of the Classic Frog, but the pelvis is not raised off the base support. BSs thorax, head and arms are all parked on the treatment

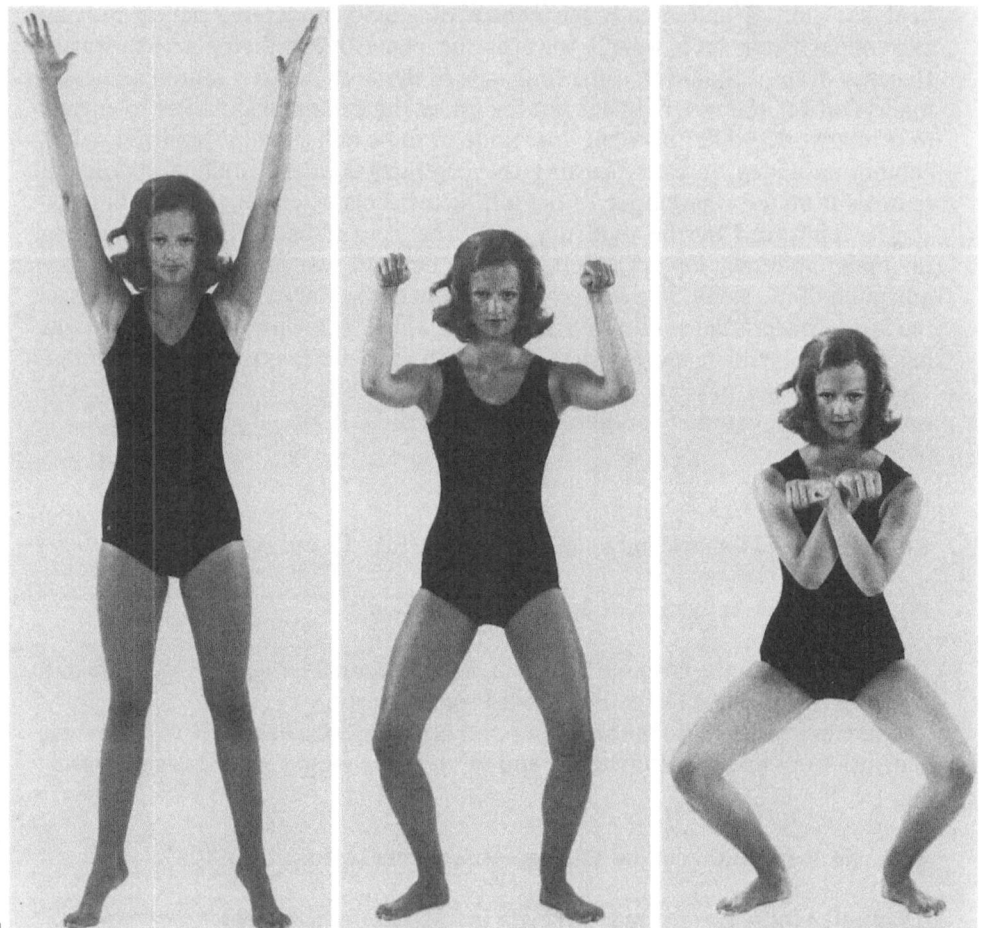

a, b   c

Fig. 12 a–c. Adaptation of the Primitive Frog. **a** Starting position, **b** middle of the sequence,
c end position

bench. The legs are in free play and are suspended extensionally at the hips from
the pelvis.

● Actio and Conditio of the Movement Sequence

Because of the flexed elbows in this adaptation, the critical distance points of the
primary arm movement are DPs right and left hands. They move footwards and
somewhat ventrally/upwards, with extension in the elbows and extension, adduction and external rotation in the shoulders by continuing movement. Because the
position in space of the long axis of the body is changing from horizontal to vertical, the long axis of the arms will in the end position be almost horizontal, slanting
slightly downwards.

42

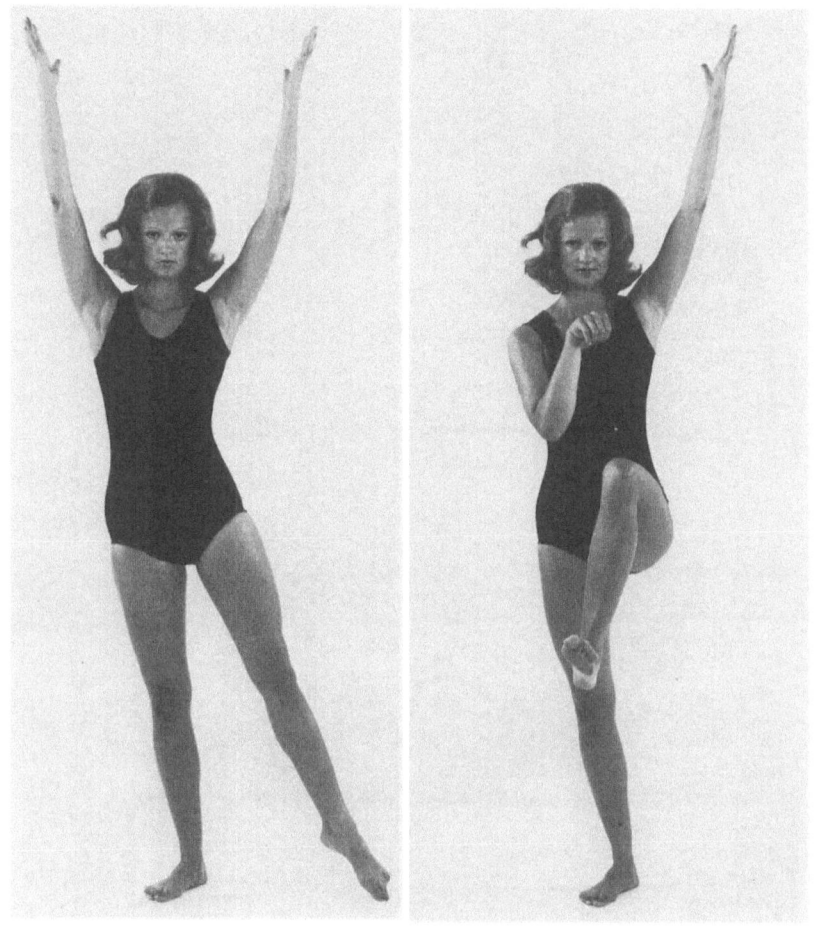

Fig. 13 a, b. Adaptation of the Diagonal Frog. **a** Mid-sequence, **b** end position

The critical distance points of the primary movements of the legs, DPs tips of the right and left feet, move downwards/dorsally/caudally. Due to their markedly horizontal direction component they act as an accelerating weight, and the same applies to the weight of the arms. Both horizontal direction components move footwards and they have a cumulative effect. The segments aligned in the long axis of the body, BSs pelvis, thorax and head, are lifted up with flexion in the hips, the abdominal muscles having to perform fall-preventing work in order to stabilize the long axis of the body.

In Fig. 14 b, moderate acceleration of the primary movement of the arms could have prevented the avoidance movement made by the head, which is reducing the length of the caudal lever by bringing about flexion in the cervical and upper thoracic spine, causing the upper abdomen to contract. If the instructions are correctly given, this fault does not arise.

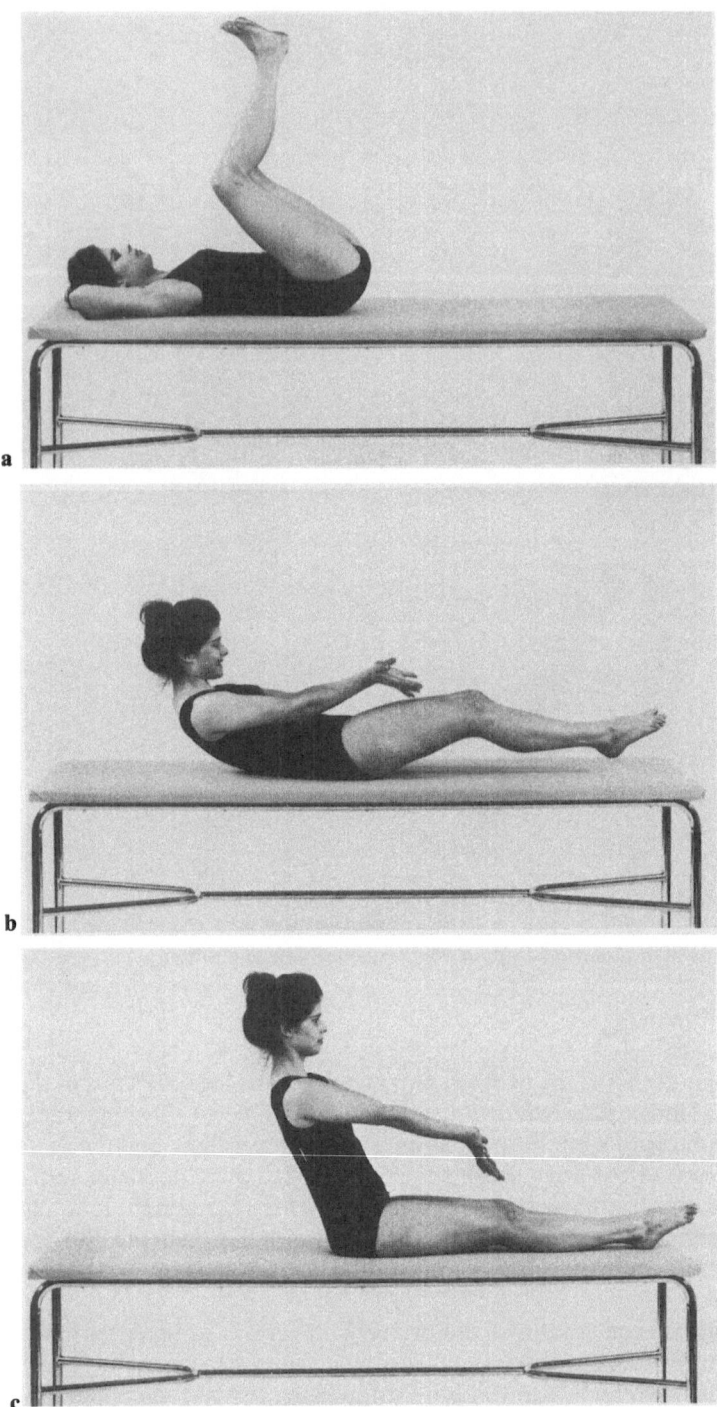

Fig. 14 a–c. Adaptation of the Classic Frog. **a** Starting position, **b** mid-sequence, **c** end position

Conclusion

We have seen how many possible adaptations to the Frogs there are, suiting every possible patient, save those whose abdominal muscles are by reason of some pathological condition nonfunctional. Once the patient has incorporated an appropriate Frog exercise into his normal movement behaviour, he can, using details of the exercise, practice contracting his abdominal muscles in every possible position throughout the day, provided that the spinal column is always brought into the optimal starting position by the alignment of BSs pelvis, thorax and head in the long axis of the body. Prolonged expiration, for instance, coupled with extensional active buttressing of the thoracic spine in its neutral position, is one abdominal muscle exercise which is very easy to practice.

Once the motor image has become imprinted in his memory, the patient will gain so much enjoyment from combining all these different elements into one smooth complete movement that he will not mind doing his exercises again and again.

2 The All-Fours Exercises: Functional Training of the Back Muscles

Functional training of the back muscles activates the back muscles as for their normal physiological function.

Note

Because, in typical human posture, the long axis of the body is vertical in space, and because it is a virtual axis that has first to be brought into being by the inherently mobile spinal column, maintaining proper posture is primarily a fight against gravity. For this reason, the kyphotically curved thoracic spine must be extensionally stabilized to prevent falling.

In these exercises we want to strengthen above all the muscles of the thoracic spine by subjecting them to positive lifting stress (i.e. making them work against gravity).

In upright posture, the different spinal segments behave in reaction to gravity in different ways. The lordotic segments – the pelvis at the hip joints and the lumbar spine, the head in the atlanto-occipital, atlanto-axial and cervical joints – are potentially mobile because their position in relation to gravity is neutral. As soon as the long axis of the body inclines forwards, however, or a leg is lifted from the floor by extension at the hip, the lordotic segments of the spine must also either become activated extensionally to prevent falling or perform positive lifting work.

An additional aim of functional training of the back muscles is to develop good mobility of the spinal column in all movement components. This is important, because good mobility of the spine is necessary for optimal alignment of the virtual long axis of the body and for economic combining of dynamic stabilization with movement or displacement through changes in the position of the joints within the different sections of the spinal column.

Function of the Autochthonous Back Muscles

The autochthonous back muscles dynamically stabilize the thoracic spine in its neutral position when the long axis of the body is vertical, in order to:
- Make available the potential movement tolerance for rotation about the long axis of the body between pelvis and thorax and in the cervical area
- Allow potential mobility of the pelvis and the head

- Provide active buttressing to the movements of respiration and of the extremities
- Protect the passive structures of the spine during positive and negative lifting

The autochthonous back muscles stabilize the entire spinal column when the long axis of the body inclines out of the vertical plane, especially forwards.

The autochthonous back muscles shorten the body appropriately for movements such as ducking, stooping or crouching, etc.

Position in Space of the Long Axis of the Body During Training of the Back Muscles

When the long axis of the body is roughly vertical, the spinal column is subjected to compressive load. Compressive loading is physiological for the spinal column, as is the extensional activity in the thoracic spine mentioned above. Compressive impulses to the roughly vertical long axis of the body, such as those occurring when we run, jump or carry heavy objects on our head, intensify this extensional activity. All distally arising movement impulses of the extremities elicit automatic and finely differentiated activation of the back muscles.

Cranially arising activation: Dorsal translations of the head in the plane of symmetry intensify the extensional activity of the thoracic spine; ventral translations activate the extensor muscles of the cervical spine. Translations in the frontal plane cannot be performed without extensional activity throughout the entire spine column.

Arm movements take place primarily in the space in front of the midfrontal plane and require activity of the back muscles in continuing movements and active buttressing.

Caudally arising activation: First and foremost, the lumbar spine is activated during walking by constant flexional, extensional and lateroflexional impulses. Leg movements performed behind the midfrontal plane require extensional activity of the back muscles.

A primary function of the back muscles is to stabilize the spinal column during vigorous movements, during active buttressing of movements of the extremities, and in order to actively buttress rib movements during forced exhalation. In stabilization of the spinal column the rotational component is very versatile: when a greater area of action is needed at the periphery (wide arm movements, big steps), it is released; when less peripheral area is needed, it is included the stabilization. Even when the spine is completely stabilized, however, the movements of the extremities and of respiration produce so much fluctuation in muscle tone that the threshold for symptoms of fatigue is astonishingly high.

Forward inclination of the long axis of the body: The automatic activity of the back muscles is easier and more primitive because now only extensional activity is required of the entire spinal column. If, however, the weights leaning forwards are too heavy or the lever too long in relation to the support area, an unavoidable avoidance mechanism to shorten the lever will occur: the pelvis will extend at the hip joints and the lumbar spine will flex, causing uneconomical stress on the spinal column.

Backward inclination of the long axis of the body: The main muscle activity occurs ventrally.

2.1 The Classic All-Fours Exercise (Fig. 15)

The name "Classic All-Fours Exercise" is an invented name. "All-Fours" refers to the starting position and "Classic" means that this exercise is the key to physiological training of the back muscles.

■ Goal of the Exercise

The goal of the exercise is for the patient to learn to functionally train the back muscles, i. e. to
– Stabilize the thoracic spine extensionally in its neutral position
– Centre lifting stress on the thoracic spine by active buttressing of rotation between the thorax and pelvis about the long axis of the body
– Mobilize the spinal column as needed
– Reduce lifting stress on the lumbar spine
– Develop skill in the back muscles by employing rotational equilibrium reactions about the stabilized long axis of the body.

▶ Functional Analysis in Therapist Language

The Classic All-Fours Exercise is suitable for training the back muscles in persons with a normal spinal column or a variant of the norm. Thoracic round back (+ TS), increased sagittotransverse diameter of the thorax and reduced lumbar lordosis (– LS) are conditions that can be improved by this exercise.

● Conception of the Exercise

In order to demand lift of the extensor muscles of the spinal column, we bring the body segments aligned in the long axis of the body – BSs pelvis, thorax and head – into the horizontal position. These segments should not touch the base support and the back must face upwards. Therefore, we choose the all-fours stance atop a box as starting position. The knees and the palms are the points of contact with the base support. The proximal joints of the extremities are in the middle position and the long axes of the arms and thighs are roughly vertical. From this starting position we can achieve the goal of the exercise. We will employ movements of the extremities that, arising distally, continue into the spinal column and stabilize it, mobilize it as necessary and, by the weight of the extremities, bring stress to bear upon it. In the starting position the weight of BS head is already suspended from the thoracic spine. Since the head must not change its position in relation to the thoracic spine, it exerts stress on the thoracic spine and thus stabilizes it.
As soon as one hand and the opposite knee leave the base support, the skill training of the spinal column begins. The moment they are lifted from the base support,

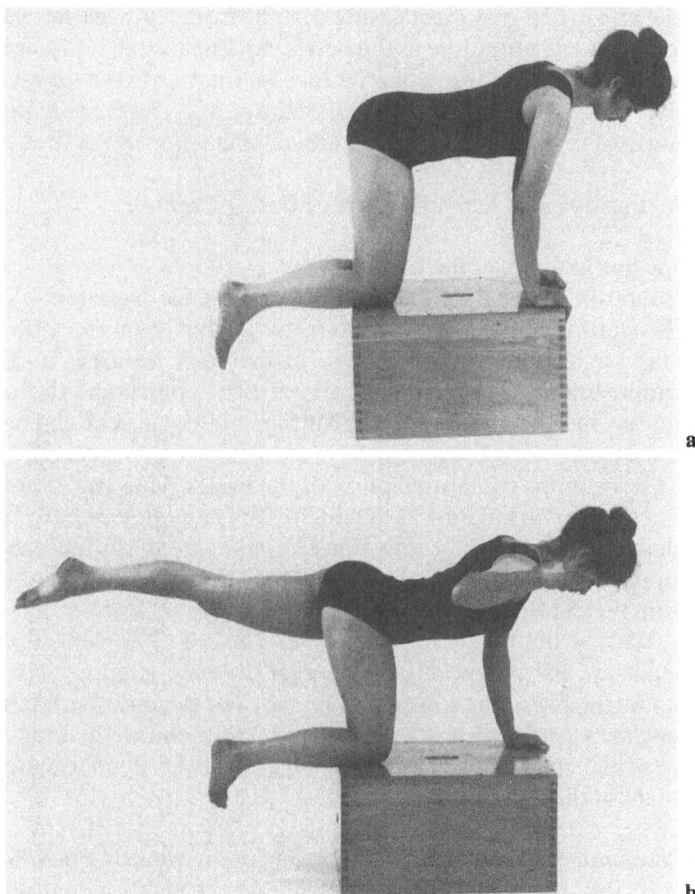

Fig. 15 a, b. Classic All-Fours Exercise. **a** Starting position, **b** end position

the weights of the arm and leg in free play become suspended from the spinal column and from the supporting arm and leg via the proximal joints of the extremities. The supporting arm and leg also have to take some of the weight of the pelvis and thorax. Because the free-play leg together with the pelvis and the free-play arm together with the thorax are so different in shape and weight, and meet the long axis of the body from right and left, the rotational components of the spinal column are unevenly stressed and are therefore unstable. Since the leg and arm in free play have sufficient movement tolerance in their proximal joints to lift their long axes into the horizontal, their weight can be utilized to increase the lifting stress (the demand for lifting work) on the extensors of the spinal column.

The movement of the leg in free play has the additional function of rotating the frontal plane of the pelvis out of the horizontal by continuing movement. In this manner, the extensional stress on the lumbar spine is reduced and the movement tolerance for rotation in the thoracic spine is mobilized, thus restoring the equilibrium.

The arm in free play must ensure that the frontal planes of the thorax remain horizontal and do not rotate as the pelvis did. The thorax remains in place as an active buttress and the movement tolerance for rotation in the thoracic spine can be completely utilized by the movement of the pelvis. The tendency of the head to translate dorsally guarantees the dynamic stabilization of the thoracic spine.

● Position and Activation in the Starting Position

Position in Space of the Critical Axes
Points of Contact Between the Body and the Environment
The starting position is on all fours atop a box (Fig. 15 a). BSs pelvis, thorax and head are aligned in the long axis of the body, which is horizontal. The patient forms a bridge, the arch being formed by BSs pelvis and thorax. BS head projects out beyond the bridge into the air like a tentacle. The patient's gaze is directed downwards.
BS arms forms the cranial pillar of the bridge, with the elbows flexed enough so that the arms are as long as the thighs. The hands are directly below the shoulders, their long axes pointing cranially. The palms are the points of contact with the base support. The olecranons point caudally. The bridge is suspended at its thoracic end from the shoulder girdle.
In BS legs the thighs form the caudal pillars. The ventral aspects of the tibial heads are the points of contact with the base support. The knees are directly below the hips. The lower legs project out beyond the box like tentacles, their long axes more or less parallel to each other and to the long axis of the body. At its pelvic end the arch of the bridge hangs suspended extensionally from the thighs at the hip joints.

Components of Movement in Relation to the Neutral Position of the Joints
In BS legs, the joints of the toes and feet are roughly in neutral position; the knees are in about 90° flexion/0° rotation; the hips are in about 90° flexion effected by the distal lever, so that the knees are directly below the hips, and 0° rotation, so that the long axes of the lower legs are in the sagittal plane of the hips.
BS pelvis is in about 90° flexion at the hip joints; the lumbar spine is in neutral position.
In BS arms, the fingers are flexed over the edge of the box. The finger tips point downwards; the thumbs joint cranially/medially; the wrists are extended to about 90°; the forearms are pronated and the elbows are flexed so far that the length of the arms is roughly that of the thighs, enabling the long axis of the body to remain horizontal. The shoulders are in 75°–85° flexion, depending on the arm length needed, and in so much adduction/external rotation that the long axes of the forearms and upper arms are in the sagittal planes of the shoulders. The plane of the scapula is almost horizontal and the scapula stays as close as possible to the thorax hanging from the shoulder girdle.
In BS thorax, the thoracic spine is in neutral position; the ribs continue to move with inspiration and expiration.
In BS head, the cervical spine is in neutral position and the atlanto-occipital and atlanto-axial joints are flexed such that the patient's gaze is directed downwards.

50

Movement Tolerances at the Critical Joints in Relation
to the Intended Primary Movement

Because the spinal column is in neutral position, it has tolerance for movement in all movement components. In this exercise rotation is needed in the area of the lower thoracic spine. Large movement excursions will take place in the arm and leg in free play and in the supporting hip.

The arm in free play needs those movement tolerances that allow the arm to be brought into the frontal plane of the thorax, now horizontal, with the elbow flexed: these are tolerances for forearm supination, elbow flexion, shoulder extension abduction/external rotation, and that movement tolerance in the sternoclavicular joint which allows the medial margin of the scapula to approach the thoracic spine by opening of the pincer jaws.

The leg in free play needs those movement tolerances that allow the long axis of the leg to be brought horizontal and more or less parallel to the long axis of the body. In the supporting hip, the pelvis is twisted upwards out of the horizontal, performing transverse abduction in the hip joint, of which it is the proximal lever, and rotation in the lower thoracic spine, of which it is the caudal lever.

Distribution of Body Weight on a Base Support or Suspension Device,
Against a Supportive Device, or over a Support Area,
and the Resulting Activity States of the Musculature

The support area in the starting position is the smallest surface encompassing the points of contact palms/base support and knees/base support – in this case, the box.

BS arms and the thighs are in supporting function. The lower legs and feet are in free play; they hang suspended from the thighs by flexional activity at the knees.

BS head is in free play. Aligned in the long axis of the body, it hangs suspended from the thorax by dorsal-translatory and extensional activity at the cervical spine. The ventral lower muscles of BSs pelvis and thorax are engaged in bridging activity. The pelvis, as the caudal end of the bridge, hangs suspended from the thighs by extensional activity at the hips. The thorax, as the cranial end of the bridge, hangs suspended from the shoulder girdle by the lemnisci of the trapezius, the rhomboids and the serratus anterior muscles.

Intensity of Muscle Activity Required with Economical Activity
Respiration

In the starting position of the Classic All-Fours Exercise, the intensity of economical activity is generally low. It is slightly higher in BS head because the long axis of the body is horizontal, and is highest in BS arms because they are not used to being in supporting function. The patient will experience resistance to normal breathing in, due to the bridging activity of the abdominal muscles.

● Actio – Reactio of the Movement Sequence

The movement sequence of the Classic All-Fours Exercise is in two parts. Only after the preparatory trot phase can the patient go into the movement sequence proper from a trot position into the end position.

Trot Phase

Actio: The Primary Movement
The actio is directed downwards. It consists of two simultaneous primary movements or primary activities.
The critical distance points of the two primary movements, DPs right knee and left palm/left knee and right palm, alternately exert increased pressure on the base support. This increased pressure raises the intensity of the economical activity of the supporting function alternately in the right leg and left arm and in the left leg and right arm.

Reactio: Activated Passive Buttressing
Although the actio is directed downwards, it evokes a reactio that is directed upwards. This is partly because the actio is a change not in the position of the joints but in the activity states within the body, and partly because it is triggered simultaneously at two different body sites located asymmetrically on opposite sides of the horizontally positioned long axis of the body.
The critical distance points of the reactio of activated passive buttressing, DPs left knee and right palm/right knee and left palm, alternately lose contact with the base support. This reactio brings first the left leg and right arm and then the right leg and left arm into free play.

Reactio: Change in the Support Area
The reactio is a drastic reduction of the support area by more than half. The support area in the starting position is a rectangle marked by the points of contact between the hands and knees and the base support. The support area in each trot position is the smallest area encompassing the points of contact between the supporting hand and supporting knee and the base support – only a narrow parallelogram. Projected onto the ventral aspect of BSs pelvis and thorax, it would be a diagonal strip running from the hip of the supporting leg to the shoulder of the supporting arm. A support area so reduced makes the rotational components of the spinal column unstable.

Actio: Accelerating Weights
Reactio: Braking Weights
Because the primary activities have no horizontal components, we cannot speak in terms of accelerating and braking weights. Nevertheless, we should watch the equilibrium reactions that, through changes in activity states, have to balance out the unequal weights of the free-play leg together with the pelvis and the free-play arm together with the thorax, without any avoidance mechanisms such as a horizontal shifting of weight occurring.
In the shift from one trot to another, horizontal avoidance mechanisms in BSs pelvis, thorax and head can be prevented because the simultaneous increase in the pressure exercised by the supporting arm and the supporting leg occurs on both sides of the long axis of the body, with the frontal planes of BSs pelvis, thorax and head horizontal. If these body segments are to remain aligned in the long axis of the body, no weight can be displaced over the supporting leg and/or arm. Weight

lying medially must therefore be connected to the relevant supporting extremity by muscle activity. In the Classic All-Fours Exercise, the medial weight attached to the supporting leg is that of the pelvis, which must be anchored to the upper thigh of the supporting leg by the muscle activity of transverse abduction, and which brings with it the weight of the free-play leg suspended from the pelvis, thus increasing the pressure on the base support. For the supporting arm, the additional weight that increases the pressure on the base support comes from the weight of the thorax and the free-play arm together with a portion of the weight of the head, which is suspended from the shoulder girdle on the side of the supporting arm.

In this exercise, then, we cannot talk of accelerating and braking weights, but rather of weights that either press down or hang. By not having a horizontal displacement of weight we have considerably increased the intensity of economical activity in the proximal joints of the supporting extremities.

Movement from the Trot Position into the End Position

This is a constant-location movement sequence. In the following description, a right supporting leg and left supporting arm are assumed (Fig. 15 b).

Actio: The Primary Movement

The actio in this movement sequence is characterized by three simultaneous continuing primary movements of the left (free-play) leg, the right (free-play) arm and BS head. The dominant direction component of the critical distance points is vertical and upwards. The horizontal components must not be allowed to compromise the dominant direction component, so that the positive lifting stress exerted by the weight of the extremities on the thoracic spine can have its full effect.

The critical distance point of the primary movement of the free-play leg, DP left patella, moves caudally/upwards/slightly to the left. The knee extends by fulcrum displacement; the left foot plantarflexes at the talocrural joint, and inverts at the subtalar and talocalcaneonavicular joints. The left thigh, as distal lever of the left hip joint, rotates in extension/very slight abduction/external rotation. By continuing movement, the pelvis, as proximal lever of the right (supporting) hip joint, rotates in transverse abduction together with the free-play leg. This is the first critical fulcrum of the continuing movement of the free-play leg. In relation to the thorax, the line connecting the iliac spines is the caudal pointer of rotation level lower thoracic spine. When the free-play leg moves and the pelvis rotates upwards out of its horizontal starting position, a pelvis-negative rotation occurs in the lower thoracic spine. This is the second critical fulcrum (or pivot) of the continuing movement of the free-play leg. The continuing movement is actively buttressed by thorax-positive rotational activation of the cranial pointer of rotation level lower thoracic spine, the frontotransverse diameter of the thorax, which is not allowed to move out of the horizontal.

The critical distance point of the primary movement of the right (free-play) arm, DP radial styloid process, moves dorsally/upwards/slightly laterally. As it moves, the extension/flexion axis of the wrist, the distal pointer, rotates into the vertical position as the forearm supinates. The wrist and digit joints are slightly flexed, the palm faces the shoulder, the long axis of the hand is held horizontal by fall-preventing radial abduction. To make this possible, DP olecranon has moved dorsally/upwards/laterally to the right/caudally into the midfrontal plane of the thorax, causing the elbow joint to flex by fulcrum displacement.

During this counter-rotational continuing movement, the upper arm, as distal lever, rotates at the shoulder joint in extension/abduction/external rotation. As the movement continues co-rotationally, DP acromion, as distal distance point of the sternoclavicular joint, moves dorsally/upwards/laterally to the right, adducting the medial margin of the scapula towards the thoracic spine. This is the critical fulcrum of the primary movement of the free-play arm. With this movement the pincer jaws open at the acromioclavicular joint.

The next lever or pointer to be caught in the "firing line" of the continuing movement of the free-play arm would be the frontotransverse diameter of the thorax, the caudal pointer of rotation level cervical spine and the cranial pointer of rotation level lower thoracic spine. However, it does not move, for thorax-positive rotational activation turns into active buttressing at the second critical fulcrum of the continuing movement of the free-play leg.

The critical distance points of the primary movement of the head, DPs right and left eyes, have a tendency to strive dorsally/upwards by flexion in the atlanto-occipital and atlanto-axial joints and by dorsal translation in the cervical spine. By continuing movement, the thoracic spine is stimulated extensionally. This extensional stimulation is selective: its effect is limited to the thoracic spine. The pelvis-negative rotation in the lower thoracic spine moves the lumbar spine out of the firing line of the continuing effect of the primary movement of the head. If the head is maintained absolutely in the starting position, the positions of the atlanto-occipital and atlanto-axial joints and the joints of the cervical spine need not change; in this case, the primary movement of the head is only a raised intensity of activity induced by the striving to move away.

Reactio: Activated Passive Buttressing
Reactio: Change in the Support Area

A reactio in the form of activated passive buttressing does not occur, because the three primary movements are in effect mutually buttressing movements.

Likewise, a reactio in the form of a change in the support area does not occur. That the movement sequence out of the trot position is a constant-location sequence is more a conditio than a reactio.

● Conditio – Limitatio of the Movement Sequence

Conditio: Constant Distances Between Body Distance Points
Limitatio: Active Buttressing and Stabilization

Conditio: The distance from DP shoulder joint to DP wrist of the supporting arm remains constant.

Limitatio: If this distance remains constant, perfect supporting function in the supporting arm is guaranteed. The triceps brachii provides the fall-preventing activity. The rotational components actively buttressing each other are pronation in the forearm and external rotation in the shoulder joint. By continuing movement, the pincer jaws open and the scapula is adducted against the thoracic spine. This movement puts the scapular plane in a good position relative to the thorax, which, as we have already mentioned, is connected to the shoulder girdle by hanging activity.

Conditio: The distance from DP point of the chin to DP jugular notch remains constant.
Limitatio: If this distance is to remain constant, BS head must remain aligned in the long axis of the body and the midfrontal plane of the thorax must remain horizontal.

Conditio: The distance from DP transverse plane through the navel to DP transverse plane through the xiphoid process remains constant.
Limitatio: This distance remains constant, even if the pelvis rotates at rotation level lower thoracic spine, provided that the thoracic spine remains stabilized in neutral in regard to flexion/extension.

Conditio: Only in the trot phase: The distance from DP shoulder joint to DP wrist of the free-play arm remains constant.
Limitatio: This distance remains constant if the arm moving into free play becomes intrinsically stabilized within itself as it leaves the base support. It is then in the best position for the supporting activity which will follow, when the shoulder girdle need only displace slightly dorsally against the thorax as the palm of the other arm, now going into free play, lifts up.

Conditio of Absolute and/or Relative Fixed Spatial Points
Limitatio by Limiting the Primary Movement, Activated Passive Buttressing and/or Change in the Support Area
In the Classic All-Fours Exercise there are absolute and relative fixed spatial points.

Conditio: The distance from the eyes to the floor is an absolute fixed spatial point.
Limitatio: This fixed point is responsible for the permanent striving of the head to translate dorsally both during the trot phase and throughout the movement sequence into the end position. It also prevents the primary activity of the head from turning into a primary movement, which would cause the thoracic spine to extend by continuing movement, and prevents the head from dropping downwards, which would shorten the distance of the eyes from the floor and cause the thoracic spine to flex.

Conditio: The unchanging horizontal position of the frontotransverse diameter of the thorax is an absolute fixed spatial point.
Limitatio: This fixed point guarantees that the continuing movement of the free-play leg is actively buttressed at the rotation level of the thoracic spine by the cranial pointer, the frontotransverse diameter of the thorax, and ensures that the movement tolerance for rotation in the lower thoracic spine is fully used up by the caudal pointer. During the trot stage, the limitatio of this active buttressing makes possible the small alternating rotational movement excursions of the caudal pointer in the lower thoracic spine.

Conditio: The head of the femur in the supporting hip and the head of the humerus of the supporting arm are absolute fixed spatial points.

Limitatio: These fixed points check the spontaneous equilibrium reaction by which the horizontal sagittofrontal axis of the supporting hip would shift laterally/downwards, causing transverse adduction, and the horizontal sagittofrontal axis of the supporting shoulder would shift laterally/downwards, causing transverse flexion.

In the trot stage, this limitation of activity facilitates the diagonal pressure activity of the supporting hand and supporting knee and stimulates pelvic rotation out of the horizontal – constituting a shortening of the pelvic lever – in the lower thoracic spine.

In the movement sequence from the trot position into the end position, this limitatio ensures that the movement tolerances at both critical fulcra of the continuing movement in the free-play leg are fully exhausted. The absolute fixed spatial point supporting shoulder keeps the thorax from dropping down with the free-play arm. Otherwise the thorax would be pulled out of the pincer jaws, these would then have to close up, and the hanging activity of the thorax from the pincer jaws on the side of the supporting arm would become a faulty stress.

Conditio: When the long axis of the free-play leg reaches the horizontal, it is more or less parallel to the long axis of the body.

Limitatio: This relative fixed spatial point limits the primary movement of the free-play leg, thereby ensuring optimal rotation of the pelvis in the lower thoracic spine by continuing movement.

Conditio: In the end position of the Classic All-Fours Exercise, all the long axes in the free-play arm are in the midfrontal plane of BS thorax, which is horizontal, and the flexion/extension axes of the elbow and wrist are vertical.

Limitatio: These relative fixed spatial points limit the mixture of movement components in the shoulder joint of the free-play arm in such a way that the movement continuing into the shoulder girdle and the activity continuing into the spinal column are precisely directed to actively buttress the rotation of the pelvis that continues from the movement of the free-play leg.

Conditio of Movement Speed
Limitatio of Economical Activity by Finding the Optimal Speed
Conditio: The trot phase of the Classic All-Fours Exercise must find its own speed gradually. The following has proved an effective way to do this. First, strictly maintaining every conditio of diagonal trotting, the patient practises the alternating trotting with the supporting arms only, then with the supporting legs only. When the two are put together, we must take particular care that the primary pressure activity in the supporting arm and the supporting leg start simultaneously.

Limitatio: The lowest intensity of economical activity in the trot phase is at 120 trots per minute. Slower or faster trotting increases the intensity of economical muscle activity. Having the patient hold the trot position is good training for balance, particularly if he then makes swiping movements out over the base support with his free-play arm and leg.

56

Conditio: The movement from the trot position into the end position of the Classic All-Fours Exercise is slow. The end position is held for a short time.

Limitatio: The ideal speed is 5 seconds for the movement sequence, 3 seconds for holding the end position. During the movement sequence, if the intensity of economic muscle activity is kept fairly low, the patient will benefit from the fine equilibrium reactions which automatically take place in order to keep the inherently mobile system of his body from losing its precarious balance and falling over. Holding the end position only serves its purpose if the patient becomes consciously aware both of the direction in which the three primary movements are pulling away and of the constant, even pressure activity of his supporting arm and leg at the points of contact with the base support.

- **Position and Activation in the End Position and Return to the Starting Position**

The way back from the end position into the starting position is through eccentric isotonic release of muscle tension. The end is reached when the right palm and the left knee resume their original places on the base support. At the moment when the support area once again becomes a rectangle, as the weight of the body becomes equally distributed over it, the muscle activity changes and becomes as it was in the starting position, described above.

▶ Instruction in Patient Language

- **Instructions Appealing to the Patient's Perception**

In the Classic All-Fours Exercise it is especially important that the patient consciously feel the increase and decrease in pressure at the points of contact between the knees and palms and the floor. In addition, he must try always to keep the proximal joints of the supporting extremities over their points of contact with the base support.

- **Verbal Instruction**   ● **Instruction by Manipulation**

Position and Activation in the Starting Position

"Kneel down on one edge of the box and support yourself with your hands on the opposite edge. Your face and stomach face the floor, trunk and head are horizontal, your bottom is over your knees, your shoulders over your hands.

You can feel your weight evenly distributed over all four limbs. Your arms have to work: make sure that your el-

It is helpful and often necessary to correct the patient's position manually, for the more precisely he takes up the position, the easier it is to achieve the specific activation successfully.

The position of the arms in particular often needs manual adjustment. Asking the patient not to resist, the therapist takes both elbows, flexes them to the de-bows point straight back and your fingers forwards. Your lower legs stick out into the air. Your trunk doesn't arch up or down and your head doesn't hang down. It's carried proudly."

gree needed, rotates the olecranons caudally, and creates the conditions for perfect weight bearing: external rotation in the shoulder and pronation of the forearm. Often, too, BS head needs to be manually aligned in the long axis of the body, slightly flexing the atlanto-occipital joint. The way the pelvis is suspended from the thighs can also be adjusted so that the lumbar spine is properly aligned in the long axis of the body.

Trot Phase

"Feel the floor under your hands. Now press downwards gently but firmly, as if the floor were spongy, first on the right, then on the left, then on the right again, and so on. Take your time but don't go too slowly. That's all you have to do.

Now do with your knees what you just did with your hands, without letting your bottom wag.

Now both together: right hand and left knee, left hand and right knee, like a perpetual motion machine set to andante con moto."

The manipulation during the trot phase consists of lightly touching the greater trochanter of the supporting leg to make the patient aware when he has displaced it too far laterally/downwards, and if necessary correct it. The same is done for the shoulder joint of the supporting arm. Such faulty lateral/downward displacements distort the alignment of the long axis of the body, jeopardizing the active buttressing of rotation around this axis.

Movement Sequence from the Trot Position into the End Position and Back into the Starting Position

"You trot slower and slower and come to a halt on your right hand and left knee.

Your left hand and right knee hover over the floor and you cautiously feel around your immediate surroundings. If everything is all right, you can start to trot again, stopping this time on your left hand and right knee, and taking time to feel around. Now make that hovering leg long, lifting it upwards, the sole facing inwards. At the same time, the hovering hand moves up alongside the shoulder. The point of the elbow is level with the hand."

During the movement phase, the therapist can manually adjust the way the free-play arm and leg are positioned in relation to the other body segments. This is an very gentle manipulation. If, however, the patient is unable to tighten the twist of BS pelvis against BS thorax, the therapist can help by pushing her one arm under the free-play leg and the side of the pelvis belonging to it and her other arm under the free-play arm and the side of the thorax belonging to it. The therapist assumes the greater part of these weights, manipulates the twist of BSs pelvis and thorax against each other and then lets the patient hold this new position.

58

"You see the floor. Imagine that the spot you're looking at is a beautiful ornament. To help you see it better, you slightly increase the distance between it and your eyes. That's fine; now your head is just where it should be, and you turn into a living, breathing statue."

"Your All-Fours is finished, even though you are only standing on two. You can whistle a little tune through your teeth and, when you run out of air, whistle back in. This four-footed creature balancing on two may sway, but it doesn't fall."

"Before you put all four limbs back on the floor, you can play with your statue a little. The marble gets a bit soft and you can move your fingers and toes. Then it gets hard again. And now go back carefully and stand on all fours again. You can start trotting again right away."

The correct end position of BS head can also be impressed upon the patient's kinaesthetic and proprioceptive awareness during this learning process by careful manipulation. Often it is enough to gently touch the critical distance points and to tell the patient in what direction they are to be moved.

The manipulation the therapist provides in the end position is limited to applying specific resistance to increase the activity of particular muscles. This resistance must be applied such that the patient is not thrown off balance, which means always applying resistance at two or more sites.

In guiding the patient back to the starting position, the therapist can help the patient by touching those skin surfaces which will eventually form the contact with the base support again and, telling the patient to keep these surfaces against her hand, guiding him along the shortest path to the correct spot on the box.

▶ Adapting the Exercise to the Patient's Constitution and Condition

● Adaptation to Constitution: Role of Lengths, Widths, Depths and Distribution of Weights

If the greater trochanters are far apart and there is overweight around the pelvis, the primary movement of the free-play leg becomes more difficult.
If the frontotransverse diameter of the thorax is wide and there is overweight in BS thorax, the primary movement of the free-play arm becomes more difficult.

● Adaptation to Condition

Poor condition in BS arms, often associated with a flat back and cubitus valgus and hyperextension of the elbows, can be improved by the Classic All-Fours Exercise.

59

The exercise is contraindicated for patients who
- Need fine movement in their hands (e. g. musicians or surgeons) or for medical reasons cannot tolerate stress to their hands (e. g. because of arthrosis etc.)
- Have hypermobility of the spinal column associated with unstable flat back or lumbar hyperlordosis and thoracic hyperkyphosis
- Have any restrictions in movement or partial stiffness of the spinal column (see adaptation Mobilizing All-Fours)

If the patient presents with muscle weakness or depressed responses, the primary movements can be performed in a supported position (adapting the exercise by padding the arch of the bridge with pillows or a ball).

● **Abnormalities of Postural Statics Requiring Adaptation of the Exercise**

See Classic Frog, p. 19.

Adaptations of the Classic All-Fours Exercise
If restricted movement and partial stiffness of the spinal column make it impossible to align the body segments in the virtual long axis of the body, we try to mobilize the spine using appropriate adaptations. These adaptations are called **Mobilizing All-Fours Exercise in Flexion/Extension** and **Mobilizing All-Fours Exercise in Lateroflexion.**
If the proximal joints of the extremities have poor stability, or if there are muscle contractions at these joints, making them unable to function well as bridge supports in the All-Fours Exercise, we can compensate these deficits with the adaptations **All-Fours Exercise for Mobilization of the Hip and Shoulder Joints** and **All-Fours Exercise for Stabilization of the Hip and Shoulder Joints.** If the weight of the pelvis, thorax, free-play leg or head is too heavy for the spinal column when the long axis of the body is horizontal, the exercise is adapted by **changing the position in space of the long axis of the body.**

2.2 Adaptation: Mobilizing All-Fours Exercise in Flexion/Extension (Fig. 16)

"Mobilizing All-Fours Exercise in Flexion/Extension" is a functional name.

■ Goal of the Exercise

The goal is for the patient to learn to move all mobile segments of the spinal column to end-stop in flexion and extension, i. e. to:

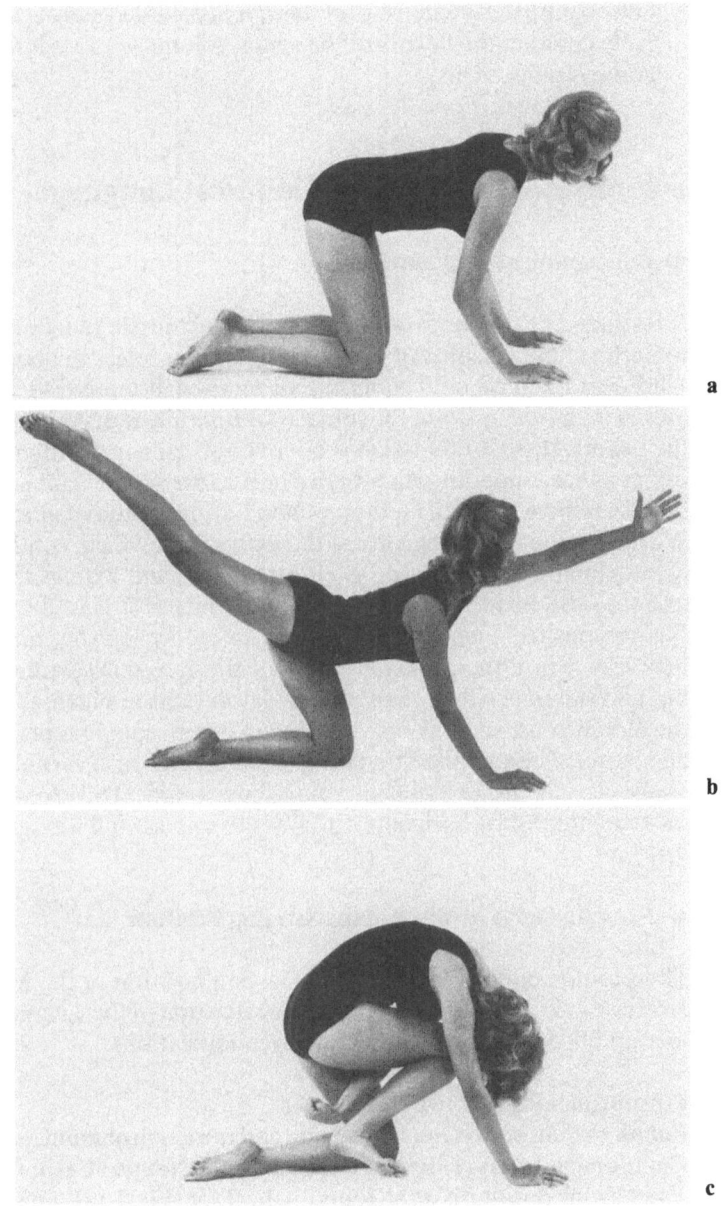

Fig. 16 a–c. Mobilizing All-Fours Exercise in Flexion/Extension. **a** Starting position, **b** end position in extension, **c** end position in flexion

- Fully contract the extensors of the spinal column against gravity (positive lift)
- Fully contract the flexors of the spinal column without having to work against gravity (reduced lift)

▶ Functional Analysis in Therapist Language

● Conception of the Exercise

If restricted flexion or extension or impaired muscle function make it impossible to perform the Classic All-Fours Exercise, we select the adaptation Mobilizing All-Fours Exercise in Flexion/Extension. Because positive lift is going to be required of the extensors of the spinal column while reduced-lift work is planned for the flexors, the All-Fours stance is a perfect starting position. This time the floor serves as base support, rather than a box, as we do not want instability of the rotational components of the spinal column during the movement sequence.

We again employ movements of the extremities which, continuing in from distal to proximal and buttressing each other, flex and extend the spinal column to end-stop. BS head is especially good for this, as it is in the plane of symmetry. For reasons of balance we choose as free-play leg the one opposite the free-play arm. Since the proximal joints of the free-play extremities (the free-play hip and shoulder) lie asymmetrically lateral to the plane of symmetry, in which the mobilization is to take place, the movement components of the free-play arm and leg must be so chosen that the flexion/extension axes of the spinal column are in the line of fire of the continuing movements. The frontotransverse axes of movement must be horizontal, in order to impose full lifting strain on the extensors.

● Position and Activation of the Starting Position

The position and activation of the starting position of the Mobilizing All-Fours Exercise in Flexion/Extension is identical to that of the Classic All-Fours Exercise (see pp. 50–51), but with the following modifications:

Position in Space of the Critical Axes
Points of Contact Between the Body and the Environment
Components of Movement in Relation to the Neutral Position of the Joints
The starting position is on all fours on the floor (Fig. 16 a). The points of contact between the body and the base support are the two palms and volar aspects of the fingers and the ventral aspects of the lower legs and dorsa of the feet.

● Actio – Reactio of the Movement Sequence

The movement sequence of the Mobilizing All-Fours Exercise in Flexion/Extension has three phases. First there is the preliminary trot stage, as in the Classic All-Fours Exercise. Next, arising out of one trot position, there is the mobilization of the spinal column in extension. Finally, arising immediately out of the end position of the mobilization of the spinal column in extension, comes the third phase, the mobilization of the spinal column in flexion. The moving levers move through space in opposite directions – head and free-play arm in one direction, free-play leg in the other – and thus buttress each other by countermovement. The movements are checked when the available movement tolerance for extension and flexion in the vertebral joints and vertebral–intervertebral disc articulations has been fully exhausted.

The movement sequence from the trot position into the end position with extension and then the end position with flexion maintains a constant location (Figs. 16 b, c). The exercise will be described for left supporting leg and right supporting arm.

Actio: The Primary Movement

The actio of the movement sequence is characterized by three simultaneous continuing primary movements: of the right free-play leg, the left free-play arm and BS head. The dominant direction component of the critical distance points is vertical/upwards. The horizontal direction components must cancel each other out and must not deflect the dominant component, so that the positive lifting stress imposed on the back muscles by the weight of the extremities has its full effect.

End Position in Extension: The critical distance point of the primary movement of the free-play leg, DP metatarsophalangeal joint of the right large toe, moves upwards/dorsally/caudally, with eversion in the subtalar and talocalcaneonavicular joints effected by the distal lever; the toes flex slightly. As the movement continues in proximally, the talocrural joint plantarflexes and the knee extends by fulcrum displacement. The distal lever at the right hip joint, the thigh, moves into extension and so much adduction that the long axis of the thigh remains in the sagittal plane of the right hip, which is vertical; it also internally rotates so far that the patella faces downwards and the sole of the foot upwards. The last lever to participate in the continuing movement of the free-play leg, the pelvis, turns in flexion as proximal lever at the left supporting hip (first critical fulcrum) and in extension as caudal lever at the lumbar spine (second critical fulcrum).

The critical distance point of the primary movement of the free-play arm, DP tip of the left thumb, moves dorsally/upwards/cranially with supination in the forearm and radial abduction in the wrist. As it does so, the wrist goes by volar flexion into the neutral position and the fingers are spread apart in abduction and extend, so that the palm now faces medially towards the plane of symmetry and the thumb points upwards/dorsally. The movement continues in proximally, causing the elbow to extend by displacement of the fulcrum. As distal lever at the left humeroscapular joint, the upper arm turns in flexion and so far in abduction that its long axis stays within the sagittal plane of the shoulder joint which is vertical; it also externally rotates. The left pincer jaws open at the sternoclavicular joint and are stabilized against the thorax, so that the medial scapular margin approaches the thoracic spine by adduction and the effect of the continuing primary movement of the free-play arm on the thoracic spine (first critical fulcrum) is purely extensional. When the thorax is securely suspended from the right pincer jaws, the latter move to cause flexion at the right supporting humeroscapular joint (second critical fulcrum) effected by the proximal lever.

The critical distance point of the primary movement of BS head, DP tip of the nose, moves dorsally/upwards/caudally in the vertical plane of symmetry by extension in the atlanto-occipital and atlanto-axial joints. By continuing movement, the cervical and thoracic spine (critical fulcrum) also extend. The primary movements of the head and the free-play arm thus have a common critical fulcrum, which intensifies the extensional mobilization of the upper thoracic spine.

End Position in Flexion: The actio of the movement sequence is again characterized by three simultaneous continuing movements: of the right free-play leg, the left free-play arm and BS head. The dominant direction component of the critical distance points is vertical/downwards. The horizontal direction components must cancel each other out and must not deflect the dominant component, so that the negative lifting stress (braking work) imposed on the back muscles by the weight of the extremities and the concentric work performed by the abdominal muscles have their full effect.

The critical distance point of the primary movement of the free-play leg, DP tip of the right foot, moves ventrally/downwards/cranially/medially. The movement continues with extension/abduction in the toes, inversion in the subtalar and talocalcaneonavicular joints, dorsiflexion in the talocrural joint, flexion and external rotation in the knee and flexion/adduction/external rotation in the hip effected by the distal lever in (Fig. 16 c there is unintentional eversion in the subtalar and talocalcaneonavicular joints and internal rotation in the hip).

The last lever to participate in the continuing movement of the free-play leg, the pelvis, turns in extension as proximal lever at the left supporting hip (first critical fulcrum) and in flexion as caudal lever at the lumbar spine (second critical fulcrum).

The critical distance point of the primary movement of the free-play arm, DP tips of digits II–IV of the left hand, moves ventrally/downwards/medially. As the movement continues, the finger joints and the wrist flex, the forearm pronates, the elbow flexes if necessary and extends again by fulcrum displacement, the shoulder extends, adducts and internally rotates. The left pincer jaws close at the sternoclavicular joint, DP acromion moves ventrally/caudally, so that the medial scapular margin is brought away from the thoracic spine and the effect of the primary movement of the free-play arm on the thoracic spine (first critical fulcrum) is purely flexional. When the thorax is securely suspended from the right pincer jaws, the latter move to cause flexion at the right supporting humeroscapular joint (second critical fulcrum) effected by the proximal lever.

The critical distance point of the primary movement of BS head, DP tip of the nose, moves ventrally/downwards/caudally in the vertical plane of symmetry by flexion in the atlanto-occipital and atlanto-axial joints. As the movement continues, the cervical spine flexes, as does the thoracic spine (critical fulcrum). The primary movements of the head and the free-play arm thus have a common critical fulcrum, which intensifies the flexional mobilization of the upper thoracic spine.

Reactio: Activated Passive Buttressing
Reactio: Change in the Support Area
A reactio in the form of activated passive buttressing does not occur, because the three primary movements can be defined as buttressing movements and take place in vertical planes.

Neither is there a reactio in the form of a change to the support area. The fact that the movement sequence out of the trot position maintains a constant location is more of a conditio than a reactio.

● Conditio – Limitatio of the Movement Sequence

Conditio: Constant Distances Between Body Distance Points
Limitatio: Active Buttressing and Stabilization
Conditio: The distance from DP shoulder joint to DP wrist of the supporting arm remains constant.
Limitatio: See Classic All-Fours Exercise (p. 54).

Conditio: The distance from DP hip joint to DP heel of the supporting leg remains constant.
Limitatio: If this distance is to remain constant, the supporting knee must be held in the starting position by first flexional and then extensional active buttressing. The extensional active buttressing is especially important, because the patient will try to make things easy for himself by try to shifting his centre of gravity caudally through flexion of the knee.

Conditio of Absolute and/or Relative Fixed Spatial Points
Limitatio by Limiting the Primary Movement, Activated Passive Buttressing and/or Change in the Support Area
In the Mobilizing All-Fours Exercise in Flexion/Extension there are absolute and relative fixed spatial points.

Conditio: The points of contact between the body and the base support and the distribution of pressure on these points of contact are absolute fixed spatial points.
Limitatio: These fixed points check the tendency to alter the distribution of pressure within the support area, i.e. to increase the pressure on the ventral aspect of the lower leg and on the dorsum of the foot. The foot remains in parking function.

Conditio: The horizontal, parallel positioning of all of the flexion/extension axes of the vertebral joints and the proximal joints of the extremities (hip and shoulder joints) is a relative fixed spatial point.
Limitatio: This fixed point guarantees the positive lifting stress on the back extensors by the weight of the extremities. It is the parallel positioning of these axes that makes possible, first, the continuing movements that mobilize the spinal column in

flexion/extension and, second, as a result, the complete exhaustion of the movement tolerances by the mutually buttressing primary movements. Including the flexion/extension axes of the proximal joints of the extremities forces the patient into the correct combination of their movement components. Even though the proximal joints of the free-play arm and leg lie lateral to the long axis of the body and the vertical plane of symmetry, it becomes possible to have a purely extensional or purely flexional continuing movement in the spinal column.

Conditio (This relative fixed spatial point applies only to the end position in extension): Although the horizontal direction components of the free-play hand and free-play foot are away from each other, because the foot moves caudally while the hand moves cranially, they must in the end position have moved closer together again.
Limitatio: This fixed point depends on the how much scope for extension is available in the spinal column. This scope is as great as the difference between the distance from DP coccyx to DP C7 when the spinal column is in neutral position and the distance between the same points in the end position of the Mobilizing All-Fours Exercise in Extension.

Conditio of Movement Speed
Limitatio of Economical Activity by Finding the Optimal Speed
Conditio: See Classic All-Fours Exercise (p. 56).
Limitatio: In the movement sequence into the flexional end position of the Mobilizing All-Fours Exercise in Flexion/Extension, as we work up to the natural optimal speed we must be sure that at the beginning of the sequence, the negative lift demanded of the extensors of the spinal column is as great as possible. The end of the movement sequence is optimal only if the abdominal muscles are fully contracted in pronounced bridging activity and the extensor muscles of the back are reflexively relaxed. If the patient is constitutionally of the appropriate build and has wide movement tolerances for flexion, his head and free-play knee will touch.

2.3 Adaptation: Mobilizing All-Fours Exercise in Lateroflexion (Fig. 17).

"Mobilizing All-Fours Exercise in Lateroflexion" is a functional name.

■ Goal of the Exercise

The goal is for the patient to be able to move all motion segments of the spinal column in lateroflexion to end-stop, i. e. to be able to contract and stretch the lateroflexors of the spinal column to the full.

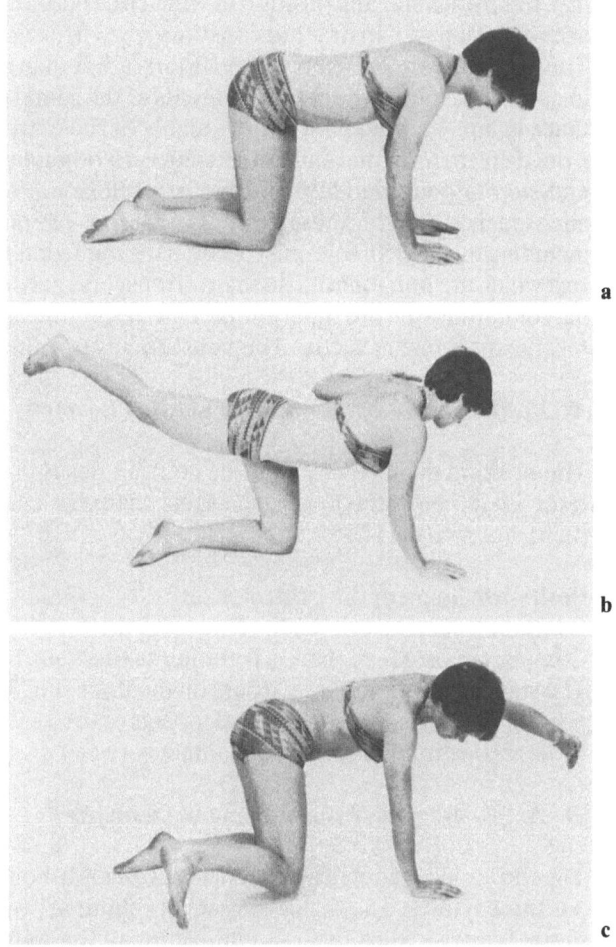

Fig. 17 a–c. Mobilizing All-Fours Exercise in Lateroflexion. **a** Starting position, **b** end position with left-concave lateroflexion, **c** end position with right-concave lateroflexion

▶ Functional Analysis in Therapist Language

● Conception of the Exercise

If the patient is unable to perform the Classic All-Fours Exercise because of restricted lateroflexional mobility or because of weakness in the lateroflexors, we choose the adaptation Mobilizing All-Fours Exercise in Lateroflexion. Since lateroflexion of the spinal column is important for the potential mobility of the lordotic spinal segments, but must at the same time be able to function undisturbed during active buttressing of costal movements in respiration, the starting position on all fours is perfect. The lateroflexors then work lift-free (i.e. not against gravity), but from a starting position in which fine coordination of flexor and extensor activity is required in order to constitute the virtual long axis of the body.

The base support will again be the floor, rather than a box, so as to avoid extreme instability of the rotational components of the spinal column.

Once again, we will employ movements of the extremities, which, continuing in from distal to proximal and buttressing each other, lateroflex the spinal column to end-stop in right- and left-concave lateroflexion. For reasons of equilibrium we choose as free-play leg the one opposite the free-play arm. The primary movements, including that of BS head, must occur in the midfrontal planes of BSs pelvis and thorax, which are horizontal. The sagittotransverse axes of movement of both the spinal column and the proximal joints of the extremities must be vertical, so that the lateroflexors do not have to work against gravity (i. e. they can work with reduced lift).

● **Position and Activation in the Starting Position**

The position and activation in the starting position of the Mobilizing All-Fours Exercise in Lateroflexion are the same as for the Classic All-Fours Exercise (see p. 50), but with the following change:

Position in Space of the Critical Axes
Points of Contact Between the Body and the Environment
Components of Movement in Relation to the Neutral Position of the Joints
The starting position is on all fours on the floor (Fig. 17 a). The palms and volar aspects of the fingers and the ventral aspects of the knees and lower legs and dorsa of the feet constitute the points of contact between the body and the base support.

● **Actio – Reactio of the Movement Sequence**

The movement sequence of the Mobilizing All-Fours Exercise in Lateroflexion has three phases. The first is the same preliminary trot stage as in the Classic All-Fours Exercise. Next comes mobilization of the spinal column in left-concave lateroflexion. Immediately arising from this end position comes mobilization of the spinal column in right-concave lateroflexion. The moving levers – one the head together with the free-play arm, the other the free-play leg – move through space in opposite directions, buttressing each other by countermovement with fulcrum displacement at about the level of T9. The movement is checked when the available movement tolerance for lateroflexion in the vertebral joints and vertebral–intervertebral disc articulations has been completely exhausted.

The movement sequence, described here from the trot position with left supporting leg and right supporting arm into the end position of left-concave lateroflexion and then into the end position of right-concave lateroflexion, maintains a constant location (Fig. 17 b, c).

Actio: The Primary Movement
The actio of the movement sequence is characterized by three simultaneous continuing primary movements: of the right free-play leg, the left free-play arm and BS head. The dominant direction components of the critical distance points are hori-

zontally footwards/headwards and lateral/medial. The vertical direction components must not deflect the dominant horizontal components, so that lift-free mobilization of the spinal column by alternating concentric isotonic muscle activity with the antagonists stretched to their maximum can take place undisturbed.

End Position in Left-Concave Lateroflexion: The critical distance point of the primary movement of the free-play leg, DP right heel, first moves dorsally/upwards/caudally/medially until it reaches the vertical plane of symmetry and fulcrum displacement has caused the knee to extend. It then moves laterally/to the left/cranially. The movement continues into the right hip joint, causing extension/adduction/very slight external rotation effected by the distal lever. The long axis of the leg moves in the midfrontal plane of BSs pelvis, thorax and head, which is horizontal. The last lever to participate in the continuing primary movement of the free-play leg, the pelvis, rotates externally as proximal lever in the left supporting hip (first critical fulcrum), and as caudal lever of the lumbar spine (second critical fulcrum) brings the latter into left concave lateroflexion. At the same time, the toes of the right foot flex/adduct, the subtalar and talocalcaneonavicular joints evert and the talocrural joint plantarflexes. The sole of the foot now faces caudally/left laterally/somewhat upwards.

The critical distance point of the primary movement of the free-play arm, DP left olecranon, moves dorsally/upwards/caudally/laterally/to the left until it is in the midfrontal plane of BSs pelvis, thorax and head, which is horizontal. As it moves, fulcrum displacement causes the elbow to flex and the upper arm, as distal lever, rotates in the shoulder joint in extension/45° abduction/external rotation to end-stop, such that the long axes of the forearm and hand reach the midfrontal plane. The movement continues with supination of the forearm, no wrist movement and slight flexion in the fingers. The palm now faces medially towards the left shoulder and the flexion/extension axes of the elbow and wrist are vertical.

By proximally continuing movement, the left pincer jaws open in the acromioclavicular and sternoclavicular joints and the medial margin of the scapula approaches the thoracic spine. As the last lever participating in the primary continuing movement of the free-play arm, the thoracic spine (first critical fulcrum) goes cranial-to-caudally into left-concave lateroflexion. When the thorax is securely suspended from the right pincer jaws, the latter, as proximal lever, bring about external rotation in the right, supporting shoulder (second critical fulcrum). The critical distance point of the primary movement of BS head, DP vertex, moves laterally/to the left/caudally in the midfrontal plane, which is horizontal, by left-concave lateroflexion of the atlanto-occipital and atlanto-axial joints. By continuing movement, both the cervical spine and the thoracic spine (critical fulcrum) go into left-concave lateroflexion. The primary movements of the head and of the free-play arm thus have a common critical fulcrum, which intensifies the lateroflexional mobilization of the upper thoracic spine.

Reactio: Activated Passive Buttressing
Due to the left-concave lateroflexion of the lumbar and thoracic spine, the critical distance point of the activated passive buttressing, DP T9, moves laterally to the right, reactively exhausting to end-stop the movement tolerance for left-concave

lateroflexion, as in buttressing mobilization. This should be seen as buttressing mobilization of a hinge-type joint, with S1/L5 as caudal DP, T1/C7 as cranial DP and T9 as fulcrum.

End Position in Right-Concave Lateroflexion: The critical distance point of the primary movement of the free-play leg, DP right heel, moves ventrally/downwards/laterally/to the right/cranially with eversion in the subtalar and talocalcaneonavicular joints. As it does so, the toes go into extension/abduction and the talocrural joint goes into dorsiflexion. By proximally continuing movement, the knee goes into flexion by displacement of the fulcrum and internal rotation effected by the distal pointer. As the distal lever in the right hip joint, the thigh moves into 90° flexion/slight abduction/considerable internal rotation. The last lever participating in the primary movement of the free-play leg, the pelvis, as proximal lever brings about internal rotation in the left supporting hip joint (first critical fulcrum), and as caudal lever brings about right-concave lateroflexion in the lumbar spine (second critical fulcrum).

The critical distance point of the primary movement of the free-play arm, DP left wrist, moves cranially/medially until it reaches the plane of symmetry and then, crossing over it, continues to move laterally to the right. As its fulcrum is diplaced, the elbow extends; the positions of the joints of the fingers and wrist remain unchanged. The long axes of the hand, forearm and upper arm move in the frontal plane of the sternoclavicular joints. By continuing movement, the upper arm, the distal lever in the left shoulder joint, rotates internally somewhat and adducts. The left pincer jaws close and move away from the thorax in the acromioclavicular and sternoclavicular joints; as they do so, DP acromion moves cranially/medially/ventrally. The last distance point to participate in the continuing primary movement of the free-play arm, C7, the cranial DP of the thoracic spine, moves medially/cranially at first, then laterally to the right/caudally, bringing the thoracic spine (first critical fulcrum) into right-concave lateroflexion. When the thorax is securely suspended from the pincer jaws, they rotate internally as proximal lever in the right shoulder joint (second critical fulcrum).

The critical distance point of the primary movement of BS head, DP vertex, moves in the horizontal midfrontal plane, first medially/cranially, then laterally to the right/caudally by right-concave lateroflexion in the atlanto-occipital and atlanto-axial joints. By continuing movement, the cervical spine goes into right-concave lateroflexion, as does the thoracic spine (critical fulcrum), cranial-to-caudally.

Because the primary movement of the head and of the free-play arm have a common critical pivot, the mobilization in lateroflexion of the upper thoracic spine is intensified.

Reactio: Activated Passive Buttressing
Reactio: Change in the Support Area
Due to the right-concave lateroflexion of the lumbar and thoracic spine, the critical distance point of the activated passive buttressing, DP T9, moves laterally to the left, reactively exhausting to end-stop the movement tolerance for right-concave lateroflexion. In this, S1/L5 should be seen as caudal DP, T1/C7 as cranial DP, and T9 as fulcrum in buttressing mobilization of a hinge-type joint.

A reactio in the form of a change to the support area does not occur. That the movement sequence out of the end position of left-concave lateroflexion of the Mobilizing All-Fours Exercise with Lateroflexion maintains a constant location is more a conditio than a reactio.

● **Conditio – Limitatio of the Movement Sequence**

Conditio: Constant Distances Between Body Distance Points
Limitatio: Active Buttressing and Stabilization
During the movement sequence from the trot position into the end position of left-concave lateroflexion and then into the end position of right-concave lateroflexion, we observe the following:

Conditio: The distance from DP shoulder joint to DP wrist in the supporting arm remains constant.
Limitatio: See Classic All-Fours Exercise (p. 54).

Conditio: The distance from DP hip joint to DP heel in the supporting leg remains constant.
Limitatio: See Mobilizing All-Fours Exercise in Flexion/Extension (p. 65).

Conditio of Absolute and/or Relative Fixed Spatial Points
Limitatio by Limiting the Primary Movement, Activated Passive Buttressing and/or Change in the Support Area
There are both absolute and relative fixed spatial points during the movement sequence first from the trot position into the end position of left-concave lateroflexion and then into the end position of right-concave lateroflexion.

Conditio: The points of contact between the body and the base support and the distribution of pressure on these points are absolute fixed spatial points.
Limitatio: These fixed points check any tendency to shift the distribution of pressure or the support area itself towards the side of the supporting leg by lateral/downward displacement of the greater trochanter on that side. This would cause transverse adduction of the supporting leg, which would impede the external rotation of the pelvis in the supporting hip and with it the lateroflexion of the lumbar spine. The limitatio consists of transverse abductional active buttressing that makes the greater trochanter of the supporting leg an absolute fixed spatial point.

Conditio: The vertical, parallel positioning of all lateroflexional axes in the vertebral column and all rotational axes of the proximal joints of the supporting extremities is a relative fixed spatial point.
Limitatio: This fixed point guarantees lift-free lateroflexion of the spinal column. The weights of the free-play extremities activate the extensors and rotators of the spinal column to fall-preventing work. It is the parallel positioning of these axes that makes possible, first, the continuing movements which mobilize the spinal column in lateroflexion and, second, the complete exhaustion of move-

ment tolerances by mutually buttressing movements. If the spinal column and the extremities participating in the primary movements all move in the same horizontal frontal plane, as planned, good lateroflexional mobilization can be achieved.

Conditio: The patient's gaze is always directed downwards and the distance from the eyes to the floor remains constant.
Limitatio: This relative fixed spatial point requires both constant dorsal-translatory fall-preventing work to hold the head and rotational stabilization to keep the head's plane of symmetry vertical.

Conditio of Movement Speed
Limitatio of Economical Activity by Finding the Optimal Speed
Conditio: See Classic All-Fours Exercise (p. 56).
Limitatio: Since the lateroflexion of the spinal column is lift-free, requiring concentric isotonic activity of the lateroflexors, it is possible to stretch the antagonistic lateroflexors by increasing the intensity of economical activity in the end positions, without sacrificing the mutually buttressing directions of movement.

2.4 Adaptation: All-Fours Exercise for Stabilization of the Hip and Shoulder Joints (Fig. 18)

"All-Fours Exercise for Stabilization of the Hip and Shoulder Joints" is a functional name.

■ Goal of the Exercise

The goal is for the patient to learn to stabilize the muscles of the hip and shoulder joints, especially by activating the rotator cuff muscles, when these muscles are subjected to stress, and still keep the long axis of the body in proper alignment.

▶ Functional Analysis in Therapist Language

● Conception of the Exercise

If the patient is unable to perform the All-Fours Exercises because of active and/or passive insufficiency of the muscles of the hip or shoulder joints, we either try to build these muscles up or switch to another exercise programme. Such muscular insufficiencies are evident as early as the preliminary trot phase,

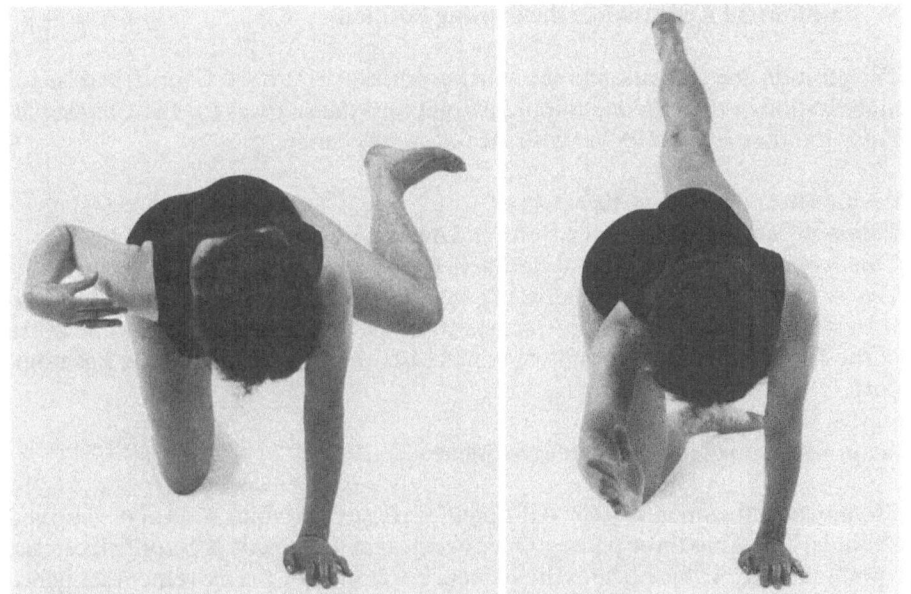

a   b

Fig. 18 a,b. All-Fours Exercise for Stabilization of the Hip and Shoulder Joints. **a** End position in abduction, **b** end position in adduction

when the patient can neither hold the pelvis by fall-preventing activity in the supporting hip nor rotate it upwards by positive lift or downwards by negative lift, nor move it horizontally. Insufficiency in the shoulder is visible when the pincer jaws are unable to anchor the thorax and/or when the pincer jaws together with the thorax cannot be moved, lifted or lowered at the supporting shoulder.

The goal of this exercise is to be attained by using an All-Fours Exercise with distal-to-proximal continuing movements of the extremities.

A condition of the exercise is that the plane of symmetry, which is vertical, must not rotate or shift in space, and that the long axis of the body, a fixed spatial point, remains in its neutral position. The head is responsible for stabilizing the long axis of the body. The free-play leg and contralateral free-play arm are given movement components which, if they continue, will rotate the long axis of the body clockwise or counterclockwise respectively if they are not checked by lift-free rotational active buttressing in the hip and shoulder joints.

The components of the two continuing movements, that of the free-play leg continuing to right-concave lateroflexion in the lumbar spine and that of the free-play arm continuing to left-concave lateroflexion of the thoracic spine, neutralize each other.

Since the flexion/extension axes of the supporting extremities are horizontal, their muscles are subject to lifting stress. The rotation axes of these extremities, however, are vertical, so the rotator cuff muscles can work lift-free.

● **Position and Activation in the Starting Position**

The position and activation in the starting position of the All-Fours Exercise for Stabilization of the Hip and Shoulder Joints are the same as for the Classic All-Fours Exercise (see p. 50), but with the following change:

Position in Space of the Critical Axes
Points of Contact Between the Body and the Environment
Components of Movement in Relation to the Neutral Position of the Joints
The starting position is on all-fours on the floor (Fig. 17a). The palms and volar aspects of the fingers, ventral aspects of the knees and lower legs and dorsa of the feet constitute the points of contact between the body and the base support.

Actio – Reactio of the Movement Sequence

The movement sequence of the All-Fours Exercise for Stabilization of the Hip and Shoulder Joints has three phases. Once again, as in the Classic All-Fours Exercise, a preliminary trot phase begins the sequence, followed by the movement sequence into the end position of abduction and then into the end position of adduction of the free-play extremities.
The movement sequence from the trot position, described here with right supporting leg and left supporting arm, into the end position of abduction and then into the end position of adduction maintains a constant location (Fig. 18).

Actio: The Primary Movement
The actio of the movement sequence is characterized by three simultaneous continuing primary movements: of the right free-play leg, the left free-play arm and BS head. The dominant direction components of the critical distance points are horizontally footwards/headwards and laterally/medially. The vertical direction components must not deflect the dominant horizontal components, so that lift-free stabilization of the rotator cuff muscles at the supporting hip and shoulder joints and fall-preventing activity in the other movement components at these joints can take place in the best possible way.

End Position in Abduction (Fig. 18a, although note that the left knee and heel are much too high in the picture): The critical distance point of the primary movement of the free-play leg, DP left heel, moves slightly upwards; as it goes, the talocrural joint dorsiflexes by fulcrum displacement and the knee flexes. In order to clear the floor, the heel moves laterally to the left/cranially, then finally the subtalar and calcaneonavicular joints evert and the toes extend and abduct. The movement continues proximally, causing the thigh to turn in the left hip (critical fulcrum) in slight flexion/slight transverse abduction/internal rotation.
The critical distance point of the primary movement of the free-play arm, DP right olecranon, moves dorsally/upwards/caudally/laterally to the right until it reaches the midfrontal plane of BSs pelvis, thorax and head, which is horizontal. The elbow flexes by fulcrum displacement and the upper arm, as

74

distal lever, turns in the shoulder joint in extension/45° abduction/external rotation to end-stop, so that the long axes of the forearm and hand attain the midfrontal plane. There is forearm supination, no wrist movement and slight finger flexion. Now the palm faces medially towards the right shoulder and the flexion/extension axes of the elbow and wrist are vertical. By proximally continuing movement, the pincer jaws open and the medial margin of the scapula moves in the sternoclavicular joint (critical fulcrum) towards the thoracic spine.

The critical distance point of the primary activity of BS head, DP vertex, strives dorsally/upwards. There is flexional activity in the atlanto-occipital and atlanto-axial joints, which continues as dorsal-translatory activity in the cervical spine and extensional activity in the thoracic spine (critical fulcrum).

End Position in Adduction (Fig. 18 b): The critical distance point of the primary movement of the free-play leg, DP left heel, moves dorsally/upwards/caudally/medially, meeting the plane of symmetry in the midfrontal plane, which is horizontal. As the heel moves, the knee extends and the thigh turns in extension/adduction/external rotation in the hip joint (critical fulcrum) such that the patella faces downwards/very slightly laterally towards the left. The talocrural joint goes into plantarflexion, the subtalar and calcaneonavicular joints into inversion and the toes into flexion.

The critical distance point of the primary movement of the free-play arm, DP right wrist, moves cranially/medially/just a little ventrally/downwards until it reaches the vertical plane of symmetry. The elbow extends by fulcrum displacement, while the fingers extend slightly into their neutral position. The long axis of the arm slants very slightly downwards and the long axis of the hand is horizontal/frontosagittal; the wrist extends and radially abducts, the forearm supinates. By proximally continuing movement, the upper arm, as distal lever in the shoulder joint, extends slightly/adducts/moderately internally rotates, the pincer jaws close in the acromioclavicular joint, and DP acromion moves ventrally/cranially/medially in the sternoclavicular joint (critical fulcrum), causing the scapula to turn in the scapular plane.

The critical distance point of the primary activity of BS head, DP vertex, strives dorsally/upwards even harder than before. The atlanto-occipital and atlanto-axial joints flex and by continuing movement the cervical spine goes into dorsal translation and the thoracic spine (critical fulcrum) into extension.

Reactio: Activated Passive Buttressing
A reactio in the form of activated passive buttressing does not occur because the horizontal components of the primary movements of the free-play leg and arm neutralize each other.

Reactio: Change in the Support Area
A reactio in the form of change in the support area does not occur because of the conditio that the movement sequence from the trot position into first the end position of abduction and then the end position of adduction maintains a constant location.

● **Conditio – Limitatio of the Movement Sequence**

Conditio: Constant Distances Between Body Distance Points
Limitatio: Active Buttressing and Stabilization
Conditio: The distance from DP symphysis pubis to DP navel remains constant.
Limitatio: This distance remains constant if the pelvis, instead of being moved as a lever by the primary continuing movement of the free-play leg, is actively buttressed in the supporting hip by extensional/transverse adductional/external rotational activity in the end position of abduction and by extensional/transverse adductional/internal rotational activity in the end position of adduction. The lumbar spine is then also stabilized in neutral position.

Conditio: The distance from DP navel to DP jugular notch remains constant.
Limitatio: This distance will remain constant if, rather than the primary continuing movement of the free-play arm moving the thorax, the movement of the pincer jaws with the thorax is actively buttressed by transverse flexional/flexional/external rotational (in the end position of abduction) or internal rotational (in the end position of adduction) activity by the distal lever in the supporting shoulder. The thoracic spine is then also stabilized in neutral position.

Conditio: The distances from DP chin to DP jugular notch and from DP jugular notch to DP navel remain constant.
Limitatio: These distances will remain constant if the tendency of the head to dorsally translate is not permitted to become a continuing movement that would lengthen the upper abdomen by extending the thoracic spine, but is instead actively buttressed by flexional activity.

Conditio: The distance from DP shoulder to DP wrist in the supporting arm remains constant.
Limitatio: See Classic All-Fours Exercise (p. 54).

Conditio: The distance from DP hip joint to DP heel in the supporting leg remains constant.
Limitatio: See Mobilizing All-Fours Exercise in Flexion/Extension (p. 65).

Conditio of Absolute and/or Relative Fixed Spatial Points
Limitatio by Limiting of Primary Movement, Activated Passive Buttressing
and/or Change in the Support Area
In the movement sequence of the All-Fours Exercise for Stabilization of the Hip and Shoulder Joints out of the trot position there are absolute fixed spatial points.

Conditio: The horizontal long axis of the body, stabilized in neutral position, is an absolute fixed spatial point.
Limitatio: This fixed point requires the continuing movement of the free-play leg to be checked at the hip joint on the side of the free-play leg and the

76

movement of the free-play arm to be checked at movement level pincer jaws/ thorax on the side of the free-play arm. This is done by active buttressing in the proximal joints (hip and shoulder) of the supporting extremities: the distal rotation pointer checks the tendency to external rotation of the proximal pointer with external rotational active buttressing, and vice versa. Since the axes of rotation of the supporting extremities are vertical, this stabilizing active buttressing is lift-free. The active buttressing also checks the tendency of the spinal column to lateroflex under the influence of the free-play extremities.

Conditio: The head of the femur of the supporting hip and the head of the humerus of the supporting arm are absolute fixed spatial points. The points of contact supporting lower leg/floor and palm of the supporting hand/floor are absolute fixed spatial points.

Limitatio: These fixed points are in fact related to each other. If the supporting hip transversely adducts laterally/downwards and the point of contact lower leg/floor displaces laterally, the pelvis would shift to the side of the supporting leg by lateral translation in the spinal column. If the shoulder transversely flexes laterally/downwards, the pressure on the point of contact palm/floor would shift too much onto the lateral aspect of the little finger, causing the thorax to shift to the side of the supporting arm by lateral translation in the spinal column. Both these translations would bring the spinal column out of neutral position and disturb the alignment of the virtual long axis of the body.

Conditio of Movement Speed
Limitatio of Economical Activity by Finding the Optimal Speed
Conditio: See Classic All-Fours Exercise (p. 56)

Limitatio: After the alternating movements of free-play leg and free-play arm have become familiar the speed can be stepped up. This is possible because the movements of the extremities continue only up to their proximal joints (hip and shoulder) and because the head and the spinal column remain fixed in space.

▶ Instruction in Patient Language

● Instruction Appealing to the Patient's Perception

It is easier for the patient to impress on his awareness a sense of his spinal column as a fixed point in space if he can imagine a mirror on the floor beneath him. In it he can see reflected the ventral aspects of his pelvis, thorax and face. These must not move even an inch.

Position and Activation in the Starting Position

"Kneel down on the floor and support yourself on your hands. Your palms touch the floor and your fingertips point forwards. Your shoulders are directly over your hands, your bottom over your knees. Your stomach faces downwards and is horizontal. You can see the floor under you but you don't let your head drop down." Continue as for the Classic All-Fours Exercise (pp. 57–58).

Minor manual adjustments to refine position and activation will be more effective if the therapist explains at the same time what it is she is correcting.

Actio and Conditio of the Movement Sequence

The trot phase is the same as in the Classic All-Fours Exercise (p. 58).

"Gradually you trot slower and slower and finally stop, resting on your left hand and right knee. Your right hand and left knee hover over the floor and feel around it a little. When you feel stable, you look down and discover that there's a mirror on the floor, and in it you see your stomach and face reflected. This reflection must not move at all during the entire exercise. Now your right hand wanders up to the right shoulder and takes a look at it. Meanwhile your left knee takes a wander out to the side, not far off the floor. Naturally your foot goes along too, in fact it goes even further out to the side. If your elbow is as high as your right hand and the reflection staring back at you hasn't moved, we're at our goal."

If the patient doesn't respond to the image of the mirror, the therapist can place a rod on the floor, directly under the long axis of the body. The patient must make sure that the long axis of his body stays exactly over the rod. To manipulate the position of the arm, the therapist grasps the patient's right hand with her one hand and his elbow with her other. Without haste, she gently moves the hand and elbow into the desired position without any resistance from the patient. For the left, free-play leg, the therapist holds on to the knee and heel and moves them into position. The abduction and internal rotation at the hip joint should not be overdone, but the 90° flexion is important.

Breathing should not be at all restricted; if the patient tends to do this, he should be asked to whistle softly while breathing both in and out.

"Now feel yourself strong, your back and neck long and immoveable – unshakable. Nothing moves anywhere except your left knee and heel pushing out to the side and your right elbow pushing out on the other side. You breathe easily and quickly; you need hardly any air."

In this end position, stabilization of the hip and shoulder joints can be increased by applying resistance. The therapist presses the right elbow in a medial and, if possible, cranial direction, i.e. in the direction of negative rotation. At the same time, she presses the left heel, which is close to the floor, in a medial/caudal direction. This should only result in

"You still don't move but now you don't need as much strength, only just enough to keep the statue from moving. The only thing that causes any movement is your breathing, for you have suddenly turned into a living pillar of salt, like Lot's wife – but you can still think. You think about the mirror on the floor, out of which a glass wall is growing; being magical, it grows up right through the middle of you. This glass wall acts like a magnet, attracting your right hand to it until your palm touches it in front of your head. What you didn't notice was that the sole of your left foot is now also stuck to the wall of glass, pretty high over the floor, about as high as your head, but of course way out back. Your right hand and left foot stick firmly to the wall of glass.

Now you get strong again. You've turned into a pillar of salt once more, but instead of being short and wide like the last time, you are now tall and thin. Don't forget to breathe."

increased activity; there should be no movement at all at the joints.

The "glass wall" may perhaps be demonstrated by gestures. Later the therapist can carefully guide the palm and the sole of the foot into the proper position, watching closely that long axis of the body maintains its fixed position in space. During this section of the exercise it has a particular tendency to negative rotation in the midfrontal plane, because hand and foot lie along the extension of the long axis of the body, and both of them, pressing against the imaginary wall of glass, seem to be striving towards negative rotation.

Firm resistance to the palm and sole of the foot in the direction of positive rotation, together with a request to the patient not to move, help to improve the stabilization of the hip and shoulder.

2.5 Adaptation: All-Fours Exercise for Mobilization of the Hip and Shoulder Joints (Figs. 19–22)

"All-Fours Exercise for Mobilization of the Hip and Shoulder Joints" is a functional name.

■ Goals of the Exercise

The first goal of the exercise is for the patient to learn to improve hip mobility, i. e.:

- In the supporting hip, to achieve transverse and frontal abduction to end-stop
- In the free-play hip, to contract and stretch to the maximum the muscles involved in flexion, abduction and internal rotation

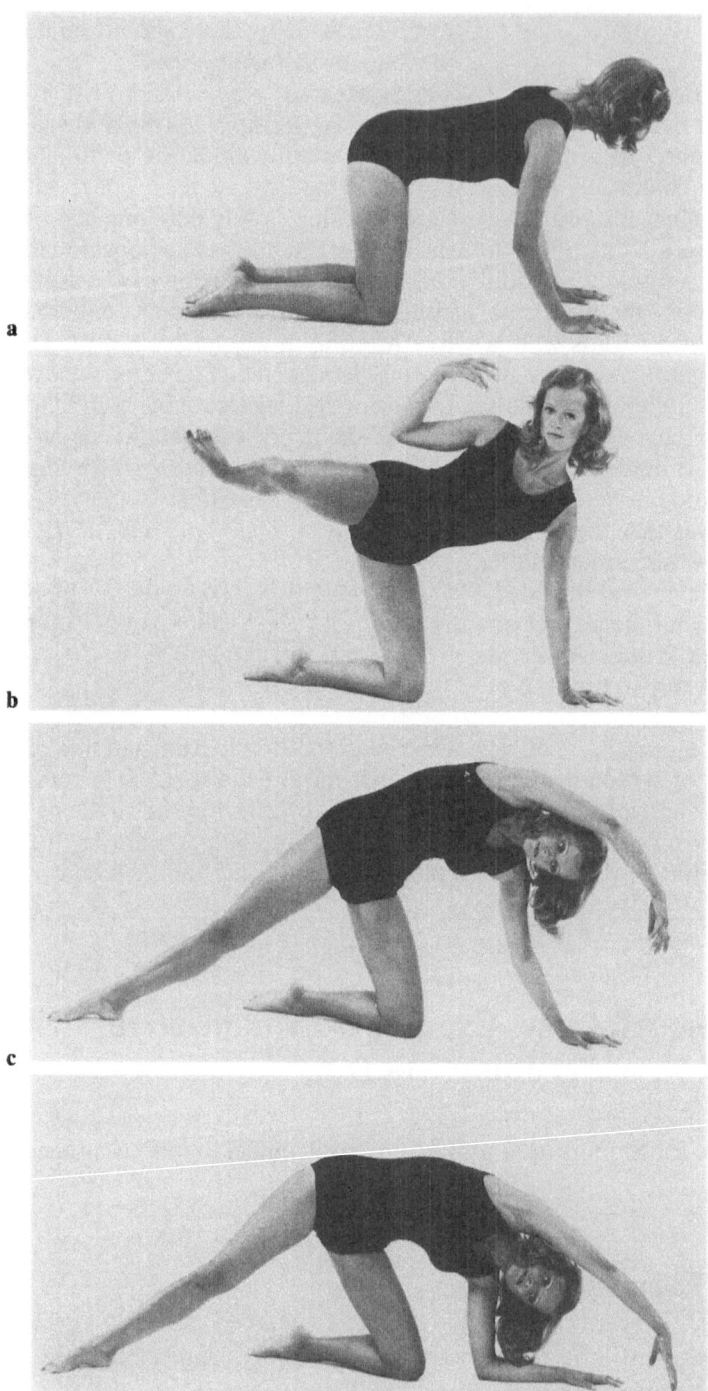

Fig. 19 a–d. All-Fours Exercise for Mobilization of the Hip and Shoulder Joints, dorsal view. **a** Starting position, **b** positive lift position, **c** stretch position, **d** increased stretch position

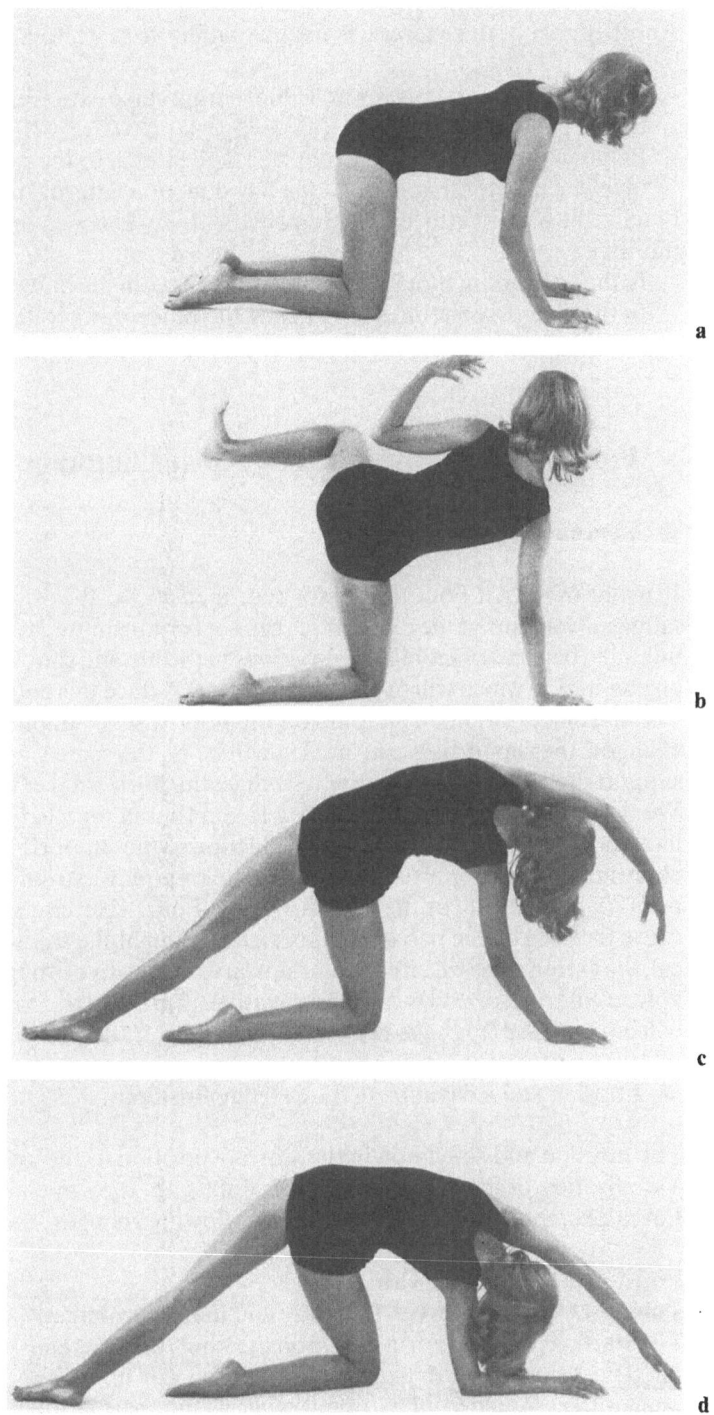

Fig. 20 a–d. All-Fours Exercise for Mobilization of the Hip and Shoulder Joints. As Fig. 19, ventral view

81

Another goal of the exercise is for the patient to learn to improve shoulder mobility, i.e.:
- In the supporting shoulder, to achieve transverse extension and flexion/abduction to end-stop
- In the free-play shoulder, to contract and stretch to the maximum the muscles involved in extension/abduction and adduction/external rotation

Finally, the patient is to learn to improve stability between the pincer jaws and the thorax, i.e.:
- In the supporting shoulder, to hold the thorax in the open pincer jaws
- In the free-play shoulder, to anchor the pincer jaws to the thorax as firmly as possible

▶ Functional Analysis in Therapist Language

● Conception of the Exercise

If, in one of the All-Fours Exercises described above, the distal-to-proximal continuing movements of the extremities cannot be transmitted to the spinal column as intended because of mobility restrictions in the hip and shoulder joints, we choose an adaptation which will overcome or at least reduce this deficiency.

The starting position on all fours on the floor will be adapted and the trot phase changed: the supporting arm and leg will be on the same side. This change to the support area makes it necessary to reduce the horizontal extension of the levers. We do this by "flapping up" the pelvis and thorax together with the extremities hanging from them, by transverse abduction in the supporting hip and transverse extension in the supporting shoulder. The free-play extremities are assigned the primary movements of the Mobilizing All-Fours Exercise in Lateroflexion. Because flapping up the pelvis and thorax has brought the frontal plane nearly vertical, the extremities will either move upwards by positive lifting, and the muscles involved contract, or downwards by negative lifting, and the corresponding muscles will be stretched (Figs. 19–22).

● Position and Activation in the Starting Position

The position and activation in the starting position of the All-Fours Exercise for Mobilization of the Hip and Shoulder Joints are the same as for the Classic All-Fours Exercise (see p.50), but with the following changes:

Position in Space of the Critical Axes
Points of Contact Between the Body and the Environment
The starting position is on all fours on the floor. BS arms constitutes the cranial pillar. The hands are symmetrically placed on the floor in the vertical transverse plane of the shoulder joints, about twice as far apart as the shoulders. The palms and volar aspects of the fingers are the points of contact between the body and the floor.

Components of Movement in Relation to the Neutral Position of the Joints
In BS arms, the shoulder joint is in about 80° flexion/transverse extension/slight internal rotation. The long axes of the arms are inclined in towards the body.

● **Actio – Reactio of the Movement Sequence**

The movement sequence of the All-Fours Exercise for Mobilization of the Hip and Shoulder Joints has three parts. First there is the modified trot phase. The patient then moves out of a trot position into the positive lift position and then, finally, out of the positive lift position into the stretch position.

Trot Phase

The trot phase in the All-Fours Exercise for Mobilization of the Hip and Shoulder Joints is a constant-location to-and-fro movement with slight shifting of the support area in the direction of the movement.

Actio: The Primary Movement
The actio is directed alternately to the right and to the left. It consists of two primary movements that begin simultaneously. A clear reactio is to be expected, owing to the dominant horizontal components of direction.
The critical distance points of the two primary movements, DP right greater trochanter and DP right acromion, move to the right (or, in the other trot step, DP left greater trochanter and DP left acromion move to the left) with transverse adduction in the hip and transverse flexion in the shoulder joints due to fulcrum displacement.

Reactio: Activated Passive Buttressing
In primary movements to the right, the critical distance points of the activated passive buttressing, DP ventral aspect of the left lower leg and dorsum of the foot and DP left palm and ventral aspects of the fingers initially cease to exert any pressure on the base support; after a few to-and-fro movements they lose contact with the base support altogether. When this happens, the left leg and left arm go into free play and become suspended from the pelvis and thorax respectively. They have become activated passive buttresses.

Reactio: Change in the Support Area
During the trot step to the right, the support area expands out to the right. DP right lateral malleolus reactively shifts to the right by internal rotation in the supporting hip and the points of contact between the lower leg and foot and the floor shift somewhat laterally (Figs. 21, 22).

Actio: Accelerating Weights
Reactio: Braking Weights
In primary movements to the right, the bisecting plane, which in the starting position was identical with the vertical plane of symmetry, shifts to the right. In the

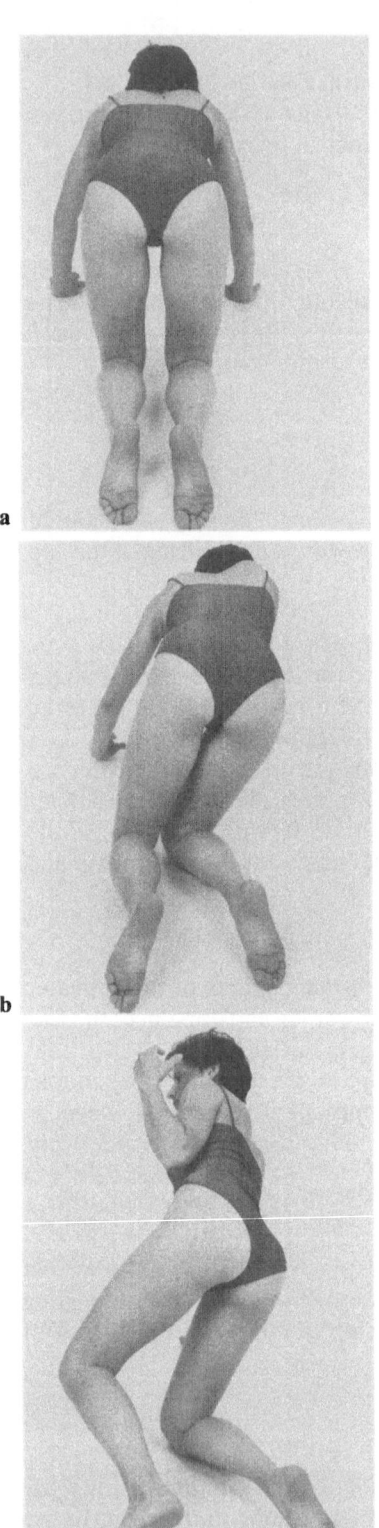

Fig. 21 a–c. All-Fours Exercise for Mobilization of the Hip and Shoulder Joints, caudal view. **a** Starting position. **b** Left arm and left leg in free play; the right leg has extended the support area to the right. **c** Shifting the hip and shoulder joints ventrally helps the patient to "flap up" into the position of positive lift

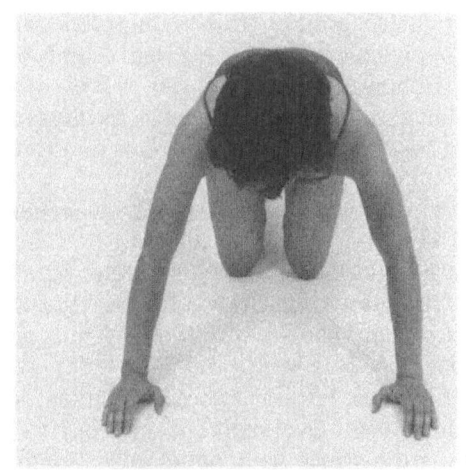

a

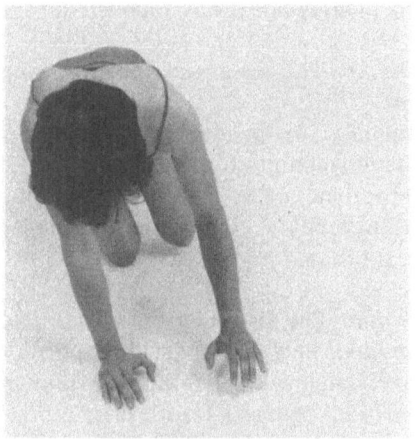

b

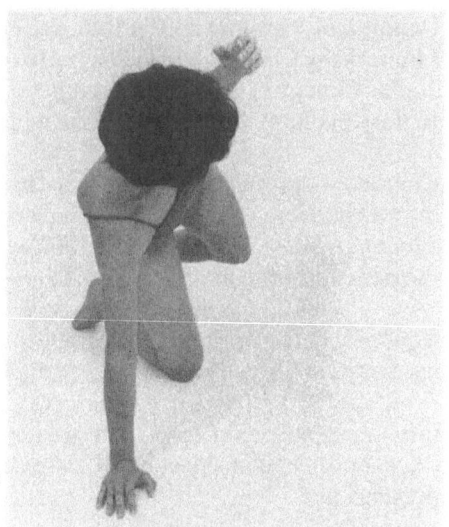

Fig. 22 a–c. All-Fours Exercise for Mobilization of the Hip and Shoulder Joints. As Fig. 21, cranial view

c

right trot position the bisecting plane runs through the right knee and the metacarpophalangeal joint of the right thumb.

All body segments or parts of body segments to the right of the bisecting plane have an accelerating effect on the movement sequence, while those to the left have a braking effect (and vice versa for primary movements to the left).

● **Conditio – Limitatio of the Movement Sequence**

Conditio: Constant Distances Between Body Distance Points
Limitatio: Active Buttressing and Stabilization
Conditio: The distance from DP right acromion to DP right earlobe remains constant.
Limitatio: If this distance is to remain constant during the supporting arm phase, movement level right open pincer jaws/thorax must be stabilized. Only then can the transverse flexional mobilization in the right shoulder the effective to end-stop. (This conditio has not been kept in Fig. 21 b.)

Conditio: The distance from DP symphysis to DP jugular notch remains constant.
Limitatio: This distance will remain constant if the critical distance point of the primary movements, DP right greater trochanter and DP right acromion, remain parallel and move the same amount to the right, and if the spinal column is stabilized at movement level upper lumbar/lower thoracic spine against lateral translation and rotation.

Conditio: The distance from DP chin to DP jugular notch remains constant.
Limitatio: This distance will remain constant if the spinal column is stabilized at movement levels upper thoracic spine/cervical spine/atlanto-occipital and atlanto-axial joints against lateroflexion/lateral translation/rotation.

Conditio of Absolute and/or Relative Fixed Spatial Points
Limitatio by Limiting the Primary Movement, Activated Passive Buttressing and/or Change in the Support Area
In the trot phase there are absolute and relative fixed spatial points.

Conditio: In primary movements to the right, the points of contact right, supporting arm and leg/floor are absolute fixed spatial points.
Limitatio: These absolute fixed points check the primary movements and prevent the patient from falling over onto his right side.

Conditio: During primary movements to the right, DP knee of the left, free-play leg moves in the vertical transverse plane of the right, supporting knee.
Limitatio: This relative fixed point prevents any caudal/downward deviation of the primary movement of the right greater trochanter. Undesired caudal shifting of the support area is checked by extensional active buttressing in the right, supporting knee.

Conditio of Movement Speed
Limitatio of Economical Activity by Finding the Optimal Speed
Conditio: The movement begins slowly with one trot about every 2 seconds, speeding up to one every second.
Limitatio: At the slow initial speed, the arm and leg that will later go into free-play maintain contact with the floor. That way transverse adductional mobilization in the supporting hip and transverse flexional mobilization in the supporting shoulder are optimal. As the speed increases, the free-play arm and leg move further and further off the floor, the primary movements become smaller and the "flapping up" of the pelvis and thorax together with the free-play leg, free-play arm and head starts the mobilization of the supporting hip and shoulder joints in transverse abduction and transverse extension.

Movement from the Trot Position into the Positive Lift Position and Then into the Stretch Position

● **Actio – Reactio of the Movement Sequence**

Actio: The Primary Movement
The critical distance points of the primary movements into the positive lift position and then into the stretch position and the primary movements themselves correspond exactly to those in the Mobilizing All-Fours Exercise in Lateroflexion. Because the patient's position in space is different, however, the free-play arm and the free-play leg are on the same side. The description below is for the movement sequence from the trot position on the right side.

Primary Movements into the Positive Lift Position: The critical distance point of the primary movements of the free-play leg, DP left heel, moves out upwards of the trot position by internal rotation/transverse abduction in the left hip, which is flexed to 90°. By proximally continuing movement, the pelvis as proximal lever rotates internally/abducts transversely in the supporting hip (first critical fulcrum), and as caudal lever brings the lumbar spine into left-concave lateroflexion (second critical fulcrum). Meanwhile, the toes extend/abduct, the subtalar and calcaneonavicular joints evert and the talocrural joint dorsiflexes (cf. p. 69).
The critical distance point of the primary movement of the free-play arm, DP left olecranon, moves dorsally/upwards/caudally/laterally to the left until it reaches the midfrontal plane of BSs pelvis, thorax and head, which is roughly vertical. With this movement, the elbow flexes by fulcrum displacement and the upper arm as distal lever turns in the shoulder in extension/45° abduction/end-stopped external rotation, such that the long axes of the forearm and hand come into the midfrontal plane. The movement continues with forearm supination, no movement in the wrist and slight finger flexion. The palm now faces medially/downwards towards the left shoulder and the flexion/extension axes of the elbow and wrist are horizontal. By proximally continuing movement, the left pincer jaws open at the sternoclavicular joint and the medial scapular margin moves towards the thoracic spine.

The final lever in the continuing primary movement of the free-play arm, the thoracic spine, goes cranial-to-caudally into left-concave lateroflexion (first critical fulcrum). When the thorax is secured in the open right pincer jaws, the latter as proximal lever move in adduction in the right shoulder joint (second critical fulcrum).

The critical distance point of the primary movement of BS head, DP vertex, moves upwards/laterally to the left/caudally in the vertical midfrontal plane by left-concave lateroflexion in the atlanto-occipital and atlanto-axial joints. By proximally continuing movement, the cervical spine goes into left-concave lateroflexion, as does the thoracic spine (critical fulcrum). The primary movements of head and free-play arm thus have the same critical fulcrum, which intensifies the lateroflexional mobilization of the upper thoracic spine (cf. p.69).

Note
Because the sagittotransverse axes of lateroflexion in the spinal column, the axis of abduction in the shoulder of the free-play arm, the flexion/extension axes in the elbow and wrist of the free-play arm, and the axes of transverse abduction and rotation in the hip of the free-play leg are horizontal, the muscles related to them have all been under positive lifting stress in contracting.

Primary Movements into the Stretch Position: The critical distance point of the primary movement of the free-play leg, DP left heel, moves downwards/caudally/dorsally/medially until its medial aspect reaches the floor in the midfrontal plane, which is roughly vertical. The toes flex and adduct, the subtalar and calcaneonavicular joints invert and the talocrural joint plantarflexes; the sole touches the floor. By proximally continuing movement, fulcrum displacement causes the knee to extend into the neutral position. The thigh as distal lever extends/adducts/externally rotates in the hip. The pelvis as proximal lever transversely abducts and externally rotates in the right supporting hip (first critical fulcrum), and as caudal lever brings the lumbar spine into right-concave lateroflexion (second critical fulcrum).

The critical distance point of the primary movement of the free-play arm, DP left wrist, moves cranially/downwards/medially in the roughly vertical midfrontal plane until it reaches the plane of symmetry and the elbow extends by fulcrum displacement. The position of the finger joints and the wrist have not changed; the palm faces caudally. By proximally continuing movement, the upper arm as distal lever turns in the left shoulder in flexion/adduction/slight internal rotation. The left pincer jaws close and move in the acromioclavicular and sternoclavicular joints away from the thorax and DP acromion moves cranially/medially/a little ventrally. The last distance point participating in the continuing movement of the free-play arm is C7: as cranial DP of the thoracic spine it moves downwards, first medially, then laterally to the right/caudally, bringing the thoracic spine into right-concave lateroflexion (first critical fulcrum). When the thorax is firmly secured in the open right pincer jaws, the latter as proximal lever move in abduction in the right, supporting shoulder (second critical fulcrum).

The critical distance point of the primary movement of BS head, DP vertex, moves downwards in the vertical midfrontal plane, first medially, then laterally to the right/caudally, by right-concave lateroflexion in the atlanto-occipital and atlanto-axial joints. By proximally continuing movement, the cervical spine goes into right-concave lateroflexion, as does the thoracic spine (critical fulcrum). The primary movements of the head and of the free-play arm thus have the same critical fulcrum, which intensifies the lateroflexional mobilization of the upper thoracic spine.

Note
Because the sagittotransverse axes of lateroflexion in the spinal column, the axis of adduction in the shoulder of the free-play arm, the flexion/extension axes in the elbow and wrist of the free-play arm, and the axis of adduction in the hip of the free-play leg, are horizontal, the muscles related to them have all stretched in negative lifting. At the same time, the muscles of the lumbar and thoracic spines involved in right-concave lateroflexion have contracted concentrically to the maximum in bridging activity. To increase the stretching, we can change the hand/floor contact into a forearm/floor contact by flexion through fulcrum displacement in the supporting elbow.

● **Conditio – Limitatio of the Movement Sequence**

Conditio of Absolute and/or Relative Fixed Spatial Points
Limitatio by Limiting the Primary Movement, Activated Passive Buttressing and/or Change in the Support Area
Conditio: In the All-Fours Exercise for Mobilization of the Hip and Shoulder Joints there is one important set of absolute fixed spatial points during the movement sequence from the trot position into the positive lift position and then into the stretch position: the points of contact between the supporting leg, the supporting arm and the floor.

Limitatio: These fixed points demand good coordination of the movements of the extremities, whose horizontal components neutralize each other, so that the lifting and braking-lowering of body segments or parts can take place over an unchanging support area.

2.6 Adaptations: All-Fours Exercises with Different Positionings in Space of the Long Axis of the Body (Figs. 23–29)

If, for whatever reason, the possible combinations of the Classic All-Fours Exercise and the adaptations so far – the Mobilizing All-Fours Exercises in Flexion/Extension and Lateroflexion, and the All-Fours Exercises for Stabilization and for Mobilization of the Hip and Shoulder Joints – with the long axis of the body horizontal in the starting position and the arms and legs supporting the body like pillars of a bridge, fail to allow functional training of the back muscles without uneconomical stress on the spinal column, we employ yet another way of adapting the All-Fours Exercise: we keep the primary movements of the extremities of the various All-Fours Exercises but alter the position in space of the long axis of the body. This way the effects of relative overweight in particular body segments or in parts of them can be neutralized. Hands and forearms need not bear weight if this is contraindicated.

Note
For the virtual long axis of the body to exist, the spinal column must be in neutral position. The intended movements in the joints of the spinal column in the Mobilizing All-Fours Exercises must occur without avoidance mechanisms even when the long axis of the body in fact no longer exists.

Adaptations with the Long Axis of the Body Slanting Downwards (Figs. 23–26)

Position and Activation in the Starting Position
The starting position is that of the Mobilizing All-Fours Exercise in Flexion/Extension (see p. 62) with the following changes: all-fours stance on the floor with the upper body now supported on the forearms. The long axes of the forearms and hands are parallel, a shoulder's-width apart, and face cranially/dorsally. The el-

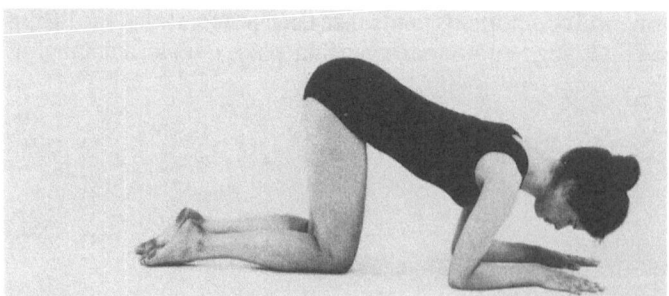

Fig. 23. Starting position for adaptations with long axis of the body slanting downwards

bows are below and caudal to the shoulder and in about 60° flexion/slight adduction/external rotation. The support area is the smallest area encompassing the points of contact between the ventral aspects of the thighs, dorsa of the feet, flexor aspects of the forearms, volar aspects of the fingers and the floor (Fig. 23).

Adaptation for – TS/ + Frontotransverse Diameter of the Thorax/ Imperfect Congruence Between the Pincer Jaws and the Thoracic Wall (Fig. 24)

Actio and Conditio of the Movement Sequence
The movement sequence of the adaptation in Fig. 24a is the same as that of the Classic All-Fours Exercise. So is the movement sequence for the adaptation in Fig. 24b, except that the primary movement of the free-play leg has its critical fulcrum in the free-play hip while the primary movement of the free-play arm continues into thorax-positive rotation in the lower thoracic and cervical spine (first critical fulcrum). If the left pincer jaws are firmly stabilized, they will have moved in transverse extension as proximal lever at the left shoulder (second critical fulcrum).

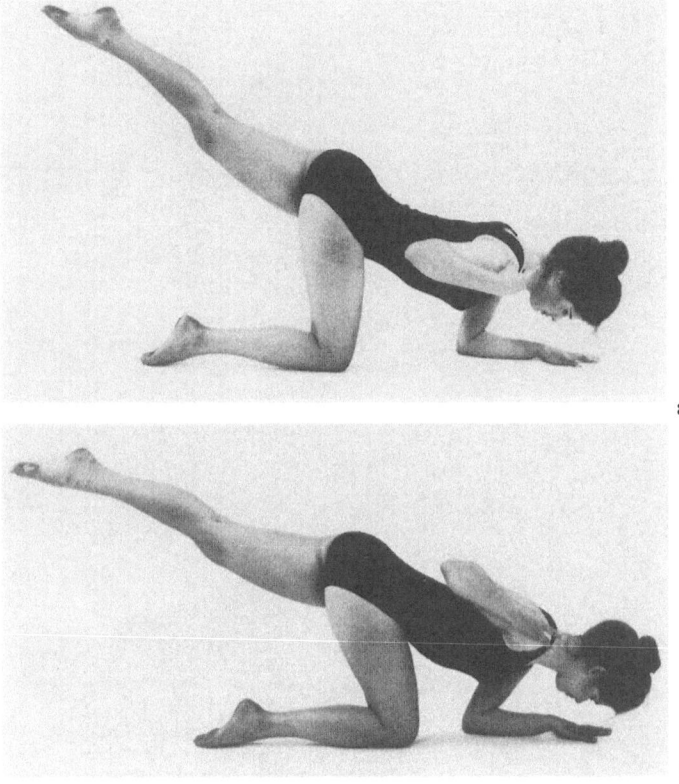

a

b

Fig. 24a, b. Adaptation for – TS/ + frontotransverse diameter of thorax/imperfect congruence between pincer jaws and thoracic wall

Adaptation When Stress to Wrists and Hands is Contraindicated or When There is Pronounced Cubitus Valgus/Insufficient Triceps Brachii/ + Width and + Weight in BS Pelvis/ + Length and + Weight in BS Legs/ Insufficient Lumbar Muscles/ + Weight in BS Thorax (Fig. 25)

Actio and Conditio of the Movement Sequence

Because of the wide and heavy thorax, we will keep both forearms for support and perform only the primary movement of the free-play leg from the Classic All-Fours Exercise with pronounced dorsal translational activity as the primary movement of the head (Fig. 25a).

By a shifting of weight cranially, the lower leg rises up easily from the base support, the support area becomes smaller and the flexion in the shoulders is reduced to about 45° (Fig. 25b). The rotational components in the vertebrae of the lower tho-

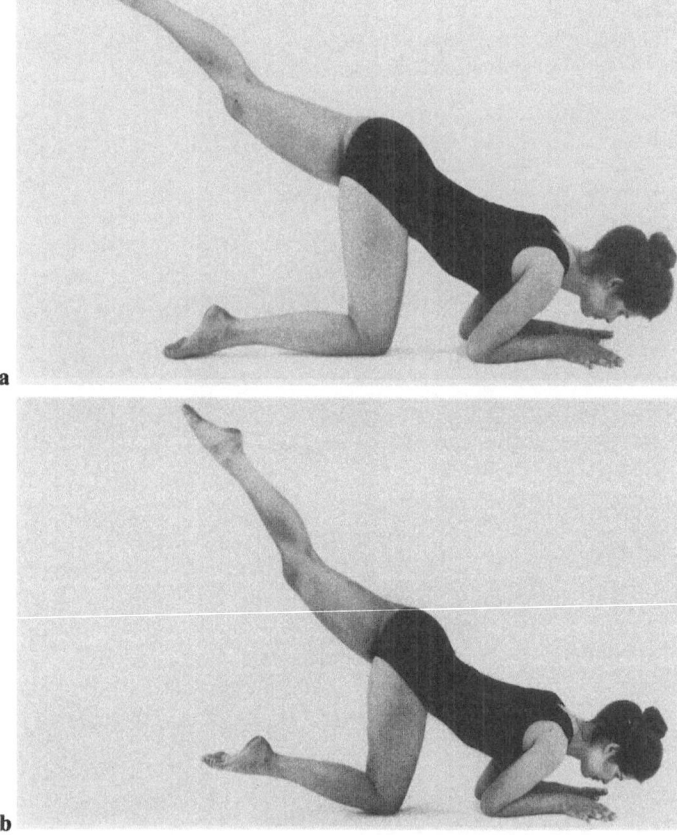

a

b

Fig. 25 a, b. Adaptation for avoiding stress to the wrists and hands/marked cubitus valgus/insufficiency of triceps brachii/ + width and + weight in BS pelvis/ + length and + weight in BS legs/lumbar muscular insufficiency/ + weight in BS thorax

racic spine are unstable and both free-play and supporting hip are trained more for strength and skill if the free-play leg performs the primary movement of the Classic All-Fours Exercise (see p. 53).

Adaptation for Pronounced – – TS/ – Sagittotransverse Diameter of the Thorax/Thoracic Scoliosis/ – – CS/Functional Cervical Kyphosis (Fig. 26)

Actio and Conditio of the Movement Sequence

By displacing weight cranially and resting the head on the floor, BS head becomes parked and this relieves the muscles of the neck. Now the activation of the back muscles comes only from the free-play leg, whose primary movement is like that in the Classic All-Fours Exercise (Fig. 26a). This type of activation is especially gentle on the passive structures of the spinal column, because the lever has been shortened by being tilted in space and slight compressive stress is exerted on the long axis of the body.

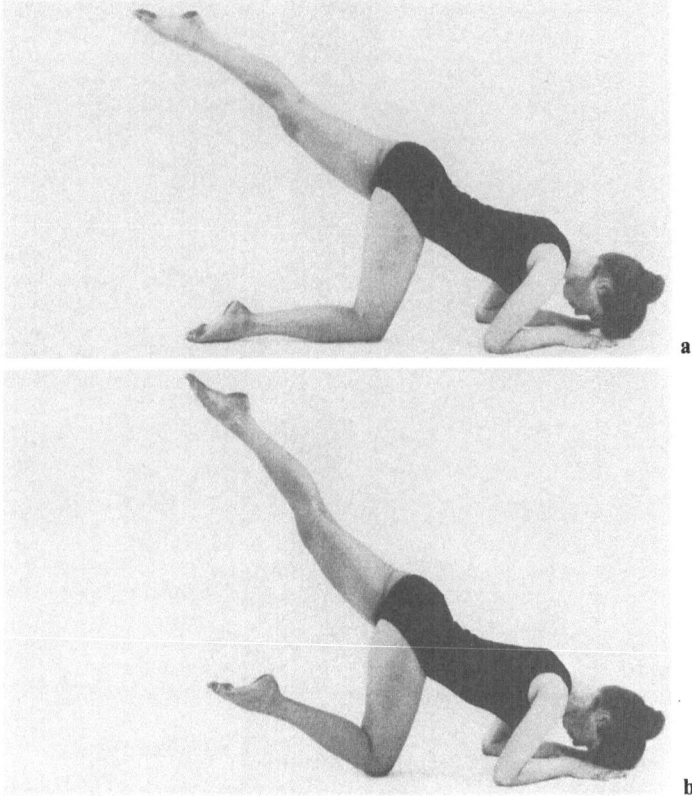

Fig. 26a, b. Adaptation for marked – – TS/ – sagittotransverse diameter of thorax/thoracic scoliosis/ – – CS/functional cervical kyphosis

93

When the supporting lower leg is lifted, the long axis of the body becomes unstable in regard to rotation (Fig. 26 b). The intensity of economical activity rises; the tilt of the long axis of the body becomes more pronounced and the compressive stress on it increases, reducing the strain on the muscles but increasing the challenge to their skill.

Adaptation with the Long Axis of the Body Inclined Forwards (Fig. 27)

This adaptation is suitable for relieving stress on BS arms, especially the shoulder girdle, or on the neck muscles. It is also a suitable exercise if a head-down position is to be avoided or when there is overwidth or overweight in BSs thorax and pelvis.

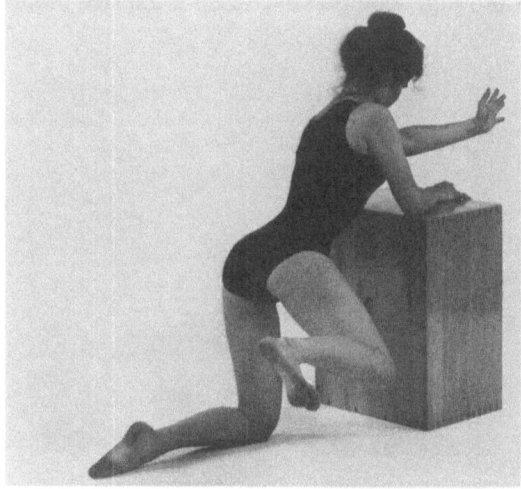

a

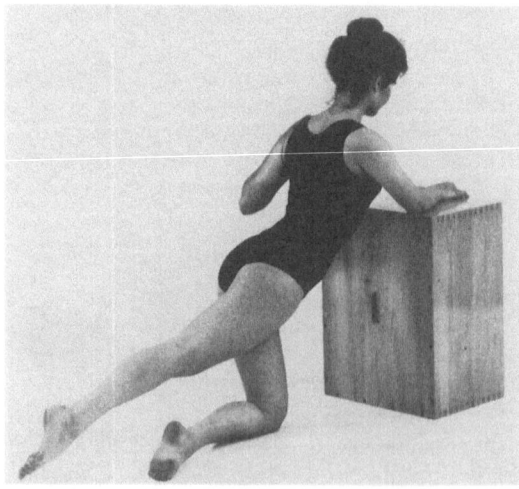

b

Fig. 27 a, b. Adaptation with the long axis of the body slanting forwards. **a** Striking out movement, **b** end position

94

Position and Activation in the Starting Position

The starting position is on all fours with the forearms supporting the body. The ventral aspects of the lower legs and the dorsa of the feet touch the floor. The flexor aspects of the forearms, the palms and the volar aspects of the fingers touch a box of a height to make the long axis of the body slant forwards about 40°. The long axes of the lower legs are below and roughly parallel to the long axes of the forearms.

The primary movements of the free-play leg, free-play arm and head are identical to those of the Classic All-Fours Exercise (see p. 53).

Actio and Conditio of the Movement Sequence

Figure 27a illustrates the striking out movement for the end position of the primary movement of the Classic All-Fours Exercise. The free-play leg is lifted up out of the trot position by transverse abduction/internal rotation in the hip; the knee remains flexed at 90°, while the subtalar and calcaneonavicular joints evert and the talocrural joint dorsiflexes. In the free-play arm the palm rotates medially by forearm supination and the shoulder joint flexes/adducts. The spinal column remains almost in neutral position with a very slight emphasis of the lumbar lordosis. The end position of the Classic All-Fours Exercise is illustrated in Fig. 27b. Before changing diagonals several to-and-fro movements should be performed.

Adaptation with the Long Axis of the Body Vertical (Fig. 28)

This adaptation is suitable for hypermobile and unstable spinal columns, for developing equilibrium with the thoracic spine dynamically stabilized in neutral position, when physiological stress on the knees is important, and when training for the back muscles with functional stress on the leg axes is desired. The starting position is upright one-legged standing.

Actio and Conditio of the Movement

Fulcrum displacement causes the knee of the right, supporting leg to flex so far that fall-preventing activity is demanded of the quadriceps. If the patient rises up on the toes of the supporting leg, this flexion should increase somewhat to ensure functional stressing of the axes of the legs. The "supporting" arm may support itself slightly against a wall, at about the level of the midtransverse plane and in the plane of symmetry. It can, however, also be stabilized in free-play without touching a wall.

The primary movements of the left, free-play leg, the right, free-play arm and the head are identical to those for the Classic All-Fours Exercise. When the toes of the free-play leg touch the floor, DP left heel rotates medially as soon as the continuing movement of the free-play leg reaches its critical fulcrum and the pelvis, as proximal lever, rotates externally in the left hip, while the rotation in the lower thoracic spine is pelvis-negative. The long axes of the free-play arm remain in the vertical midfrontal plane and bring about thorax-positive active buttressing of the pelvic rotation in the lower thoracic spine (Fig. 28a).

Now we can switch to the end position of the Mobilizing All-Fours Exercise in

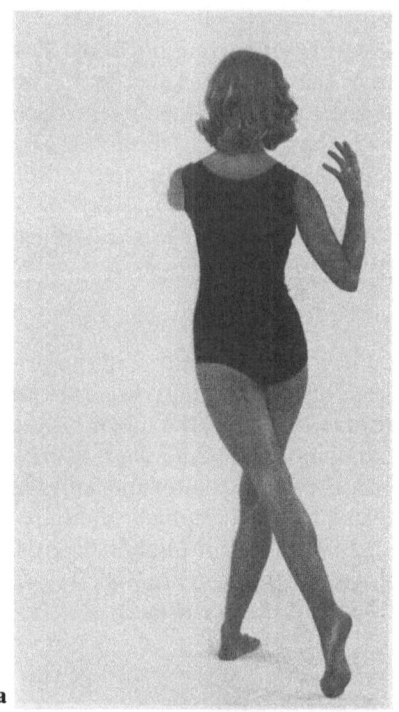

a

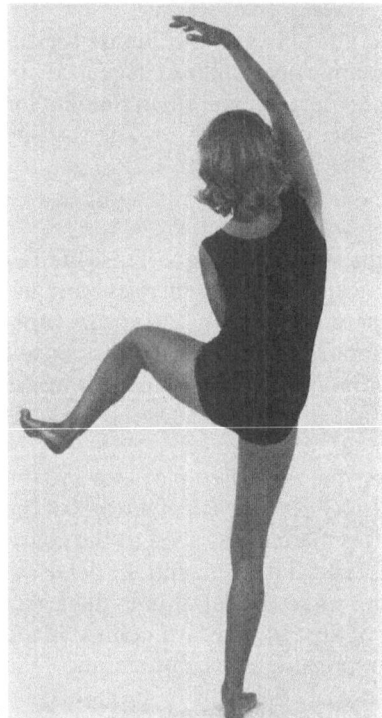

b

Fig. 28 a, b. Adaptation with the long axis of the body vertical

Lateroflexion (Fig. 28 b) by performing the primary movements of the free-play leg and arm in pure antagonistic countermovements and allowing these movements to continue on into the spinal column.

Instead of returning to the end position of the Classic All-Fours Exercise, we can now allow the movements of the free-play leg and arm to continue in the midfrontal plane, bringing the patient into the end position of right-concave lateroflexion. However, the left, free-play foot must cross well over behind the right, supporting foot on the floor, which causes the pelvis to slant forwards with flexion in the right, supporting hip; with it go BSs thorax, head and arms, moving in the midfrontal plane.

Adaptation with Direct Lateral Support of BSs Pelvis and Thorax in Sidelying (Fig. 29)

This adaptation is suitable for patients in whom stress on the supporting extremities is contraindicated, for older patients, for patients in poor general condition, or for those who have pain, especially in the lumbar region. It can be used as an exercise to reduce cardiac stress, and as a starting-up exercise in bed in the morning.

Position and Activation in the Starting Position

The starting position is left sidelying (Fig. 29 a). BSs pelvis, thorax and head, their frontal planes vertical, are aligned in the horizontal long axis of the body.

In BS legs, the long axes of the thighs are sagittotransverse, those of the lower legs are frontosagittal. In BS arms, the left arm provides support for the head. The long axis of the right forearm is frontosagittal and the forearm rests with its flexor aspect on the floor. DP elbow is in the transverse plane of the shoulder.

BSs pelvis and thorax and the right arm are parked on the floor; the head is parked on the left arm, the right leg is parked on the left leg.

Actio and Conditio of the Movement Sequence

The primary movements of free-play leg, free-play arm and head correspond to those of the All-Fours Exercise for Mobilization of the Hip and Shoulder Joints (see pp. 87, 88).

The left hand can support the head if there is uncomfortable stress on the neck in the positive lift position (Fig. 29 b).

In the stretch position (Fig. 29 c), pressure activity by the sole of the right foot, right palm and left side of the head on the floor and external rotation in the left shoulder (effected by the distal pointer, the flexion/extension axis of the left elbow) can increase the stretching on the upper side of the body by the bridging activity going on on the lower side. The yawning reflex can also be triggered in this way to get the respiration going well.

A good movement sequence is for the patient to roll over from the left-side stretch position into supine and then into the right-side stretch position, changing over the extremity movements as he rolls. The head need never leave the base support, but simply roll over on the floor.

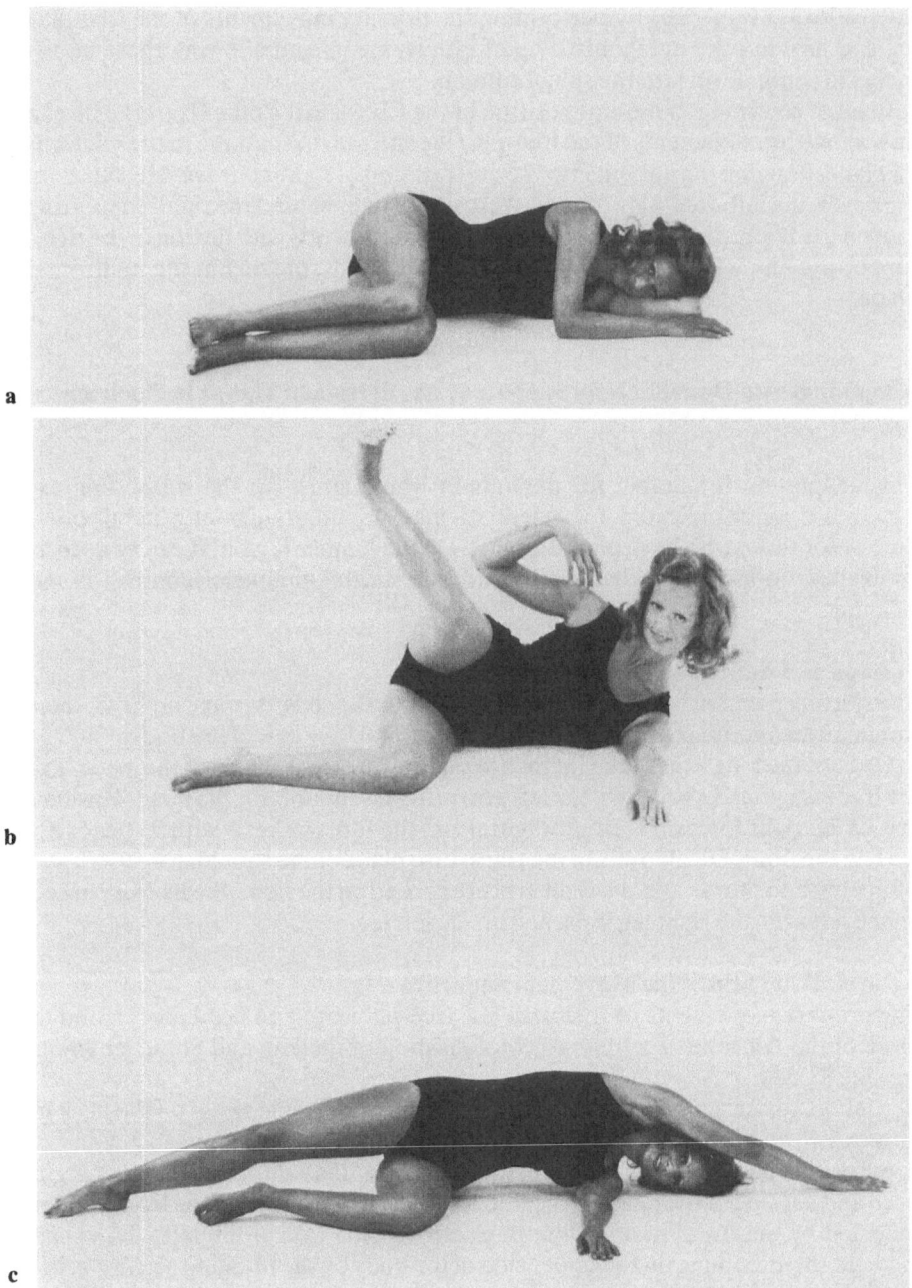

Fig. 29 a–c. Adaptation with BS pelvis and BS thorax laterally supported. **a** Sidelying, **b** positive lift position, **c** stretch position

3 Functional Training of Rotation About the Long Axis of the Body and the Long Axes of the Thighs

Functional training of rotation about the long axis of the body and the long axes of the thighs gives practice in activating and mobilizing these components of movement as part of economical movement behaviour.

Note

Because in typical human upright posture the long axis of the body and the long axes of the thighs are vertical, rotation about them is essential for economical locomotion and for skilful use of the hands.

Because the long axis of the body is the rotation axis of the inherently mobile spinal column, the motion segments which constitute the rotation level must be capable of dynamic stabilization in their neutral position, otherwise rotation cannot take place in the best way. Since the long axis of the body is only a virtual axis (rather than an actual one), dynamic stabilization of the rotation levels is particularly important, because rotational movements are the only movements to take place in the spinal column during which the virtual long axis of the body is not lost.

When there is rotation in the hip joints about the frontosagittal functional long axis of the thighs, either both pointers or only the distal pointer or only the proximal pointer may rotate. Since rotation of the proximal pointer, the line connecting the right and left iliac spines, is extremely important for economical stressing of the hip joints during walking and standing, pelvic rotation in the hip joint will be discussed in detail.

Position in Space of the Long Axis of the Body and the Long Axes of the Thighs During Functional Rotation Training

When the long axis of the body and the long axes of the thighs are vertical, rotation about them is lift-free. The rotation levels in the spinal column are the atlanto-occipital and atlanto-axial joints, the cervical spine and, normally, the lower thoracic spine. To be capable of rotation, these must be dynamically stabilized.

Dynamic stabilization in the area of the spinal column is primarily the function of the autochthonous vertebral muscles. They have the coordination to be able to meet the continually changing demands of posture. Consequently, lift-free rotation in the spinal column is inseparable from maintaining the virtual long axis of the body.

That we nevertheless perform the exercise Turn Again, Whittington with the long axis of the body horizontal, so that the economical forward movement resulting from rotation has to take place through the body's turning on the base support, is for the following reasons: first, we are training the rotation under conditions of lifting stress (against gravity), which constantly changes as the body turns on the floor; second, we can keep the speed of movement low and thus bring the different phases of the movement better under control, despite the increased stress. We are thus training both skill and strength.

3.1 Turn Again, Whittington (Figs. 30, 31)

Turn Again, Whittington is suitable as rotation training for patients with normal spinal columns and hip joints or variants of the norm. Incipient and moderate restrictions in movement in these areas are pathological deviations that can be improved by this exercise.

"Turn Again, Whittington" is an invented name, an anglicization of the German "Who Turns, Gains", and refers to the legendary medieval Lord Mayor of London, Richard Whittington, who as a poor young apprentice was on the point of leaving the capital in discouragement when he heard the bells of London calling him back, and "turned again" to find fame and fortune.

■ Goal of the Exercise

The goal is for the patient to learn to coordinate the rotational movements and/or the muscular activities of rotation in the hip joints with those of the spinal column as in walking. We aim to reach this goal by training the muscles of rotation in the hip and vertebral joints for strength and skill.

The patient is to learn to roll his body across a base support under steady control, without any involuntary acceleration or slowing down.

▶ Functional Analysis in Therapist Language

● Conception of the Exercise (Fig. 30)

To strengthen the rotational muscles of the vertebral and hip joints by imposing positive lifting stress, and to train their equilibrium reactions by placing the patient in a position of precarious balance, we choose a starting position in supine.

To ensure that the rotational demands made on the spinal column as the body turns are the best possible, the spinal column must be in the neutral position.

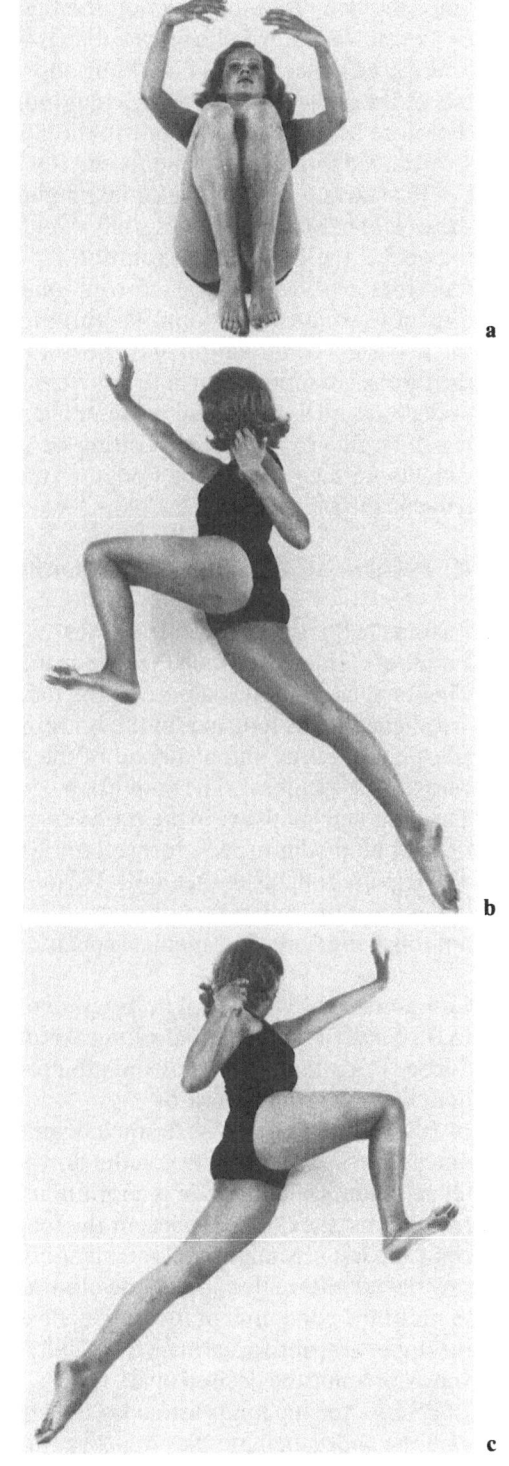

Fig. 30 a–c. Turn Again, Whittington.
a Starting position, **b** end position after
turn to the right, **c** end position after turn
to the left

101

Since the body is to turn over on the base support without involuntary acceleration or slowing down, the arms and legs will be used as potential accelerating and
braking weights, although without allowing BSs pelvis, thorax and head to get
out of their alignment in the virtual long axis of the body. Arms and legs must
therefore be potentially mobile in the starting position and their weights must be
so arranged that these segments can function independently.

For the starting position we choose supine with arms and legs lifted off the floor,
the weight of each resting neutrally over its proximal joint (hip or shoulder). Since
the goal is the coordinated rotation typical of normal gait, BSs pelvis and head
must rotate in one direction (co-rotational) while BS thorax rotates in the opposite
direction (counter-rotational). In turning over to the right, the positive rotation of
the pelvis is a continuation of the legs' movements, while the negative rotation of
the thorax is continuation of the movements of the arms. As long as the rotation is
underway and until the end position over the new support area is reached, the left
leg and right arm act as accelerating weights, the right leg and left arm as braking
weights. In the process, the body has turned over on the floor from supine into
lying on the right side.

● **Position and Activation in the Starting Position**

Position in Space of the Critical Axes
Points of Contact Between the Body and the Environment
The starting position is supine on the floor (Fig. 30 a). BSs pelvis, thorax and head
are aligned in the long axis of the body, which is horizontal. The dorsal aspects of
BSs pelvis, thorax and head and of the scapulae constitute the points of contact
with the base support. The patient's gaze is directed upwards.

The arms and hands are in the transverse plane of the shoulder joints, which is vertical. Their medial aspects form an upright oval; the fingers do not touch.

The legs are roughly in the sagittal planes of the hip joints, which are vertical. The
knees are more or less over the navel and the heels over the hip joints; the feet do
not touch the floor. The medial aspects of the legs may touch.

Components of Movement in Relation to the Neutral Position of the Joints
In BS head, DP vertex is in the long axis of the body. Cervical lordosis is slightly reduced. The atlanto-occipital and atlanto-axial joints are so far flexed that the patient looks ventrally/upwards.

In BSs thorax and pelvis, thoracic kyphosis and lumbar lordosis are reduced so
much that the contact between the dorsal aspects of these two sections of the vertebral column and the floor is continuous.

In BS arms, the dorsal aspects of the scapulae touch the floor; consequently DPs
right and left acromions are dorsally positioned. The shoulder joints are transversely flexed/internally rotated, the elbows flexed (the forearms supinated) and the
joints of the hands and of the fingers flexed just so much that the flexor aspects of
the upper arm and forearm face medially and those of the fingers and palms downwards, forming the desired oval.

In BS legs, the hip joints are so far flexed that the weight of the legs does not activate the abdominal muscles to prevent the legs from falling, and so far adducted

that the medial aspects of the legs touch. The knee joints are so far flexed that the lower legs are suspended from the thighs without quadriceps activity; the joints of the feet and toes are not activated against gravity.

**Movement Tolerance at the Critical Joints in Relation
to the Intended Primary Movement**
Since the spinal column is roughly in the neutral position, the full movement tolerance for rotation is available.
The starting position of the extremities, both by their position in space and by the positions of the joints, also offers the potential mobility needed.
In order to turn to the right on the floor, we need:

- Head-positive rotation in the cervical spine; pelvic-positive rotation in the thoracic spine
- Full extension/internal rotation/some adduction in the right hip; extension in the knee joint
- Flexion/external rotation in the left hip; flexion in the knee joint
- Flexion/internal rotation in the right shoulder; extension in the elbow joint
- Extension/abduction/external rotation in the left shoulder joint; flexion in the elbow joint

**Distribution of Body Weight on a Base Support or Suspension Device,
Against a Supportive Device, or over a Support Area,
and the Resulting Activity States of the Musculature**
The support area in the starting position is the smallest area encompassing the points of contact between the pelvis, thorax, head and shoulder girdle and the floor. The muscle activity which links BSs pelvis, thorax and head and makes their base support a support area is the pulling away of DPs vertex and coccyx from each other. The spinal column is stabilized, BS legs is in free play. In BS arms the shoulder girdle is supported by the floor, the arms are in free play.

**Intensity of Muscle Activity Required with Economical Activity
Respiration**
In the starting position of Turn Again, Whittington, the intensity of economical activity is low in the extremities and a little higher in BSs pelvis, thorax and head. If the effort of stabilization causes any inhibition of respiration, the patient should whistle softly as he breathes in and out.

**Potential Accelerating and Braking Weights in Relation to the Bisecting Plane
of the Intended Primary Movement**
Because we plan for the body to turn over on the floor from supine into sidelying, the bisecting plane in the starting position coincides with the plane of symmetry, which is vertical.
During rotation to the right, the bisecting plane also moves right. To the observer standing at the patient's feet, however, this plane has moved left. Thus, to the observer, the accelerating weights are to the left and the braking weights to the right

of the bisecting plane. The patient will perceive the accelerating weights as front weights and the braking weights as back weights (see p. 116).

- ● **Actio – Reactio of the Movement Sequence**

Turn Again, Whittington is a location-changing movement sequence.
As a prelude to the exercise, the head is lifted just off the base support into free play and becomes suspended from the thorax by the ventral muscles of the neck. The thorax becomes linked to the pelvis by the abdominal muscles.

Actio: The Primary Movement

The actio is characterized by simultaneous primary movements of all five extremities, which initiate the rotation from supine to right sidelying using buttressing movements. In doing so, the buttressing movements of the free-play legs bring about pelvis-positive rotation in the thoracic spine, those of the free-play arms bring about thorax-negative rotation in the thoracic and cervical spines, and the head rotates positively in the cervical spine.

The critical distance point of the primary movement of the right free-play leg, DP right patella, moves dorsally/caudally/downwards (in regard to the supine body)/against the direction of movement (in regard to the side position), which is towards the right, with extension of the knee by fulcrum displacement. The joints of the feet plantarflex and invert and the toes flex. By proximally continuing movement, the thigh as distal lever turns in extension/slight adduction/external rotation in the right hip joint; the pelvis and thorax rotate on the floor (the pelvis more than the thorax) onto their right sides, with pelvis-positive rotation in the lower thoracic spine (critical fulcrum).

Simultaneously, the critical distance point of the primary movement of the left free-play leg, DP left patella, is transported to the right/downwards/ventrally (in regard to the body)/somewhat laterally to the left. The thigh as distal lever turns in slight horizontal abduction/external rotation in the left hip joint. By proximally continuing movement, the pelvis as proximal pointer rotates internally in the right hip joint (first critical fulcrum) and as caudal pointer rotates pelvis-positively in the lower thoracic spine (second critical fulcrum). Simultaneously, the joints of the feet dorsiflex and invert and the toes extend and abduct. The flexion in the hip and knee joints remains unchanged. In the sidelying position the left heel is almost on the floor.

The critical distance point of the primary movement of BS head, DP tip of the nose, moves laterally to the right/dorsally/downwards by rotation in the atlanto-occipital and atlanto-axial joints. The movement continues caudally with head-positive rotation in the cervical spine (critical fulcrum).

The critical distance point of the left free-play arm, DP radial styloid process, moves laterally to the left/dorsally/downwards (in regard to the supine body) and against the direction of the movement (in regard to the side position), which is to the right. The forearm supinates and the elbow flexes by displacement of its fulcrum. The upper arm as distal lever turns in extension/up to about 40° abduction/external rotation in the humeroscapular joint, such that in the right sidelying position the palm is facing the left shoulder and the joints of the hand and fingers have barely changed position. By continuing movement, the pincer jaws open in the acromioclavicular joint and the medial scapular margin moves in the sternoclavicular joint towards the processes of the thoracic spine, such that the frontotransverse diameter of the thorax, as cranial pointer in the lower thoracic spine and as caudal pointer in the cervical spine, actively buttresses the continuing movements of the left, free-play leg and of the head by thorax-negative rotation.

Simultaneously, the critical distance point of the primary movement of the right free-play arm, DP ball of the thumb, moves to the right/downwards/ventrally (in regard to the body)/ cranially, while the forearm pronates and the elbow extends by displacement of its fulcrum. The upper arm as distal lever turns in flexion and internal rotation in the right humeroscapular joint. By continuing movement, the pincer jaws close up in the acromioclavicular joint and DP acromion moves cranially/ventrally/medially in the sternoclavicular joint. Meanwhile the extensor aspect of the upper arm has come to touch the floor. The wrists have extended; no significant change has occurred in the position of the finger joints.

Reactio: Activated Passive Buttressing
In Turn Again, Whittington, activated passive buttressing arises in the economical form of a location-changing movement sequence, in that parts of body segments are lifted off the base support. As soon as the left side of BSs pelvis and thorax have left the floor during the body's turn towards right sidelying, they become activated passive buttresses. As soon as their frontal planes become vertical, however, only parts of the left arm and right leg are still able to act as activated passive buttresses. Once the frontal plane of the pelvis starts to incline in the direction of movement, some of the weight of the pelvis becomes accelerating weight.

Reactio: Change in the Support Area
Turn Again, Whittington, is a location-changing movement sequence: the support area in the starting position is abandoned completely and moves to the right. In the end position of right sidelying this area is the smallest area encompassing the points of contact between the right side of the pelvis, thorax and right arm (the shoulder joints being activated) and the floor.

Actio: Accelerating Weights
Reactio: Braking Weights
Since all the extremities are performing primary movements, the turning of the body on the base support causes the weights of some extremities to act as braking weights or activated passive buttressing and the weights of others to act as accelerating weights. The bisecting plane, identical in the starting position to the plane of symmetry, moves to a greater or lesser extent to the right. When the right upper arm touches the floor and becomes parked, it ceases to act as an accelerating weight. In this case, and even when the right arm is able to remain in free play in the end position and continue to act as accelerating weight, the bi-

secting plane in the end position roughly coincides with the midfrontal plane of BSs pelvis and thorax. However, if the right upper arm goes into supporting function on the base support and there is bridging in the shoulder joint, the bisecting plane will be that much further to the right and fewer (or smaller) braking weights will be needed.

All weights in front of and ventral to the bisecting plane are accelerating, all weights behind and dorsal to it are braking weights.

● **Conditio – Limitatio of the Movement Sequence**

Conditio: Constant Distances Between Body Distance Points
Limitatio: Active Buttressing and Stabilization
Conditio: The distance between the transverse plane in which the cranial pointer of cervical rotation rotates and the transverse plane in which the caudal pointer of cervical rotation rotates remains constant.
Limitatio: If the line connecting the eyes and the frontotransverse diameter of the thorax are to rotate in parallel planes, the virtual long axis of the body must be dynamically stabilized in the area of the cervical and thoracic spine. This can be achieved by keeping the head in the long axis of the body by dorsal translational/left-concave lateroflexional/left lateral translational active buttressing in the cervical spine.

Conditio: The distance between the transverse plane in which the cranial pointer of thoracic rotation rotates and the transverse plane in which the caudal pointer of thoracic rotation rotates remains constant.
Limitatio: If the frontotransverse diameter of the thorax and the line connecting the right and left iliac spines are to rotate in parallel planes, then the virtual long axis of the body must be dynamically stabilized in the thoracic and lumbar spine. This can be achieved by keeping the pelvis in the long axis of the body by right-concave lateroflexional/dorsal translational/right lateral translational/flexional active buttressing in the lumbar spine.

Conditio: The distance between DP C2–C1 and DP S1–L5 remains constant.
Limitatio: If the entire length of the spinal column is to remain unchanged, the movements occurring within the spinal column must be limited to rotation. Any other deviations out of the neutral position of the spinal column must be prevented by active buttressing. Since the physiological curvatures of the spinal column were somewhat reduced in the starting position, the return of the segments of the spine to their neutral position is desirable.

Conditio of Absolute and/or Relative Fixed Spatial Points
Limitatio By Limiting the Primary Movement, Activated Passive Buttressing and/or Change in the Support Area
Conditio: The critical distance points of the primary movements of the legs, DPs left and right patellae, which move farther and farther apart during the movement sequence, must maintain the distance they have reached in the end posi-

tion. DP right patella must have moved at least as far as the midfrontal plane of the pelvis.

Limitatio: These spatial relationships can only be maintained if the right hip joint reaches end-stop in extension, if the right foot with the knee extended crosses the midfrontal plane dorsally, and if the muscle activity of the counter-rotational leg movements is kept up even in the end position. In this way the lumbar spine remains potentially mobile and is stabilized in its neutral position, checking the continuing positive rotation of the pelvis in the lower thoracic spine perfectly.

Conditio: When the body turns on the base support, the ventral aspects of BSs pelvis and thorax must not touch the floor.

Limitatio: This relative fixed spatial point limits the changing of the support area. It can only be maintained by either increasing the support area in the direction of movement, by touching the floor with the right upper arm; or by intensifying the active buttressing activity acting against the direction of movement, provided by the left free-play arm and the negative rotation of the thorax; and/or by reducing the internal rotation of the pelvis in the right hip joint, by internally rotating the right free-play leg in the end position; and/or by reducing the accelerating weight of the left free-play leg, by increasing the transverse abduction of the thigh in the left hip joint (i.e. shortening the left-leg lever).

Conditio: In the end position, the patient's gaze is directed downwards, but the distance between the eyes and the floor must not get any smaller.

Limitatio: This relative fixed spatial point means that the head must be constantly pulling away as if for dorsal translation in the cervical spine, thus ensuring that the virtual long axis of the body is maintained despite the rotation in the thoracic and cervical spines.

Conditio of Movement Speed
Limitatio of Economical Activity By Finding the Optimal Speed
Conditio: The exercise should remain slow. Movement should be smooth and even. The end position should be held and breathing remain natural.

Limitatio: As a guideline, the speed of the exercise should be about 3 seconds from the starting position into right sidelying, 2 seconds holding in the end position and 2 seconds to move back into the starting position or 5 seconds to move from right into left sidelying.

● **Position and Activation in the End Position and Return to the Starting Position**

The goals of the exercise have been fulfilled when the end position is reached. The return to the starting position is by coordinated lowering of the intensity of economical activity. From the position of right sidelying, only the right leg needs to be pulled in.

If turning over from right into left sidelying is desired, BS head must remain in free play and go straight into the new turning movement. As soon as the right leg has been brought back in, the primary movements of the arms and legs begin, with roles reversed. If this form of the exercise is chosen, the movement can gradually be speeded up.

▶ Instruction in Patient Language

● Instruction Appealing to the Patient's Perception

The patient will be able to learn all five primary movements with precision in a relatively short amount of time if time is taken before beginning the exercise to feel the five critical distance points and imagine their counter-rotational movements (right knee counter-rotational to left knee, right hand to left hand; which knee and hand move co-rotationally with the head and which counter?).

● Verbal Instruction

● Instruction by Manipulation

Position and Activation in the Starting Position

"Lie on the floor like a beetle on its back with its legs in the air. Your head is also lying on the floor.
Make your back broad and quite long. Feel the floor, not only with your back, but also with the back of your head, your neck and your waist. Pretend that you're holding a big balloon in your arms. The insides of your legs touch; it's no effort at all to hold this position."

The therapist can adjust BSs head, arms and legs as the patient is taking up the starting position.
During this activation, the therapist watches the economical activity and makes sure that the intensity is highest in the spinal column. This can be stimulated by gently applying compression on the vertex. The therapist also keeps an eye on the patient's breathing.

Actio and Conditio of the Movement Sequence

"Lift your head up a little from the floor and look over your right shoulder. When you can see the floor, keep your nose away from it. You will roll over onto your right side as if on ball bearings if you can thread your right foot through under your left leg and then make a large step backwards, until your right leg is long and stretched out. At the same time,

For this exercise to fulfill its goal, the coordination of the displacement of weights of the body segments and the corresponding activation of the muscles must be established for each patient individually. The manipulative cues that the therapist provides, therefore, consist of lifting and holding parts of weights and of stimulating activity by applying guiding resistance.

your left hand is drawing a bowstring. If you start to feel as if you're going to roll onto your stomach, pull the handbrake with your left hand, or the footbrake, by pushing your right heel against the floor. You even have a headbrake; it works by your keeping your nose away from the floor. When everything's okay, you turn into a breathing statue."

If this is not enough, it can be helpful to break the exercise down into smaller steps. Before doing the whole exercise, the patient lies in the end position and the therapist allows him to experience particular buttressing resistances separately: e.g. compression to the right arm and traction to the left, or compression to the right leg and traction to the left, or traction to the left arm and left leg, or compression to the right arm and right leg, or positive-rotation resistance to the pelvis and negative-rotation resistance to the thorax, etc.

End Position and Return to the Starting Position

"The statue is holding up well. Try to breathe naturally, or quietly whistle a tune. For example, 'Row, row, row your boat' as you breathe out, 'Gently down the stream . . .' as you breathe in, etc.

You start to look back to where you came from. The tension in the bow subsides, and the right leg returns to join the left leg. Now you're back where you were at the beginning. The beetle is lying on its back again with its head on the floor. Look up and let your legs hang comfortably, with their insides touching. Hold onto the balloon again. It's oval-shaped and very light."

In the end position, the therapist can make minor adjustments by tapping and saying, "A little shorter here, longer there. Move your hands a little," etc.

The therapist makes sure that now too there is not too much acceleration in the movement. The pelvis usually needs to be held back, especially if constitutionally the distance between the greater trochanters is wide. Using gentle guiding resistance to the arms and legs the therapist directs the patient back into the starting position without any deviations.

Transition from Right into Left Sidelying

"Look to the left, over your left shoulder, until you see the floor again. But keep the tip of your nose away from it. Your arms have let the bow relax, only to draw it again to the left. Now you have to thread your left foot under your right leg and take that large step backwards with your left leg until it's stretched out. You have the same brakes, but use your right hand and left heel now.

Here too the therapist giving the manipulative cues must pay attention to the weight of BS pelvis. If several to-and-fro movements are performed consecutively, the long axis of the body easily starts to turn in the horizontal plane. The therapist must make sure that the long axis of the body remains parallel to itself as it moves from side to side in space. The cause of turning in the horizontal plane is usually that

Your headbrake still works too, of course." the activated passive buttressing leg has not fully extended in the hip and knee joints. The knee and foot are then no longer dorsal to the midfrontal plane.

► Adapting the Exercise to the Patient's Constitution and Condition

● Adaptation to Constitution: Role of Lengths, Widths, Depths and Distribution of Weights

Increased weight in the pelvis and legs and increased widths in BS pelvis, especially a wider than normal span between the greater trochanters, often make it necessary to raise up BSs thorax and head with a support, which must be wide enough not to disturb the body's roll into sidelying.

● Adaptation to Condition

Poor Physical Fitness or Wish to Increase Performance
Very often the patient lacks the muscle condition to lift his legs, which act as counterweights on the spinal column, and still maintain the virtual long axis of the body as he rolls over.
The patient begins in sidelying and brings the extremities into the necessary joint positions as far as possible without the movement components requiring positive lift. Thus, the lower extremities are parked on the base support. The head and left leg are then brought into the end position; the left heel should be supported on the floor. The counterscrew of the thorax is activated by the arms and the patient then attempts to lift his heels from the floor.

Restricted Movement and/or Hypermobility
Restricted movement and/or instability of the rotation levels in the spinal column are frequent.
In such cases, the patient sits upright and practices the counterscrew of the thorax with the aid of his arms (Fig. 31 a, b). The opposing arm movements are in response to either an imagined or an actual resistance manually applied to the hands by the therapist.
The countermovement of the legs and the rotation of the pelvis in the lower spinal column are also practised sitting upright on the edge of a chair. The legs take up the end position of Turn Again, Whittington. Activation is again in response to either an imagined or an actual resistance applied by the therapist to the knees. The thorax remains in the neutral position.
Finally the two exercises can be combined, including now the head movement (Fig. 31 c, d). The movement sequence is now lift-free for the rotations in the spinal column and the lift demanded of the extremities is reduced.

This way of doing the exercise has the additional advantage that it can practised easily and often during the day.

Muscular Weakness or Depressed Reactivity
Depressed muscle reactivity is often seen when an unfamiliar movement sequence is demanded of the body.
The patient lies in the starting position of Turn Again, Whittington, with the pelvis close to the edge of a short end of the treatment bench. During the movement se-

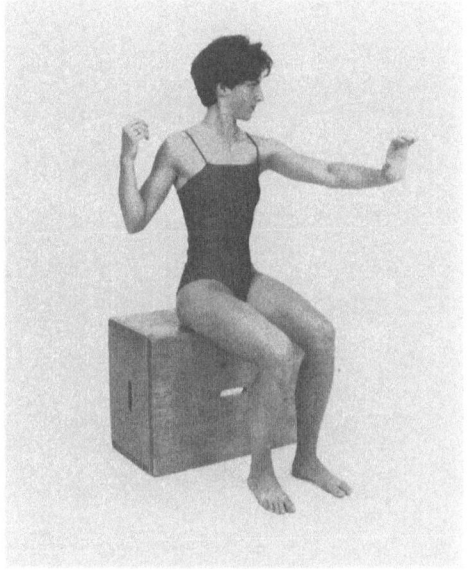

a

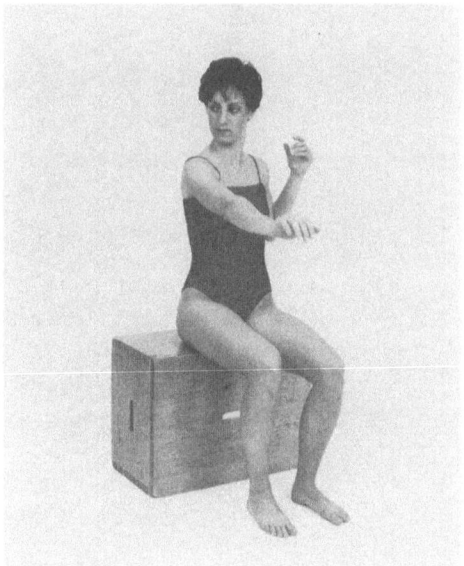

Fig. 31 a–d. Turn Again, Whittington, seated. During turning to the right (**a**) and left (**b**), the hands move in the transverse planes of the shoulder joints.

b

111

quence and in sidelying, the legs hover over an "abyss". The depressed muscle reactivity is then "dangerous" and the body will automatically try to overcome it.

Problems Requiring Special Adaptations

If we are unable to reach the goal of the exercise with Turn Again, Whittington, because of:

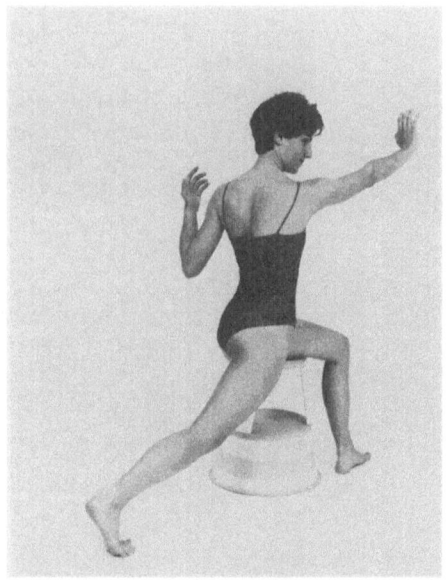

c

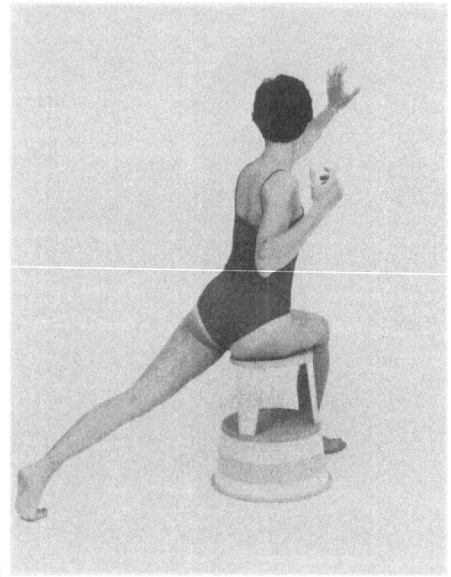

d

Fig. 31 c, d. Coordinated arm, leg and head movement turning to the right (**c**) and left (**d**)

- Pain arising during the exercise
- Critical movement deficits caused by muscle contractures in one or both hip joints
- Inability to achieve even a rough alignment of BSs pelvis, thorax and head to form the long axis of the body
- Dizziness caused by the turning of the head in the cervical spine

we can resort to the following alternatives:

Adaptations of Turn Again Whittington

If the functional status of the patient for any reason contraindicates rotation of the spinal column, we restrict the functional rotation training to the hip joints. This adaptation is called **The Dreaming Traffic Policeman.**
If the functional status of the patient indicates that rotational training in the spinal column should be concentrated on, we block the possibilities of movement in the hip joints. This adaptation is called **The Yogi.**

3.2 Adaptation: The Dreaming Traffic Policeman (Fig. 32)

"The Dreaming Traffic Policeman" is an invented name suggested by the way the arms in the end positions look like a policeman directing traffic.

■ Goal of the Exercise

The goal is for the patient to learn, with his spinal column roughly stabilized in the virtual long axis of the body, to

- Control turning the aligned BSs pelvis, thorax and head at the hip joint as in walking
- Control turning the legs at the hip joints as in walking

▶ Functional Analysis in Therapist Language

● Conception of the Exercise

In order to train the roughly stabilized spinal column in its neutral position for all the components of movement of this inherently mobile system, as required by the

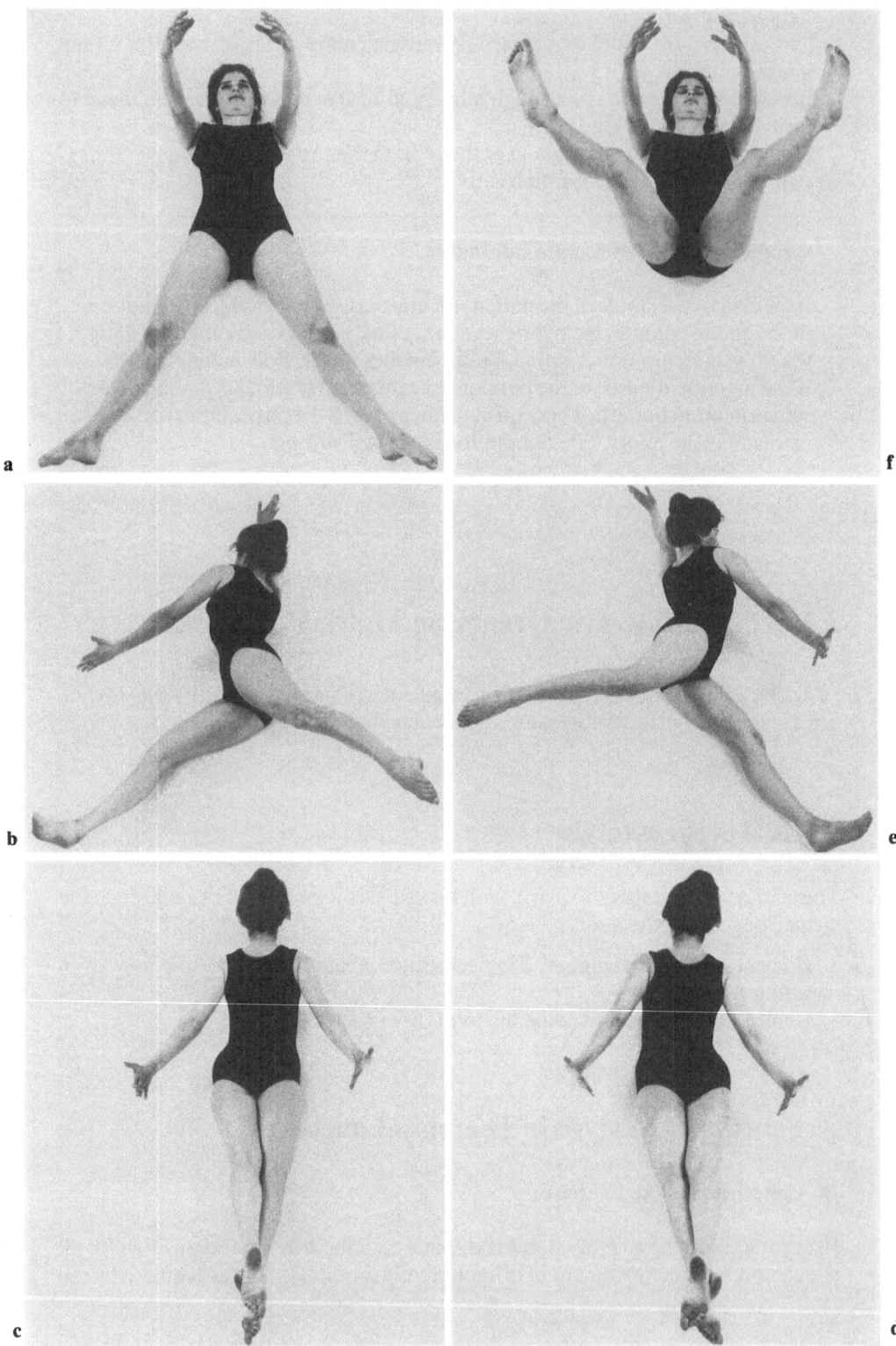

goal of the exercise, we position the spinal column horizontally and turn the body on the floor. In this way, even with only small changes in the positions of the joints in the spinal cord, all of the relevant muscles are in a position to suppress possible movements by stabilizing fall-preventing activity.

If one were to attempt rolling the body over on the floor without using arms and legs, one would find it impossible to keep the movement under control, without unwanted accelerating and/or slowing down, especially with the spinal column roughly in the neutral position. For this reason, we use the arms and legs as accelerating and/or braking weights when they are in free play and to start the roll-over by pushing off or braking it by supporting themselves on the floor.

We start in supine, roll over on the floor first onto one side, then onto the stomach, onto the other side, and finally end up on the back again – the end position. The long axis of the body should keep parallel to itself as it moves.

In addition to the turning of the body on the base support, the pelvis with the thorax and head rotate each time en bloc at the underlying hip.

● **Position and Activation in the Starting Position**

Position in Space of the Critical Axes
Points of Contact Between the Body and the Environment
The starting position is supine on the floor. BSs pelvis, thorax and head are aligned in the horizontal long axis of the body. The dorsal aspects of these body segments and of the scapulae touch the base support. The patient's gaze is directed upwards (Fig. 32 a). The arms and hands are in the transverse plane of the shoulders, which is vertical. Their medial aspects form an upright oval; the fingers do not touch.

The legs are symmetrically positioned in a wide frontal straddle on the floor; they touch the floor dorsally and slightly laterally.

Components of Movement in Relation to the Neutral Position of the Joints
In BS head, DP vertex is in the long axis of the body. The cervical lordosis is somewhat flattened. The atlanto-occipital and atlanto-axial joints are so far flexed that the gaze is directed upwards.

Because of the way the body is positioned, the thoracic kyphosis in BS thorax is reduced. In BS pelvis, the lumbar spine is in neutral position.

In BS arms, the dorsal aspects of the scapulae touch the floor. The shoulder joints are so far transversely flexed, the elbow joints so far flexed, the forearms supinated, the wrists and the joints of the fingers so far flexed that the medial aspects of the arms and hands form the desired upright oval without the fingers touching.

In BS legs, the hip joints are in extension/almost maximum abduction/moderate external rotation, the knee joints are in neutral position, the joints of the feet in

◄───

Fig. 32 a–f. The Dreaming Traffic Policeman. **a** Starting position, **b** right sidelying, **c, d** prone, **e** left sidelying, **f** end position

plantarflexion and inversion, the joints of the toes in flexion such that DPs right and left patellae face laterally/upwards and the soles of the feet face medially/downwards.

Movement Tolerances at the Critical Joints in Relation
to the Intended Primary Movement

Because the spinal column is in its neutral position, it has tolerance for movement in all movement components. This requires a high capacity for stabilization, since the Dreaming Traffic Policeman requires stabilization in neutral throughout.

In the starting position, the hip joints are more or less at end-stop in extension and abduction and are slightly externally rotated. Thus, the tolerance for internal rotation in the hip joint by both the distal and proximal pointer is sufficient for beginning the movement sequence.

Distribution of Weight on a Base Support or Suspension Device,
Against a Supportive Device, or over a Support Area,
and the Resulting Activity States of the Musculature

For activation of the starting position, DP vertex, DP right toes and DP left toes pull away from the body centrepoint. In this way a support area is formed, the smallest area encompassing the points of contact between the activated BSs legs, pelvis, thorax and head and the base support. The shoulder girdle is parked on the floor and the arms are in free play.

Intensity of Muscle Activity Required with Economical Activity
Respiration

The intensity of economical activity in the starting position of the Dreaming Traffic Policeman is only slightly above that of resting. The therapist should check that the patient is breathing normally.

Potential Accelerating and Braking Weights in Relation to the Bisecting Plane
of the Intended Primary Movement

The intended rolling movement of the body on the base support is continuously to the right or to the left as perceived by the patient in the starting position and the therapist when observing from the patient's head.

In the movement to the right, the bisecting plane shifts to the right as the patient rolls over; it will be identical to the vertical plane of symmetry when the patient is in supine and prone and almost identical to the vertical midfrontal plane when the patient is lying on his side. As seen by the observer, the weights to the left of the bisecting plane are braking weights and those to the right are accelerating weights.

● **Actio – Reactio of the Movement Sequence**

The Dreaming Traffic Policeman is a location-changing movement sequence. The dominant direction component out of the supine starting position is horizontal and to the right. We will therefore expect a clear reactio.

For our analysis, we differentiate four movement stages, the first and fourth stages being the most important therapeutically.

Stage 1: From the starting position in supine into right sidelying
Stage 2: From right sidelying into prone
Stage 3: From prone into left sidelying
Stage 4: From left sidelying into the end position in supine.

Stage 1: From the Starting Position in Supine into Right Sidelying (Fig. 32 a, b)

● **Actio – Reactio of the Movement Sequence**

Actio: The Primary Movement
The actio is characterized by three simultaneous, coordinated primary movements. For a roll-over to the right, the left leg starts the roll by pushing off and the left arm, in free play, brings accelerating weight into the direction of movement. The right arm moves against the direction of movement, but its weight has a neutral effect because it becomes aligned parallel to the cranial projection of the long axis of the body, and by striving in a dorsal direction intensifies the extensional stabilization of the latter.

In sidelying, the large frontal straddle of the starting position has turned into a large step across the midfrontal plane. Ideally, the lower right leg only rotates onto its lateral aspect.

The prelude to the primary movement of the left leg is a moderate medial rotation of the patella by internal rotation in the hip. Then DP left heel pushes off from the floor downwards/to the left, causing the left side of the pelvis to lift up off the base support. The talocrural joint plantarflexes, the knee joint extends and the hip joint extends/abducts/internally rotates; at the right hip the proximal lever effects internal rotation (critical fulcrum). The pelvis turns on the base support onto its right side.

Simultaneously, the critical distance point of the primary movement of the left free-play arm, DP ulnar margin of the hand, moves medially/caudally and to the right/downwards. The joints of the fingers and the wrist extend into their neutral positions, the forearm supinates, the elbow joint extends. By proximally continuing movement, the upper arm turns as distal lever in extension/slight adduction/external rotation in the shoulder joint and DP acromion moves caudally/dorsally in the sternoclavicular joint, while the pincer jaws have opened in the acromioclavicular joint and the external rotation in the shoulder has brought the medial scapular margin towards the spinal processes of the thoracic spine (critical fulcrum), counterstabilizing them extensionally. The thorax, together with the head, which has pushed off from the floor, and with the pelvis, turns on the base support onto its right side.

Meanwhile, the critical distance point of the primary movement of the right free-play hand, DP radial margin of the hand, has moved dorsally/cranially/downwards. The joints of the fingers and the wrist extend, the forearm supinates and the elbow joint extends. As the movement continues proximally, the upper arm as distal lever turns in the shoulder joint in flexion/slight adduction/external rotation and DP acromion moves cranially/medially/dorsally in the sternoclavicular joint (critical fulcrum).

Reactio: Activated Passive Buttressing

When the critical distance point of the activated passive buttressing, DP left heel, lifts up off the base support, the left leg becomes an activated passive buttress. This is the economical formation of a counterweight in location-changing movement sequences. The left leg goes into free play and becomes suspended from the pelvis in abduction/internal rotation at the left hip joint; the pelvis in turn becomes suspended as proximal lever from the right thigh in internal rotation at in the right hip joint, and as caudal lever from the thorax. The right leg has also lifted from the base support, reactively, has gone into free play, and is now suspended in flexion and adduction from the pelvis and becomes an accelerating weight.

Reactio: Change in the Support Area

The support area has become smaller cranially by the lifting of the head, caudally by the legs' lifting reactively up off the base support, and laterally by the patient's rolling from supine into right sidelying. Changing its location, it has moved to the right.

Actio: Accelerating Weights
Reactio: Braking Weights

In the starting position, the bisecting plane is identical to the plane of symmetry, which is vertical. During the movement sequence it moves, keeping parallel to itself, to the right. In right sidelying it more or less transects DP right greater trochanter and DP right acromion.

All weights lying to the left of – in relation to the movement direction, behind – the bisecting plane have a braking effect on the movement sequence; all weights lying to the right – in front – of the bisecting plane have an accelerating effect.

● Conditio – Limitatio of the Movement Sequence

Conditio: Constant Distances Between Body Distance Points
Limitatio: Active Buttressing and Stabilization

Conditio: The distances from DP jugular notch to DP point of the chin and from DP jugular notch to DP navel remain roughly constant.

Limitatio: If these two distances are to remain constant, BSs pelvis, thorax and head must turn en bloc from supine into sidelying: pelvis and thorax, for instance, must not rotate relative to each other. For this to happen, the pushing off of the left heel from the floor with the accompanying internal rotation by the distal pointer in the left hip joint and the external rotation by the distal lever and internal rotation by the proximal lever in the right hip joint must be properly coordinated with the lifting of the head from the base support and the primary movement of the left arm.

118

Conditio of Absolute and/or Relative Fixed Spatial Points
Limitatio by Limiting the Primary Movement, Activated Passive Buttressing
and/or Change in the Support Area
Since the Dreaming Traffic Policeman is a location-changing exercise, it can only
have relative fixed spatial points.

Conditio: In right sidelying, the right knee does not touch the floor.
Limitatio: This relative fixed spatial point checks the primary movement, because
if too much weight is brought in the direction of movement the support area will
increase on the right side by the right thigh leaning against the base support. In
order for the right leg to be in the free-play activity state, the counterweight of the
left free-play leg and the counterstabilization of the pincer jaws by the left free-
play arm must balance each other out. Having the frontal planes of BSs pelvis, thorax and head vertical is one factor that helps this to be achieved.

Conditio: From supine into sidelying, the angle formed in the horizontal plane by
the long axes of the legs does not narrow.
Limitatio: This relative fixed spatial point means that, as the patient rotates from
supine into right sidelying, the component of abduction in the right hip joint
becomes one of flexion pulling towards further flexion and that in the left hip joint
becomes one of extension pulling towards further extension.

Conditio: The distance from DP right medial malleolus to DP left medial malleolus must not become smaller as the patient turns over into sidelying.
Limitatio: In order for this distance to remain constant as the patient rotates from
supine into sidelying, the patient must widen the step by an amount equal to the
frontotransverse distance between the hips.
The reason for this is as follows. In supine, the long axes of the legs abducted in the
hip joints lie in the midfrontal plane, which is horizontal and in which the hips are
also aligned. The distance between the malleoli is thus augmented by the frontotransverse distance between the hips. In sidelying, however, the long axes of the
legs lie in the sagittal planes, now horizontal, of the right and left hip, one flexed,
the other extended. The frontotransverse distance between the hips is vertical and
perpendicular to these two sagittal planes. If he did not widen his step, therefore,
the patient would narrow the distance between the malleoli by the distance between the hips as he turned.

Conditio: In right sidelying, the long axes of the right leg and left arm should be
parallel and meet the bisecting plane at a caudal angle of about 40°.
Limitatio: These relative fixed spatial points facilitate stabilization of BSs pelvis,
thorax and head in the neutral position as desired. With the left arm at this angle of
flexion in the shoulder joint, there is good counterstabilization by the pincer jaws
without the hand having to forego pulling in the direction of movement. Having
the right leg at this same angle of flexion in the hip, with the right foot pulling in the
direction of movement, counteracts the tendency of the lumbar spine to hyper-
extend. This angle also stimulates the innervation of the oblique muscles of the abdomen and the back.

Conditio: The frontal planes of the BSs pelvis and thorax should be vertical in side-lying.

Limitatio: This relative fixed spatial point neutralizes the weights of these body segments and thus limits how much they modify the effect of the accelerating and braking arm and leg weights on the movement sequence.

Stage 2: From Right Sidelying into Prone (Fig. 32 b, c)

● **Actio – Reactio of the Movement Sequence**

Actio: The Primary Movement

The actio is characterized by four simultaneous coordinated primary movements. The direction of movement continues to the right. The upper, left leg, together with BSs pelvis, thorax and head, initiates the roll out of sidelying into prone lying. The arms and the right leg have the task of bringing the roll to a halt, which they do by lifting their weights against gravity off the floor, symmetrically to the bisecting plane, thus abandoning the direction of movement for the time being. In the end position the spinal column has given up being in neutral in favour of total extension. If the transition from sidelying into prone is not smooth with all of the extremities in free play, the left hand should temporarily lean on the base support so as to keep the movement sequence under control.

The critical distance point of the primary movement of the left free-play leg, DP left heel, moves to the right, in the direction of the movement; in the right hip, the movement is internal rotation by the proximal lever, during which the pelvis and BS thorax rotate together on the base support into prone lying. With the thorax goes the head, which by dorsal translation in the cervical spine and (continuing movement) extension in the thoracic spine keeps the face a good distance away from the floor. The positions of the joints of the left leg and of the lumbar spine should hardly change. However, the extensors, adductors and external rotators of the hip joints and the extensors of the lumbar spine, some of them with the joints at end-stop, must be activated at a high intensity of economical activity to prevent falling.

Simultaneously, the critical distance point of the primary movement of the right free-play leg, DP ball of the right great toe, moves somewhat to the left, against the direction of movement, as the hip extends and the right foot crosses under the left foot. As it goes, the right talocrural joint plantarflexes and the subtalar and calcaneonavicular joints evert.

As soon as BSs pelvis and thorax together with the head start to rotate right/downwards into the prone position, the critical distance point of the primary movement of the left free-play arm, DP tip of the left thumb, moves to the left/upwards, against the direction of movement, and in relation to the body it moves caudally/dorsally, by extension/adduction/external rotation in the shoulder joint.

By proximally continuing movement, DP left acromion moves caudally/dorsally/laterally in the sternoclavicular joint, due to the pincer jaws opening in the acromioclavicular joint and the medial scapular margin moving towards the spinal processes of the thoracic spine. If the movement sequence is not smooth, the left palm can temporarily lean against the base support at about the level of the navel,

120

with the forearm pronated, the elbow joint flexed and the shoulder joint slightly internally rotated. Having prevented an anticipated uncontrolled flop onto the stomach, the hand can then take up the position described above.

Meanwhile, the critical distance point of the primary movement of the right arm, DP tip of the right thumb, was moved left, against the direction of movement; in relation to the body it moves caudally/laterally/dorsally. There is supination in the forearm and the movement continues with extension/external rotation until the right arm is positioned symmetrically to the left arm.

Reactio: Activated Passive Buttressing

The counterplay between accelerating and braking weights is suspended during the movement sequence from sidelying into prone lying. All activity is vertical and directed upwards. Because of the way in which they relate to the plane of symmetry, which in the prone position is vertical, the horizontal directional pulls cancel each other out.

Reactio: Change in the Support Area

In relation to the starting position, the support area has now moved right, the long axis of the body having undergone a parallel shift to the right. It has become wider, but has shortened cranially because BS arms no longer touches the floor at any point.

If the patient needed to lean his left hand on the floor during the movement sequence, the support area temporarily became larger. Many patients with deficient movement tolerance for extension in the spinal column and/or insufficiency in the extensor muscles of the back need to do this.

● **Conditio – Limitatio of the Movement Sequence**

Conditio of Absolute and/or Relative Fixed Spatial Points
Limitatio by Limiting the Primary Movement, Activated Passive Buttressing and/or Change in the Support Area

The relative fixed spatial point in this phase is the following:

Conditio: In the end position of prone lying, the plane of symmetry is vertical, the arms are symmetrical and the legs are crossed in the plane of symmetry.
Limitatio: The symmetry of this end position, with the plane of symmetry vertical, has no directional tendencies other than the upward pull of the fall-preventing activity. The intensity of this activity can therefore be increased ad libitum.

Stage 3: From Prone into Left Sidelying (Fig. 32 c–e)

● **Actio – Reactio of the Movement Sequence**

Actio: The Primary Movement

In order to continue rotating to the right from prone into left sidelying, the legs first cross over the other way so that the right leg is on top.

The actio of the third stage of the Dreaming Traffic Policeman is characterized by three simultaneous coordinated primary movements. The right hand pushes off, initiating the rolling over, and the right leg in free play brings accelerating weight in the direction of the movement. The left arm moves against the direction of movement, but its weight has a neutral effect because it becomes aligned parallel to the cranial projection of the long axis of the body and stimulates stabilization of the latter.

In sidelying, the legs that were crossed when prone now make a wide step across the midfrontal plane.

The primary movement of the right arm begins with the right palm touching the base support at about the level of the waist. The fingertips point cranially. Then, as the right palm pushes off downwards/to the left with extension and radial abduction by the proximal lever in the wrist accompanied by forearm pronation, elbow extension, and shoulder adduction, via the pincer jaws the right side of the thorax is lifted up off the base support, and the thorax rolls over on the base support to the (observer's) right into left sidelying.

Simultaneously, the critical distance point of the primary movement of the right free-play leg, DP ball of the right little toe, moves to the right, in the direction of the movement, and slightly upwards; in relation to the body it moves dorsally/cranially. As it goes, the pelvis, as proximal pointer, rotates externally in the left/lower hip joint and moves en bloc with the thorax, which takes with it the free-play head, into left sidelying. It will help the patient to make the change of the head's position in space if he concentrates on the change in the direction of his gaze. In the end position, the right hip joint is extended but not rotated.

Before BSs pelvis and thorax begin to rotate from prone into left sidelying, the critical distance point of the third primary movement, DP tip of the left thumb, moves cranially/laterally at first, then medially. The shoulder joint flexes/first abducts then adducts/externally rotates. By proximally continuing movement, DP acromion moves cranially/medially in the sternoclavicular joint and the pincer jaws close in the acromioclavicular joint (critical fulcrum) until the long axis of the left arm is roughly parallel to the cranial projection of the long axis of the body.

Reactio: Activated Passive Buttressing

As the critical distance point of the activated passive buttressing, DP right palm, is lifted from the base support, the right arm becomes an activated passive buttress. This is the economical formation of a counterweight in location-changing movement sequences. When the right arm moves into free play, it becomes suspended from the shoulder girdle by transverse extension/flexion/external rotation in the shoulder joint, and, with the pincer jaws open, the shoulder girdle becomes suspended from the right side of the thorax. The primary movement of the right leg and the rotation of the pelvis onto the left side make the lower left leg into an activated passive buttress too. It is already in free play and moves left by flexion in the hip, against the direction of movement. Its long axis should be parallel to the long axis of the actively buttressing right arm.

Reactio: Change in the Support Area
The support area has become smaller because of the change from prone to side-lying and has been displaced to the right, in the direction of movement.

Actio: Accelerating Weights
Reactio: Braking Weights
In the prone position, the bisecting plane is identical with the vertical plane of symmetry. During the continued roll to the right it moves, keeping parallel to itself, to the right. In left sidelying it more or less transects DP left greater trochanter and DP left acromion.
All the weights to the left of the bisecting plane – in relation to the direction of movement, behind; in relation to the body, ventral – have a braking effect on the movement sequence, while all those to the right of it – in relation to the direction of movement, in front; in relation to the body, dorsal – have an accelerating effect.

● **Conditio – Limitatio of the Movement Sequence**

Conditio of Absolute and/or Relative Fixed Spatial Points
Limitatio by Limiting the Primary Movement, Activated Passive Buttressing and/or Change in the Support Area
Since the Dreaming Traffic Policeman is a location-changing exercise, it can only have relative fixed spatial points.

Conditio: In left sidelying, the long axes of the left leg and the right arm should be parallel and meet the bisecting plane at an angle of about 40°.
Limitatio: When the patient turns out of prone lying into left sidelying, these relative fixed spatial points belong to the activated passive buttresses. After pushing off, the right arm, extending at the elbow and externally rotating in the shoulder, moves into the optimal position in space for counterstabilizing the pincer jaws and (by continuing movement) stabilizing the thoracic spine in its neutral position. This position also puts the left leg at a good angle to act as counterweight to the right leg without risking that the ischiocrural brake will flex the lumbar spine in a continuing movement and thus destroy the integrity of the virtual long axis of the body.

Conditio: In sidelying, the frontal planes of BSs pelvis and thorax should be vertical.
Limitatio: This relative fixed spatial point neutralizes the weights of these body segments and thus limits how much they modify the effect of the accelerating and braking arm and leg weights on the movement sequence.

Stage 4: From Left Sidelying into Supine (Fig. 32 e, f)

● **Actio – Reactio of the Movement Sequence**

Actio: The Primary Movement
The actio is characterized by three simultaneous, coordinated primary movements. The direction of movement continues to the right. The right arm moves in

this direction and starts the roll-over of the thorax into supine lying. The left arm is aligned symmetrically with the right. The right leg coordinates the turn of the pelvis into the supine position. The left leg is reactively positioned symmetrically to the right.

The critical distance point of the primary movement of the right free-play arm, DP tip of the right thumb, moves to the right, in the direction of movement, cranially/laterally/ventrally in relation to the body. It is brought into the transverse plane through the sternoclavicular joint by flexion in the right shoulder joint, which also goes into slight transverse extension and rotates internally until it reaches rotational neutral. As it does, the finger joints and wrist flex and the forearm pronates slightly to form the erect oval that characterized the arm position in the starting position (see p. 115). The thorax also rolls over the base support from left sidelying into supine lying.

Simultaneously, the critical distance point of the primary movement of the right free-play leg, DP right heel, moves slightly downwards (orientation in space), ventrally/medially (orientation within the body). The right hip externally rotates, the long axis of the thigh rotating where it is in the air. By continuing movement, the pelvis as proximal pointer in the left hip glides in external rotation and transverse abduction and together with the thorax and the head en bloc rolls over the base support into supine lying. The right hip flexes by dorsal displacement of the fulcrum.

Meanwhile, the critical distance point of the primary movement of the left hand, DP left ulnar margin, moves ventrally/caudally/laterally up to the transverse plane of the sternoclavicular joints and positions itself symmetrically to the right arm.

Reactio: Activated Passive Buttressing

DP left heel, the critical distance point of the activated passive buttressing by the left free-play leg, which during left sidelying was already suspended from the pelvis by flexion and adduction in the hip joint, is transported upwards (orientation in space), cranially/laterally (orientation within the body), as the pelvis rolls over, until the left leg is in the transverse plane of the hip joints, which is vertical. This change in its position in space reduces the effect of its weight as an activated passive buttress.

Reactio: Change in the Support Area

The support area has become larger again and moved to the right. In the end position, the head touches the base support and moves out of free play into parking function.

Actio: Accelerating Weights
Reactio: Braking Weights

During the movement sequence, the bisecting plane moved further to the right, parallel to its previous position, and in the end position coincides with the vertical plane of symmetry. The symmetry of the arms and legs and of BSs pelvis, thorax and head aligned in the long axis of the body provides a well-balanced position that can be held by the activity of the transverse adductors and hip flexors and of the straight and oblique abdominal muscles.

124

- **Conditio – Limitatio of the Movement Sequence**

Conditio: Constant Distances Between Body Distance Points
Limitatio: Active Buttressing and Stabilization
The conditio and limitatio under this heading are the same as for Stage 1 of the exercise (see p. 118).

Conditio of Absolute and/or Relative Fixed Spatial Points
Limitatio by Limiting the Primary Movement, Activated Passive Buttressing
or Change in the Support Area
Conditio: The angle between the long axes of the legs in left sidelying projected onto the plane of symmetry, and the angle that they form in the vertical transverse plane through the hip joints in the end position in supine, are the same.
Limitatio: If this fixed spatial point is to be maintained, the critical distance point of the primary movement of the right leg, DP right heel, must not slide to the left during the movement sequence, against the direction of movement. Moreover, the pelvis must make a true transverse abduction/external rotation in the left hip, so that the left leg can be brought in to balance the right.

Conditio of Movement Speed
Limitatio of Economical Activity by Finding the Optimal Speed
The requirement stated in the goal of the exercise that the movement sequence be performed with control gives the speed. It is slow, smooth, and there is a stop at the end of each stage. The four intermediate stages should be brought into a resting equilibrium by appropriate coordination of the muscle activities, particularly fall-preventing.
Except in the starting position, the intensity of economical activity is quite high, being highest in the prone position.

▶ Instruction in Patient Language

- **Instruction Appealing to the Patient's Perception**

In the starting position, the direction of movement must be well impressed on the patient. The best method is to orientate the exercise to an object in the room, e. g. a window or door.
In rolling over into sidelying, the patient will find it helpful to imagine taking a large step forwards or backwards.
Although the head will not change its position in relation to the thorax, it will nevertheless rotate 360° through space. The patient will be looking upwards when supine, downwards when prone, horizontally in sidelying.

Position and Activation of the Starting Position

"Lie on the floor with your feet wide apart. Your knees face outwards, but not too much. Stretch your feet. The soles of your feet face each other a little but they also face downwards. There can be a little tension in the crutch, but not too much. You are looking up, holding a large oval balloon in your arms. It rests against your sternum on its end and is so big that when your palms rest on it your fingers don't touch. You breathe freely and easily."

The therapist checks to make sure the straddle is symmetrical. If there is too much tension in the adductors, resistance to the abductors can be applied to both legs.

The position of the arms may be corrected by manipulation if necessary.

Actio and Conditio of the Movement Sequence

"Your left leg rotates a little to the right and you push off from the floor with your left heel. Your left arm moves diagonally across your stomach and your head comes with it as you roll onto your right side, taking a wide step with your legs. Your right leg is under you and in front of you, the sole of the foot faces forwards, and so does your left hand. Your right arm has moved backwards. Your left leg is on top and behind you with its sole facing backwards. Both legs are floating in the air. Now you roll onto your stomach and your legs cross. The left leg is still on top. You can support yourself with your left hand on the floor until you are lying on your stomach. Now you don't need to support yourself any more. Your arms float in the air alongside your body, palms facing out; you keep your eyes well away from the floor. Now cross your legs the other way, bringing the right leg on top. You push off a little from the floor with your right hand, again taking a big step with your legs, and you are lying on your left side. Now the right leg is on top and behind you. Your left arm stretches your back and your right arm is now in front of you. Rolling on further,

If the timing of the movement sequence is not coordinated properly, the therapist can apply manual resistance to either the left heel or to the abductors of both legs; in sidelying this resistance then becomes resistance against flexion/extension in the hip joints. The patient performs the arm movements and positions the head by himself. Just as we can adapt the push-off from the floor to the patient's capacities by providing manual resistance as he rolls over into sidelying, so we can provide manual support to the left palm as he rolls into the prone position. As he rolls further into left sidelying we change our manual support to the right palm, finally applying resistance to the right heel as he rolls into supine. Another method of manual aid is for the therapist carefully to guide both legs through the entire movement sequence, lifting the weight or holding it back, etc.

you land on your back again. Make sure
that it goes smoothly and comfortably,
without jerking. Your legs are straddled; they point upwards like the arms,
but they also face outwards."

3.3 Adaptation: The Yogi (Fig. 33)

"The Yogi" is an invented name: the position aimed at is reminiscent yoga
(Sanskrit for "harness").

■ Goal of the Exercise

The goal is for the patient, by blocking mobility at the hip joints, to learn to mobilize the spinal column in rotation and stretch to their maximum the rotators at
movement level lower thoracic spine and the extensors, abductors and rotators of
the hip joints.

▶ Functional Analysis in Therapist Language

● Conception of the Exercise

We bring the legs into such a position relative to the long axis of the body, which is
vertical, that any impulses arising cranially for rotation about this axis are firmly
blocked from continuing into the hip joints, because this would be an avoidance
mechanism.

● Position and Activation in the Starting Position

Position in Space of the Critical Axes
Points of Contact Between the Body and the Environment
Components of Movement in Relation to the Neutral Position of the Joints
The starting position is sitting on the heels on the floor. BSs pelvis, thorax and head
are aligned vertically in the virtual long axis of the body.
In BS arms, the long axes are parallel to the long axis of the body. The arms are in
slight supporting function, palms touching the floor. Thumbs point forwards/lat-
erally, the other fingers point backwards/laterally.
In BS legs, the ventral aspects of the lower legs and feet touch the floor. Knees are
fully flexed, dorsal aspects of the lower legs and thighs are pressing together. The

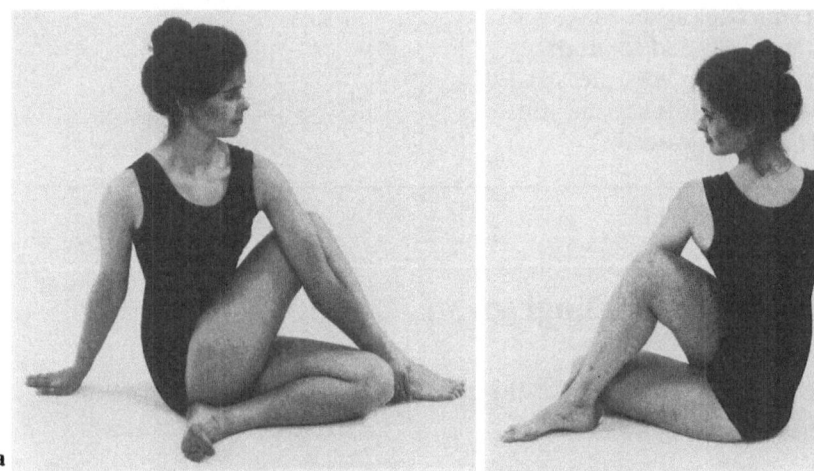

Fig. 33a, b. The Yogi. End position: **a** ventral view, **b** dorsal view

feet bear most of the weight of BSs pelvis, thorax and head. If the patient's arms are not long enough to allow him to support himself on his palms, he can use his fingertips.

● **Actio – Reactio of the Movement Sequence**

We cannot analyse the Yogi the same way we would other movement sequences. In the Yogi, the patient moves by stages into an end position in order to himself manipulate joint positions in the inherently mobile system of his body, some of which are at end-stop, and so to stretch the muscles that span these joints. The only reactive events, if they can be regarded as such, are the aftereffects of the exercise. The most important element is the conditio that will lead to fulfilment of the goal.

● **Conditio – Limitatio of the Movement Sequence**

To perform this adaptation the patient must have good flexibility in the hip joints. If he does not, the Corkscrew (p. 280) will be found more suitable.
The Yogi goes through three stages.

Stage 1
By a shifting of the sitting surface to the left, alongside the heels, the supporting function of the left arm increases and the right hand lifts off the floor. The weight is now off the right leg and this is crossed over the left thigh. The sole of the right foot touches the floor. The right heel is to the left of the left thigh. The long axis of the foot is roughly sagittotransverse. The hip joints are blocked.

Stage 2
The rotations around the long axis of the body flow as co-rotational continuing movements. As cranial lever, the head rotates positively in the cervical spine, to

the right. By continuing movement, the thorax as cranial pointer rotates positively in the lower thoracic spine; as it does, the pressure on the right ischial tuberosity increases. The arms moves with the thorax; the left arm goes into free play and the right arm into supporting function. The points of contact between the palms or fingertips and the floor are slightly behind the right greater trochanter. The left arm now crosses over the right thigh, pressing against it and causing it to flex and transversely adduct in the hip against the pelvis and thorax. The left hand grasps the lateral malleolus of the right leg from cranially. This movement securely blocks the hip joints.

Stage 3

The head, as cranial pointer, now rotates negatively in the cervical spine, performing a buttressing rotational movement to the thorax. Due to buttressing, both levels of rotation in the spinal column are now rotated to end-stop. The muscles relating to each are stretched.

This position is held for several seconds, until economical normal breathing has been resumed despite the extreme torsion of the position.

▶ Instruction in Patient Language

● **Verbal Instruction**   ● **Instruction by Manipulation**

Position and Activation in the Starting Position

"Sit back on your heels. Your back is long, you are slim and your stomach is relaxed; your breathing is easy. Imagine you are a puppet. There's a thread going through the top of your head and this thread is being gently pulled all the time. Your fingers are on the floor next to your feet. Your thumbs point forwards, the index and middle fingers point outwards and the ring and little fingers point outwards and backwards."

The therapist makes sure that the spinal column is straight and vertical. Exerting light compression on the vertex helps to maintain the long axis of the body and to correct the patient's position if necessary. It is important to be careful that the activity of the abdominal muscles is not too great; this would restrict normal respiration.

If the feet hurt in heel sitting, a cushion may be placed under them.

Actio and Conditio of the Movement Sequence
Stage 1: Blocking the Hip Movement

"The puppeteer starts to pull a little harder on the thread on your head and he moves you to the left until you are sitting beside your heels. To keep your back long, you turned your left hand so that the fingers point forwards and you

When the patient is sitting to one side beside the heels, the compensating lateroflexion of the spinal column should be economical. On no account should the patient collapse to the side. We can prevent this by watching the way the

can now support yourself easily on your arm. Now the right leg crosses boldly over the left. It is then firmly planted on the floor and points forwards."

left arm supports the weight: when the hand rotates to bring the fingers to point forwards, only the forearm should pronate – the shoulder must not internally rotate but remain externally rotated. In this manner we can achieve normal supporting function, which helps the position of the spinal column.

Stage 2: Rotation About the Long Axis of the Body

"Now comes the exciting part. Don't forget that during the entire exercise, someone is always pulling on that thread on your head. No matter how much your back is twisted, it stays long. You look over your right shoulder. As soon you feel that your shoulder is starting to turn backwards as well, you must settle down well on your right buttock and maybe make room with your left foot. Lean on your right arm; it has already moved backwards and won't let your right knee take part in the rotation. On the contrary: the left arm now crosses over the right thigh and, if it can, the hand rests on the outside of the right ankle. More important than that, though, is that the left upper arm keeps the right knee where it is, or even pushes it back a little. If you're really flexible this is a gentle brake, but if you're stiff you'll need lots of strength."

The therapist can guide the rotation in the spinal column by gently twisting the head. Alternatively, she can guide the right arm backwards/laterally with external rotation and place the palm on the floor. Or, she may help by manipulation to ensure that the stress on the right half of the pelvis is correctly placed.

The crossing of the left arm over the right thigh can also be manipulated, especially until the patient has acquired the movement. Coming from in front of/medial to the patient, the therapist grasps the back of the patient's left arm with her left hand. At the same time she pushes the patient's right knee to his left with her right hand, asking the patient to place his left palm on the outside of his right ankle.

Stage 3: Counter-rotation of the Head

"Last of all, you look over your left shoulder and you feel the complete Yogi.

Although you're now held as if in a vice, try to keep on breathing easily and smoothly without dropping any height or undoing the rotation at all. Try to lose that feeling of effort, as if you could stay like that for hours."

The therapist watches especially that BS head does not translate forwards as it counter-rotates.

Fine adjustment of the end position by manipulation: the better the vertical position of the spinal column, the more effective the rotation in terms of the scope of the movement excursion and hence the more intense the stretch on the autochthonous rotators of the spinal column.

4 Functional Respiration Training

Functional respiration training is directed at economical coordination of posture, respiration and movement.

Note

Functional respiration training is used when there is:
- A functional respiratory disorder resulting from postural and motor deficits
- A functional respiratory disorder resulting from postural statics that deviate from the norm
- Uneconomical distribution of activity, such as in the case of autonomic dystonia (it is irrelevant whether these are symptoms of stress or decreased motivation)
- Functional aerophagia (air gulping)
- Functional hyperventilation
- Any specific syndrome involving a respiratory disorder that can be improved by the regulation of function

---

To train functional respiration we have to practice coordinating the respiratory processes the therapist can see with signals the patient perceives in his body, and bring these together into simple, easily memorized verbal cues.

Normal Breathing

Visible Respiratory Processes
During inspiration: The epigastric angle widens, the intercostal space expands; the frontotransverse and sagittotransverse diameters of the thorax increase; the abdomen, especially the upper abdomen, swells out; *no* hyperactivity in the scalene muscles.
During expiration: The epigastric angle narrows; the intercostal space narrows; the frontotransverse and sagittotransverse diameters of the thorax decrease; abdominal volume decreases; *no* hyperactivity in the abdominal muscles.

Perceptible Body Signals
During the pause before inspiration begins: The flow of saliva increases; the tongue is warm and relaxed and can feel the inside of the lower teeth with its outer edges;

the upper lip is soft, long and relaxed; the beat of the pulse can be felt, especially in the upper abdomen; suddenly a need to inhale arises.

During inspiration: There is a coolness induced by evaporation in the nose as the inspired air flows past the moist nasal mucous membranes; a clear, high-pitched sound caused by the inflowing air; perceptible stretching of the thoracic and abdominal walls, which explains the breather's feeling of physical lightness.

During the pause at the peak of inspiration: The flow of saliva increases; there is a feeling of lightness, of floating; pleasant tickle in the back of the throat and a desire to yawn.

During expiration: Gradually the air is allowed to flow away; the emitted air feels warm in the nose; the air flows out with a low sound; there is a slow caving in of the thorax and sinking down of the abdomen; the length of the spinal column does not change (the thoracic spine should not become rounded); the air flow gradually subsides.

Verbal Cues

During the pause before inspiration begins: "You are very quiet. Your tongue is warm. It lies quite relaxed in your mouth. Your tongue is swimming in saliva. It can feel your lower teeth. Your upper lip is soft and long. Your heart is beating quietly. You're not in a hurry. Wait until your body demands air."

During inspiration: "Smell the air. Smell the aroma of coffee (red wine, the mountains, etc.). The air flowing into your nose is cool."

During the pause of the peak of inspiration: "Now you have time to think about things, to be amazed. You almost have to yawn. You feel light and good."

During expiration: "The air wants to to flow away, but only let it out very slowly. Now it flows all by itself. Let it go until the flow subsides. The air flowing out is warm."

Interpretation of Verbal Cues

"You are very quiet" – prevents hyperventilation.

"Your tongue is relaxed in your mouth. Your tongue can feel your lower teeth" – the larynx relaxes.

"Your tongue is warm. It is swimming in saliva" – parasympathetic reaction.

"Your upper lip is soft and long" – lengthening and narrowing of the "air inlet" of the nose.

"Your heart is beathing quietly. You're not in a hurry" – no hyperventilation.

"Wait until your body demands air!" – patient waits until the rising level of carbon dioxide in the blood triggers the inspiration reflex.

"Smell the air!" – as the patient smells the air, the nostrils flare and the nose, the inlet for the inflowing air, becomes narrower. The suction must increase to get air in through the narrowed inlet. This happens reflexively by the diaphragm lowering and the thorax widening, resulting in a drop in interpleural pressure.

"The air flowing into your nose is cool." This cue will have the same effect as smelling, only now it is the command to feel the coolness caused by the air flowing past the moist mucous membranes that causes the air inlet to narrow.

"You have time to think about things, to be amazed" – the respiratory phase favourable to oxygen uptake is prolonged.

"You almost have to yawn" – prevents any swallowing of air.

"You feel light and good" – inspiratory expansion prevents glottal closure.

"The air wants to flow away, but only let it out very slowly" – by slowing down the initial expiration, we elicit eccentric isotonic (braking) work from the muscles of inspiration and facilitate lowering of the ribs.

"Now the air flows all by itself" – the elasticity of the lung can take over.

"Let the air go until the flow subsides" – there is unimpeded expiration to the intermediate stage of respiration.

"The air flowing out is warm" – in feeling the warmth of the air flowing out, the patient will regulate and increase the volume of expired air, which has been warmed in his body.

Respiration Under Physical Stress

> **Note**
> In functional respiration training, "respiration under physical stress" means respiration with increased expiratory and consequently also increased inspiratory volume. We bring about the stress not by increasing the burden on the circulation, but rather by voluntarily prolonging expiration. To avoid any symptoms of hyperventilation, we breathe "in slow motion".

Visible Respiratory Processes

During inspiration: The epigastric angle widens; the intercostal space expands; the frontotransverse and sagittotransverse diameters of the thorax increase; the abdomen, especially the upper abdomen, swells out.

These movements are all greater than during normal breathing.

The activity of the scalene muscles increases.

During expiration: The epigastric angle narrows; the intercostal space narrows; the frontotransverse and sagittotransverse diameters of the thorax decrease; the abdominal volume decreases.

These movements are all greater than during normal breathing.

With the prolongation of expiration, the activity of the abdominal muscles becomes evident, causing the abdomen to flatten further, the waist to narrow and the extensional active buttressing of the thoracic spine in its neutral position to increase.

Perceptible Body Signals

During expiration: Initially this is the same as for normal breathing. As expiration is prolonged beyond the midrespiratory stage, tension in the abdominal muscles increases and the thoracic spine will stabilized in extension.

During the pause at the end of expiration: Abdominal tension is maximal; saliva flows; the beating of the pulse can be clearly felt in the thoracic cavity.

During inspiration: The tension in the abdominal wall slowly fades as cool air flows in through the nose.

NB: If the tension in the abdominal muscles is released too quickly, inspiration will be inhibited. The patient can perceive this without difficulty.

Inspiration sounds louder; the air flows in without any effort. Otherwise, the perceptible signals are the same as during normal breathing at rest.

Verbal Cues

During expiration: "The air wants to flow out, but only let it out very slowly" (just as in normal breathing). "Now the air flows all by itself" (just as in normal breathing). "Make sure that the air continues to flow out smoothly. Your stomach becomes tense and hard. Your back stays long. Stop the flow of air before it gets weaker."

During the pause at the end of expiration: "The tension in your stomach is normal; keep it that way. Your throat is relaxed and warm."

During inspiration: "Gently let your stomach relax. Just as gently, the cool air flows in through your nose. Smell the air" (etc., just as in normal breathing).

Interpretation of Verbal Cues

"Make sure that the air flows out smoothly" – the concentric isotonic activity of the abdominal muscles comes into play: in order to expire more air, the body reduces the respiratory space.

"Your stomach becomes tense and hard" – through activity of the oblique abdominal muscles, the ribs drop and the waist narrows considerably.

"Your back stays long" – the thoracic spine stabilizes extensionally in its neutral position in order to actively buttress the movement of the abdominal muscles, preventing active insufficiency, particularly of the oblique muscles.

"Stop the flow of air before it becomes any weaker" – forcible expulsion of air, which easily leads to air swallowing, is avoided.

"The tension in the stomach is normal; keep it that way" – the long respiratory pause averts any risk of hyperventilation.

"Your throat is relaxed and warm" – a relaxed throat prevents glottal closure.

"Gently let your stomach relax" – if the glottis is open, the onset of inspiration becomes coordinated with the eccentric isotonic release of the muscles of expiration.

"Just as gently, the cool air flows in through your nose" – the transition into the concentric phase of inspiration is smooth.

Note

Inspiration at rest involves concentric isotonic work of the muscles of inspiration. **Inspiration under physical stress** involves eccentric isotonic work of the muscles of expiration during the first phase; not until the second phase does concentric isotonic work of the muscles of inspiration begin.

Expiration at rest involves eccentric isotonic work of the muscles of inspiration. **Expiration under physical stress** involves eccentric isotonic work of the muscles of inspiration during the first phase; not until the second phase does concentric isotonic work of the muscles of expiration begin.

4.1 The Lion (Fig. 34)

The Lion is an exercise for training normal breathing. It is appropriate for any patient who is able to sit upright and unsupported on a chair.
There is a story behind the name "the Lion". The exercise was developed for a certain Madame Lion, and helped her so much that it was named after her.

■ Goal of the Exercise

The goal is for the patient to learn to trigger normal breathing by economical activity with the long axis of the body vertical, and to be able to achieve a state of relaxation and well-being by economical coordination of posture, respiration and movement.

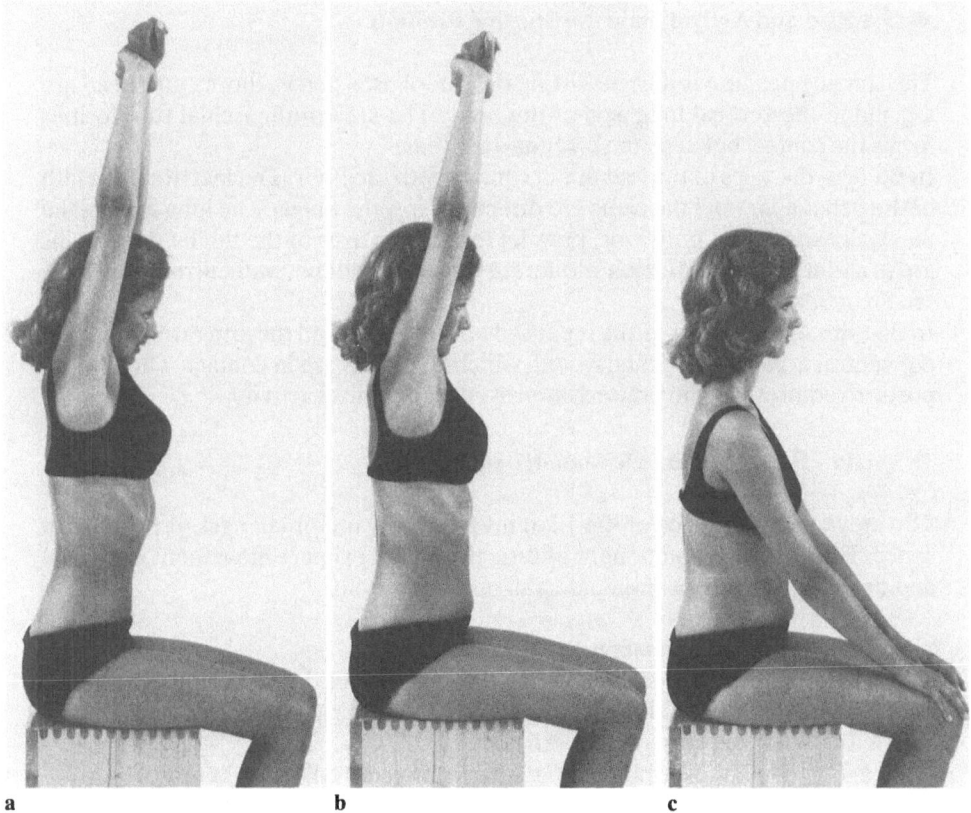

a   b   c

Fig. 34 a–c. The Lion. **a** Primary movement of the arms, **b** mid-sequence with relaxed stomach muscles, **c** end position with normal quiet breathing

▶ Functional Analysis in Therapist Language

● Conception of the Exercise

To achieve normal physiological breathing with the help of the Lion, through economical activity in the vertical spinal column, we must remember the following: neither the start of normal breathing nor the activity of economical upright posture can be perceived in the form of effortful activity. Therefore, these activities cannot be called forth in response to a direct movement instruction – we have to proceed indirectly. We will give instructions only for consciously controllable, voluntary movements, even if these movements only relate to part of the goal. Some mistakes will be unavoidable, but we must reverse them without sacrificing what has already been achieved. This toing-and-froing will continue until the goal has been attained. We will always succeed in this, because following the various instructions for voluntary movement in combination ultimately leads automatically to the goal. The patient easily perceives this goal as a state of general relaxation and pleasant, effortless breathing.

● Position and Activation in the Starting Position

The starting position is upright sitting on a stool. BSs pelvis, thorax and head are aligned in the vertical long axis of the body. The area of the ischial tuberosities forms the contact between the body and the seat.
In BS legs, the soles of the feet are in contact with the floor. The feet are the width of the pelvis apart and the heels are directly below the knees. The long axes of the feet point somewhat outwards, parallel to the long axes of the thighs. The thighs are in about 90° or less flexion/moderate transverse abduction/neutral rotation in the hip joints.
In BS arms, the shoulder girdle is parked on the thorax and the arms are parked on the ventral aspects of the thighs, with which the palms are in contact. The upright posture requires a slightly raised intensity of economical activity.

● Actio – Reactio of the Movement Sequence

The movement sequence of the Lion involves only minor changes of position in space. The dominant component of direction of the primary movement is vertical and upwards. We do not anticipate a significant reactio.

Actio: The Primary Movement
The actio is characterized by the primary movement of the arms, which by continuing movement brings about a lengthening of the virtual long axis of the body. This is a necessary detour towards our goal.
Critical DP right hand, gripping the left wrist from dorsally, moves upwards in the plane of symmetry slightly in front of the ventral tangential frontal plane which is vertical, causing the wrists and elbows to flex and the forearms to supinate: The movement continues proximally with, counter-rotationally, extension in the elbows

136

and flexion and internal rotation in the shoulders; co-rotationally, the right and left acromions move cranially/medially in the sternoclavicular joint and the pincer jaws close in the acromioclavicular joint. By caudally and co-rotationally continuing movement, the ribs lift up in the costovertebral joints on inspiration. The thoracic spine extends cranial-to-caudally, extension in the lumbar spine increases and the pelvis as the proximal lever brings about flexion in the hip joints (critical fulcrum). At the end of the primary movement, the forearms are pronated and the wrists extended so that the palms face upwards, making the pull on the shoulder girdle and the spinal column greater.

Reactio: Change in the Support Area
The slight parallel displacement forwards of the long axis of BSs thorax and head, with flexion of the pelvis in the hip joints and extension in the lumbar joints, causes the support area to shift forwards somewhat, and BS legs goes into supporting function.

● Conditio – Limitatio of the Movement Sequence

In the actio we described a detour that led to overshooting reactions which must be neutralized. As a result of the intensive upward pull of the hands on the shoulder girdle, the neck has disappeared. The potential mobility of the cervical spine and of the atlanto-occipital and atlanto-axial joints is gone. Glottal closure evokes hyperactivity in the scalene muscles on inspiration, elevating the thorax.

Any extension of the lumbar and thoracic spines is always accompanied by a pulling in of the stomach. The conditio must now reverse the detour described in the actio, so that, through the limitatio, the goal can be fulfilled.

Conditio: Constant Distance Between Body Distance Points
Limitatio: Active Buttressing and Stabilization
Conditio: In the end position of the Lion the spinal column should return to its neutral position, as it was in the starting position. To regain the activity state of potential mobility in the cervical spine, the patient should gently nod his head as if to say, "Yes," shake it as if to say "No," and tilt it from side to side as if asking a question. To release the hold of the scalene muscles on the thorax and loosen the glottal closure, the patient should sigh as if relieved.

For the lumbar spine to return from hyperextension to the neutral position, DP coccyx must move somewhat downwards. At this moment, the extensional anchoring of the pelvis in the lumbosacral spine is released and the pelvis extends slightly in the hip joints. The lumbar spine flexes back into its neutral position, causing the long axis of BSs thorax and head together with the arms to make a corresponding parallel movement backwards, without abandoning its vertical position in space.

To release the hyperactivity of the abdominal muscles, the patient must at the same time allow the abdomen to "flop down". To allow the thoracic spine to return to its neutral position and attain the desired activity state of dynamic stabilization, the hands must stop pulling upwards, because this causes the thoracic spine, one of the movement levels affected by the continuing movement, to deform extensionally.

The pull, with its upward direction tendency, is therefore carefully relaxed and the cranial distance point of the thoracic spine, DP jugular notch, moves very slightly forwards/downwards by the thoracic spine's flexing into the neutral position. The distal distance point of the sternoclavicular joint, DP acromion, moves downwards/caudally/laterally, the pincer jaws open, and the shoulder girdle moves into the neutral position in the activity state of parking, provided the thoracic spine is properly dynamically stabilized. In the meantime, the hands, still clasped, have moved downwards by flexion in the elbows and extension/abduction/external rotation in the shoulder joints. The hands then part and return to their starting positions.
Limitatio: After all of these elements of the conditio "Return of the spinal column to its neutral position with the long axis of the body vertical" have been fulfilled in proper coordination, the limitatio of all overshoot reactions shows, in the up and down costal movements of the ribs on inspiration and expiration in coordination with the excursions of the diaphragm and the visible outward swelling and expansion of the upper abdomen during inspiration, that the desired physiological, normal breathing has begun. The patient feels good and relaxed. He should experience and enjoy this state, so that he is motivated to reproduce it often during the course of a day.

Conditio of Movement Speed
Limitatio of Economical Activity by Finding the Optimal Speed
Conditio: The fine differentiations involved in bringing about and releasing hyperactivity, and the necessity of finding economical coordination of muscle tone in the area of BSs pelvis, thorax and head means that all elements of the exercise have to be practised carefully. The speed is therefore slow; the patient needs time for conscious perception of each change so than he can duplicate it later.
Limitatio: In the stretch position after the "detour" is over, the intensity of economical activity has increased markedly. When the conditio "Return of the spinal column to its neutral position" has been fulfilled, it is low. Normal breathing begins automatically if the conditio has been fulfilled exactly: the thoracic spine remains in neutral, there is absolutely no hyperactivity in the muscles of the abdomen, neck or shoulder girdle, and the long axis of the body is vertical. If all this is the case, the thoracic spine is dynamically stabilized and normal respiration begins.

▶ Instruction in Patient Language

● Instruction Appealing to the Patient's Perception

See conditio pp. 137–138.

● Verbal Instruction   ### ● Instruction by Manipulation

Position and Activation in the Starting Position
"Sit on the stool. Your legs are just comfortably straddled and your knees

The therapist checks the height of the seat. The distance from the patient's

and toes face in the same direction, a little outwards. Your hands rest on your thighs, or you can fold them if you like. The stool is hard and you can feel your bones pressing down on it. Your rib cage is directly above your pelvis and your head directly above your rib cage. You are looking straight ahead."

hips to the floor should be greater than the distance from the knees to the floor. There must always be room for the hips to flex with the long axis of the body vertical. The axes of each thigh and the ipsilateral foot are in the same plane. The head is in the virtual long axis of the body.

Actio and Conditio of the Movement Sequence

"Your right hand comes from above, grips your left wrist and pulls your left arm straight. Your joined hands pull upwards together until they are above your head, nice and central. You pull on your arms until your neck disappears between your shoulders. You are now tall and thin. Your stomach and your back are also long."

"You've been holding your breath but now you breathe again. Now relax the small of your back; you'll notice that you sway backwards a little. Naturally your head goes with it. You relax your head as well, and now it's easy to nod as if to say "Yes," or to shake your head as if to say "No" or to tilt it from side to side as if to say "Maybe." Now comes the best part. Did you notice how you pulled in your stomach? Now let it go, very slowly. When your stomach is relaxed you can feel how when you breathe your rib cage moves without your doing anything. You feel good and relaxed. You must keep breathing this way when you let your arms slowly down until your hands rest again on your thighs and your shoulder girdle has dropped gently onto your rib cage."

The therapist can adjust the pull of the arms and make sure that the joined hands move in the plane of symmetry. If there are any restrictions in shoulder flexion, only the shoulder girdle should be actively moved upwards. If extension in the thoracic spine is not satisfactory, the therapist can help by physically fixing the thoracic spine dorsally with one hand and lifting the weight of the thorax ventrally with the other (see Fig. 80).

As the anchor of the lumbosacral muscles is released, the therapist can lightly touch the skin in this area. The potential mobility of BS pelvis in the hips can be manually facilitated by turning the pelvis to and fro about the flexion/extension axis. Achieving potential mobility of BS head can also be facilitated by gentle manipulation. Special care must be taken that the head stays in the long axis of the body and the patient keeps looking to the front.

As the patient relaxes his abdominal muscles, the therapist watches the costal respiration and the drop in the activity of the scalene muscles, and repeats the instructions to relax. If normal breathing does not begin as it should, the therapist can augment the pull of the arms or support the weight of the thorax as described above. This manipulation is always effective in evoking spontaneous normal breathing.

4.1.1 Adaptation: The Sleeper (Fig. 35)

If we are unable to attain the goal – spontaneous automatic normal breathing associated with a feeling of well-being – by practising the Lion, the first thing to be sacrificed is the vertical position of the long axis of the body with the thoracic spine economically stabilized in its neutral position. Instead, we will place the patient in a position in which normal breathing starts automatically, thus fulfilling an important part of the goal.

"The Sleeper" is a descriptive invented name: the starting position is a good position for sleep.

■ Goal of the Exercise

The goal is to evoke spontaneous normal breathing by appropriate positioning of the patient with the long axis of the body horizontal.

▶ Functional Analysis in Therapist Language

● Conception of the Exercise

We are looking for a position that will permit the spinal column to be horizontal and approximately in the neutral position, and in which it has enough tolerance for reduced-lift movements so that the vertebral joints are never at end-stop. In such a position the muscles do not have to engage in fall-preventing stabilizing activity, and it is interesting to study the beneficial effect this position has on the abdominal muscles and on cardiac activity. The ideal position is one about halfway between prone and right sidelying, with plenty of cushioning under BSs pelvis and thorax, the spinal column in neutral position and the arms and legs lying naturally.

● Position and Activation in the Starting Position

The starting position is halfway between prone and right sidelying. BSs pelvis and thorax, whose midfrontal plane is at an angle of about 45° to the horizontal base support, are resting on enough cushions that no activity against the force of gravity

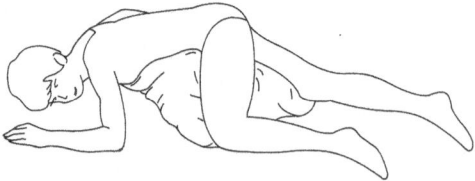

Fig. 35. The Sleeper

140

is triggered. Cushions may also be placed under the cervical spine. The head normally lies comfortably on the floor without a pillow. It is often impossible to keep the head from coming ventrally out of alignment with the long axis of the body, and this must be accepted.

The right arm rests comfortably on the base support behind the back. The cushions in front must be placed under the thorax such that there is no uncomfortable pressure on the right shoulder which would displace it dorsally. BSs pelvis, thorax and head are aligned in the horizontal long axis of the body.

Cushions are also placed under the medial aspect of the left upper arm and the ventral aspect of the left shoulder to keep the left elbow from slipping ventrally. The forearm rests on the base support, its long axis roughly parallel to the long axis of the body.

The right leg lies with its ventrolateral aspect on the base support and is comfortably flexed at the hip and knee. There are cushions under the medial aspect of the left thigh to counteract any tendency of the left knee to slide ventrally. The left hip and knee are well-flexed in a comfortable position.

In this position, normal breathing starts spontaneously because the coordinated buttressing and stabilizing activities of the thoracic spine are not necessary before the costal respiratory movements can occur.

The cushions under the stomach exert a compression that provides a buttress for the diaphragmatic movements of respiration, often needed especially by patients with a flaccid abdominal wall and/or a distended stomach. If this is still not enough, the compression can be increased using a foam rubber bandage.

Cushions under the thorax are essential above all in patients with flat backs in the thoracic area, otherwise the weight of the thorax would hang actively suspended from the cervical spine, immediately triggering "stress respiration."

● **Actio and Conditio of the Movement Sequence**

In the starting position described above the patient has already reached the goal. The movement event is therefore concerned with intensifying the patient's awareness of the position and preparing him to practise on his own.

Guided by the verbal cues for normal breathing (see. p. 132), the patient experiences the perceptual signals his body is giving him.

In this semisidelying position, practically all of the joints can be given reduced-lift mobilization. The therapist can now decide what movements are to be made. She tells the patient in what direction the manipulation will be carried out, and at first the patient passively allows the therapist to move him. Then he carefully begins to join in, until the movement is so easy that the therapist thinks the patient is doing the work and the patient thinks the therapist is. Now the patient takes over completely, moving as if automatically. After the patient has performed a few variations, including ones which involve the extremities, the therapist begins to manipulate two such movements at the same time. These kinds of movement sequences help the patient to become more and more relaxed. Breathing functions without any special instructions. The unfamiliar movement combinations take up the whole of the patient's perceptual capacity, leaving no room for private thoughts. In a very short time the patient is able to perform the Sleeper entirely without the help of the therapist. In it he has also discovered a good remedy for insomnia. Moreover, as he sleeps, he will begin to stretch more again whenever he feels uncomfortable and therefore have less pain from sleeping in a bad position.

▶ Instruction in Patient Language

Instruction Appealing to the Patient's Perception

See p. 132.

● **Verbal Instruction**

● **Instruction by Manipulation**

Actio and Conditio of the Movement Sequence

"You are lying comfortably. You can feel the insides of your lower teeth with your tongue. Your breathing comes automatically. You feel a little current of cool air in your nose. It carries the smell of coffee. You almost have to yawn. Let the air out, slowly – you have plenty of time. Now you feel comfortable and quiet again."

The therapist's right hand rests lightly and flatly on the patient's left side. Her left hand rests flatly on his left iliac crest. As the patient breathes in, the therapist gently pushes the ribs ventrally/cranially while simultaneously pulling gently dorsally/caudally on the pelvis to buttress the movement. During the inspiratory pause, the therapist changes her grip (left hand on the thorax, right hand in the middle of the thoracic spine), and as the patient begins to exhale she gently pushes the ribs dorsally/caudally and gently presses the thorax ventrally/cranially to extend the thoracic spine.

"Now I'm going to take your shoulder for a walk along your rib cage. First it goes up to the tip of your nose and then it moves away again. It goes easily to and fro. Now you join in, you know the way. Don't try too hard, don't go too fast. Now do it all by yourself. And let the movement just fade away. Now it's my turn again. I'm going to take your shoulder for a walk down to your navel and then away from it again." And so on.

The therapist pushes her left hand under the patient's left upper arm and grips his shoulder joint from in front. Her right hand comes to rest dorsally on the scapula and pushes the left pincer jaws along with the arm, whose weight now rests on her left arm, cranially/ventrally/medially and, on the way back, caudally/dorsally/laterally. The other way is to move caudally/ventrally/medially first, then back cranially/dorsally/laterally.

4.1.2 Adaptation: Sitting Like a King (Figs. 36, 37)

If the patient can perform the Sleeper with ease, but still has trouble with the Lion, we try another exercise with the patient sitting on a chair with a back support. "Sitting Like a King" is an invented name indicating that, sitting in a chair with a back and armrests, the patient is as comfortable and contented as a king being waited on hand and foot.

■ Goal of the Exercise

The goal is to evoke spontaneous normal breathing in a position in which the back and the arms are supported and the long axis of the body is roughly vertical without dynamic stabilization of the thoracic spine.

▶ Functional Analysis in Therapist Language

● Conception of the Exercise

To fulfil the conditions set out in the goal we must find the most comfortable sitting position possible (Fig. 36). For this we need a chair with a shaped back that supports the physiological curvature of the lumbar spine and follows the curves of the lower and midthoracic spine which press against it. Now all we have to do is find a base support for the arms, so that their weight doesn't pull at the body.

In this position we can keep the spinal column in neutral and roughly vertical, while reducing the need for muscular fall-preventing stabilization of the thoracic

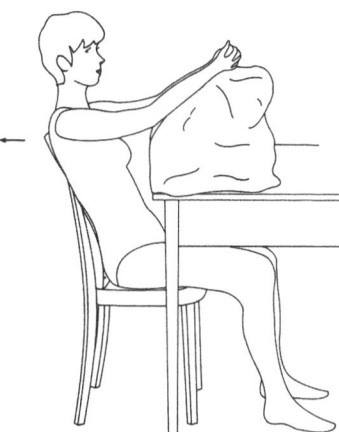

Fig. 36. Sitting Like a King. Optimal sitting position using the moulded Abo back support and arms comfortably supported

143

spine. The desired normal breathing with economical coordination of the costal movements and diaphragmatic excursions can now take place.

● **Position and Activation in the Starting Position**

Position in Space of the Critical Axes
Points of Contact Between the Body and the Environment
Components of Movement in Relation to the Neutral Position of the Joints

The starting position is sitting on a chair with a backrest and, if possible, armrests. If the chair doesn't have a backrest that can conform to the shape of the back (with the spinal column in neutral position) we can modify it to fit, using pillows or the very effective Abo-back Support (Thergofit, Bad Ragaz, Switzerland). The seat is flat and horizontal or inclines slightly backwards. The height of the seat allows the hips to be flexed to 90° or a little more.

The long axis of BSs pelvis and thorax inclines moderately backwards. The long axis of BS head is vertically above T1. The ischial area and the dorsal/cranial aspects of the thighs touch the seat. The dorsal aspects of BSs pelvis and thorax are in continuous contact with the back of the chair up to about T4.

In BS legs, the soles of the feet are in contact with the floor. They are about the width of the pelvis apart and the thighs are comfortably straddled.

In BS arms, the weight of the arms rests either on the armrests of the chair, on a table of an appropriate height or on the thighs.

Distribution of Body Weight on a Base Support or Suspension Device,
Against a Supportive Device, or over a Support Area,
and the Resulting Activity States of the Musculature

BS legs is parked. The thighs use the seat as base support; the feet and lower legs use the floor.

BS pelvis has the seat for base support and the back of the chair as supportive device; it has reduced potential mobility.

BS thorax has the back of the chair as supportive device and exerts only a little of its weight on the pelvis. It bears the weight of BS head, whose position in space makes possible the neutral position of the thoracic spine.

BS head balances in free play over T1.

In BS arms, the shoulder girdle is parked on the thorax. The arms are parked on the armrests of the chair or on a table as base support.

Intensity of Muscle Activity Required with Economical Activity
Respiration

The intensity of muscle activity is very low. Because the weights of the body are supported by base supports and supportive devices, the patient can breathe normally without his spinal column having to work very hard to maintain posture.

If the patient cannot reach the goal in the way described, the therapist gets behind him, puts her arms around his thorax and gently lifts the weight of the thorax, causing slight extension in the thoracic spine. The patient can place his arms, hands folded over each other, around the therapist's neck while she is lifting and rest his head against her stomach. Now the patient has to let his abdomen "go flop". After

144

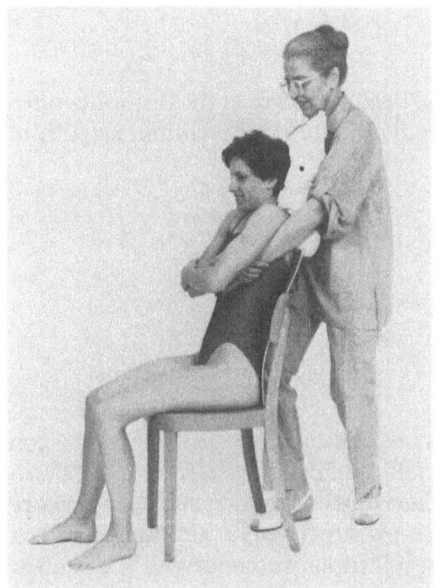
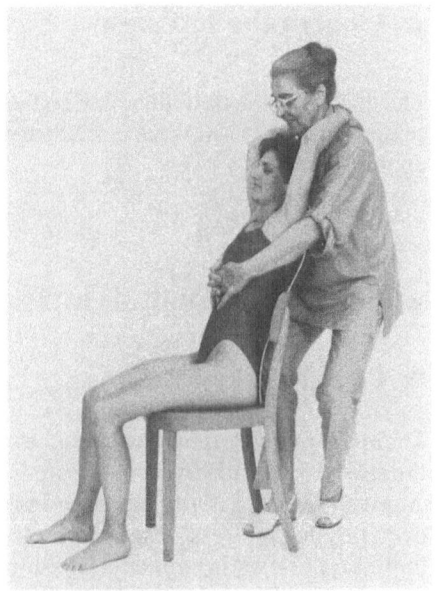

a   b

Fig. 37 a, b. Sitting Like a King. **a** The therapist lifts the weight of the patient's thorax and arms. The patient's head is supported by a pillow. **b** The therapist lifts the weight of the thorax. The patient wraps her arms around the back of the therapist's neck and leans her head against the therapist's chest

a short while, normal breathing begins with visible costal respiratory movements (Fig. 37).

● **Actio – Reactio of the Movement Sequence**

There is no movement sequence in Sitting Like a King. Everything depends on correctly assuming the position described above. Hearing the verbal cues for normal breathing (see p. 132), the patient can become aware of the signals his body is sending him.

4.2 Slow Motion Breathing

Slow Motion Breathing trains respiration under stress. It is appropriate for all patients who have mastered normal breathing. "Slow Motion Breathing" is a name we invented; in this exercise a full breath taken at slow motion speed is used to clarify the processes of respiration to the patient.

■ Goal of the Exercise

The goal is for the patient to understand and become aware of the respiratory processes that occur when the circulatory system is under stress, without actually inducing this stress.

▶ Functional Analysis in Therapist Language

● Conception of the Exercise

There are many patients who need to train respiration under stress but for whom the stress to the cardiovascular system normally entailed in such training, or the increased physical activity employed to produce it, is contraindicated. Since, moreover, physically stressful activity undertaken to trigger deeper respiration will not improve pre-existing functionally faulty respiration, we conceived the exercise Slow Motion Breathing.

In this exercise, the physiological respiratory processes that occur when the cardiovascular system is stressed are simulated, but the physical exertion that generally triggers these processes is missing. Since the body doesn't really need this deep breathing, we may, or, rather, we must, take a lot of time in order to avoid hyperventilation. So we just breathe in slow motion, and make ourselves physically aware of the different phases of prolonged inspiration and expiration.

● Position and Activation in the Starting Position

The starting position is subject to only one condition: the long axes of BSs pelvis, thorax and head should constitute the virtual long axis of the body in the best possible way. Maintaining the long axis of the body upright demands stabilizing activity from the autochthonous muscles of the spinal column.

In the analysis below, it is assumed that the long axis of the body is either vertical or leaning forwards.

● Actio, Conditio – Limitatio of the Movement Sequence

For the purpose of our analysis there are six phases of respiration:
Phase 1: Concentric isotonic inspiration starting in the respiratory middle position
Phase 2: Pause at the peak of inspiration
Phase 3: Eccentric isotonic expiration
Phase 4: Concentric isotonic expiration
Phase 5: Post-expiratory pause
Phase 6: Eccentric isotonic inspiration

Phase 1

In the respiratory middle position the patient waits calmly for his body to signal a need to inhale. When he breathes in, through his nose, he is aware of the coolness due to evaporation in his nose, of the flow of his saliva and of the widening of his thorax and upper abdomen. The ribs lift up, the intercostal spaces expand, the diaphragm drops, the abdomen broadens and the thoracic spine becomes actively flexionally buttressed in its neutral position.

Phase 2

The pause at the peak of inspiration requires the intercostal muscles and the diaphragm to keep the abdomen as broad as it was in phase 1. The glottis stays open: if it closes, the activity of the inspiratory intercostal muscles ceases. This pause lasts for a few seconds.

Phase 3

The air escapes slowly, braked by the eccentric isotonic work of the intercostal muscles. Extensional stabilization of the thoracic spine begins. Expiration continues until the patient is back at the respiratory mid-position, i.e. as far as the expiration stimulated by the elastic recoil of the lungs continues. The ribs drop and the abdomen collapses.

Phase 4

To make sure that the air does not cease flowing out, the patient continues to breathe out by concentric isotonic work of the abdominal muscles and the intercostal muscles of expiration. The extensional active buttressing of the thoracic spine increases. The epigastric angle narrows, the abdominal muscles contract concentrically, the upper abdomen narrows, the lower abdomen shortens. The intensity of economical activity is now at its highest.

Phase 5

The post-expiratory pause can be held as long as the patient likes. The tension in the muscles of expiration must be sustained. There must be no glottal closure.

Phase 6

Inspiration starts with the eccentric isotonic release of the abdominal and intercostal muscles of expiration and the simultaneous flow of air in through the nose. The extensional active buttressing of the thoracic spine ceases and flexional active buttressing is about to start. This phase ends when the patient once again reaches the respiratory mid-position.

Note
There is little risk of hyperventilation if the respiratory pauses are held for long enough. Nevertheless, a break after five repetitions of Slow Motion Breathing is recommended.

▶ Instruction in Patient Language

● **Verbal Instruction**   ● **Instruction by Manipulation**

Actio and Conditio of the Movement Sequence

Phases 1 and 2

"You are quiet, waiting for your body to need air. When it does, let the air flow gently in and the widening of your rib cage and stomach make you feel as if you are floating. The air flowing in feels cool in your nose. You can float like this as long as it feels good."

Phases 1 and 2 occur only at the beginning of Slow Motion Breathing. When the patient performs the five repetitions recommended as one exercise unit, each repetition will consist only of phases 3, 4, 5 and 6.

Phases 3 and 4

"Let the air flow away slowly; at first you have to keep the brakes on it. The air tickles a little in your nose. Now it flows away easily, let it go on that way. Don't let the smooth flow run out. You are becoming taller and thinner and the tension you feel in your stomach is good. Hold the tension in your stomach when the air runs out. Your tongue is relaxed and warm and swimming in saliva."

It can be very helpful if the therapist places her hands on the patient's thorax so that she can follow the respiratory movement of the ribs when expiration begins and then, during the prolongation of expiration, help lower the ribs with one hand while exerting extensional pressure on the thoracic spine at the same time with the other. The manipulation to help lower the ribs is a curving movement and is directed caudally/dorsally.

Phases 5 and 6

"You have plenty of time to wait until your body says it wants to breathe in. Gently relax your stomach and make sure that the air doesn't flow in too fast through your nose; you have to take time to feel the coolness of the breeze in your nose. As your body gets wider, you turn into a balloon floating in the air. The tension in your stomach is completely gone. Your nose is tickling; you almost have to yawn. Let your tongue feel your teeth. You have time to wait again."
Phases 3 and 4, 5 and 6, etc.

When inspiration begins, the therapist takes her hands away, but only as far as if she wanted to draw the thorax with a magnet. During the prolongation of inspiration, manipulation to lift the ribs is directed cranially/ventrally and is supported by a diagonal counterpull on the pelvis caudally/dorsally. The manipulation should cause the thoracic spine to flex slightly. Pressing the patient's upper lip towards the centre from the sides and pulling forward on it is also helpful.

4.2.1 Adaptation: Rhythmic Breathing

If the patient's expiratory volume per second is too low, making it impossible for him to reproduce an adequate percentage of his vital capacity during forced expiration, his respiration is inefficient. Although the vital capacity can be improved with Slow Motion Breathing, another exercise is needed to improve expiratory volume per second, hence tidal volume per minute, the basic measurement of respiration. The name "Rhythmic Breathing" refers to the fact that, for practice purposes, we use rhythm to structure the breathing.

■ Goal of the Exercise

The goal is for the patient to be able to increase his expiratory volume per second by using rhythmic structuring of inspiration and expiration.

▶ Functional Analysis in Therapist Language

● Conception of the Exercise

In order to train rapid exhalation of as much air as possible, we decide on a given unit of time during which the air will be exhaled a varying number of times and hence in amounts of varying sizes. Our ultimate goal is for all the air to be exhaled quickly in one single go. In this way the patient will learn to divide up the same quantity of air in different ways and to manage, despite the required interrupted inspiration and expiration, not to close the glottis and to do without extra breaths. The speed indicated is too fast for these mistakes to occur anyway.

● Position and Activation in the Starting Position

The starting position is upright sitting on a stool. BSs pelvis, thorax and head are aligned in the long axis of the body, which is vertical. Another possibility is to sit at a table with the arms resting on the table and BSs pelvis, thorax and head aligned in the long axis of the body, which is either vertical or leaning slightly forwards. Lastly, upright standing can be selected as the starting position, with the feet the width of the pelvis apart and BSs pelvis, thorax and head vertically aligned in the long axis of the body. In all three starting positions, the thoracic spine is dynamically stabilized in neutral position and BSs pelvis and head are potentially mobile. The intensity of economical activity is low.

● Actio and Conditio of the Movement Sequence

The basic neter for Rhythmic Breathing is 4/4 time at 100 beats/minute and a phrase length of two bars.
The first bar and the first quarter of the second are for expiration; the remaining three-quarters of the second bar are for inspiration. We begin by breathing out

through the mouth. The lips are positioned as if to whistle. Pitch is around concert A (440 oscillations/second). The sound is very soft and is a fricative somewhere between "h" and the German "ch".

The patient always breathes in through his nose if it is open enough. If the nasal passages are obstructed, the patient may breathe in by sucking air through his mouth with his lips puckered as for whistling, making the same sound as he made to breathe out.

	out	in	out	in
1) 4/4	♪♪♪ ♪♪♪ ♪♪♪ ♪♪♪	♩' ↑↑↑	♪♪♪ ♪♪♪ ♪♪♪ ♪♪♪	♩' ↑↑↑
2) 4/4	♫ ♫ ♫ ♫	♩' ↑↑↑	♫ ♫ ♫ ♫	♩' ↑↑↑
3) 4/4	♩ ♩ ♩ ♩	♩' ↑↑↑	♩ ♩ ♩ ♩	♩' ↑↑↑
4) 4/4	♩ ♩	♩' ↑↑↑	♩ ♩	♩' ↑↑↑
5) 4/4	o	3' ↑↑↑	o	3' ↑↑↑

Basic Rhythm Pattern, To Be Varied Ad Libitum

The two-bar phrase units should be repeated about four or five times without the patient running out of breath. After about five repetitions, the patient should pause in breathing and wait until he feels the body signal "Air please" as described in the section on normal breathing (see p.132). This keeps him from hyperventilating.

It is advisable to practice patterns 1, 2 and 3 first for a while, then add 4, and only when these have been mastered add pattern 5. The goal has then been fulfilled.

4.2.2 Adaptation: Double Panting

If the patient is not yet ready for Rhythmic Breathing or becomes out of breath during the exercise, we choose something simpler as a preparatory or partial substitute exercise.

"Double Panting" means that the patient pants in the usual way except that each time he performs *two* inhalations and *two* exhalations.

150

■ Goal of the Exercise

The goal is for the patient to functionally train the muscles of the diaphragm, larynx, pharynx, tongue, abdomen and intercostal area by skill exercises.

▶ Functional Analysis in Therapist Language

● Conception of the Exercise

To develop skill in the muscles involved in respiration, Double Panting should be practised during the ordinary activities of daily living. We try to keep an even speed of 120 units/minute. The direction for dynamics in Double Panting is "piano" (quietly); rhythmically it should be "staccato" (each breath short and sharp).

● Position and Activation in the Starting Position

There are no restrictions to the starting position. Double Panting can be done all the time, while cooking, going up stairs, walking, playing the piano or violin, typing, etc.

● Actio and Conditio of the Movement Sequence

The basic measure is a 2/4 bar at a speed of 80 beats/minute. The coordination of the rapid shift from two exhalations to two inhalations trains skill.
Keeping the panting "piano" reduces the danger of "pressured breathing". The patient does not have time for his glottis to close up or for the flow of air to be too much impeded by inappropriate glottal constriction.
The "staccato" requires another precise skill, namely breathing in short bursts. Each burst of inhalation or exhalation is followed or punctuated by a short break. During this break, no air is allowed to flow in after the brief inspiratory burst and no air is allowed to flow out after the expiratory burst. Since, during the short break, the glottis should not close – and indeed cannot close, because of the slow speed and the dynamic required – the muscles of respiration must perform skilfully.
After each expiratory burst, the muscles of expiration have to hold the respiratory space at the constriction just reached for the duration of the break; after each inspiratory burst the muscles of inspiration must keep the respiratory space at the expansion just reached.
Inspiration and expiration are through the mouth, which is again puckered as if to whistle. The dynamic is constant at "piano" and the rhythm is even, staccato quavers (eighth-notes). The patient may instead breathe in through his nose and out through his mouth, or in and out through his nose.

♫   ♫♪ │ ♫   ♫♪ │ ♫   ♫♪ │ ♫   ♫♪ │ ♫   ♫♪ │ ♫   ♫♪ │ ♫   ♫♪ │ ♫   ♫♪ │
out   in │ out   in │ out   in │ out   in │ out   in │ out   in │ out   in │ out   in │

Basic Rhythm Pattern
The tempo can vary.
Double Panting should be performed around the respiratory mid-position. The quantity of air that the patient breathes in and out should be small and always remain the same. Double Panting should never cause dyspnoea or hyperventilation; if either of these occurs, the exercise should be interrupted and the return of normal breathing awaited. There need be no time limit to Double Panting if it is performed correctly.

▶ Instruction in Patient Language

● **Verbal Instruction**

● **Instruction by Manipulation**

Actio and Conditio of the Movement Sequence

"Pout your lips to make a pointed snout. Stay quite calm and wait until your body wants to breathe. Now suck in two thimblefuls of cool air through your mouth, then blow both thimblefuls back out through your mouth:

In/in, out/out, in/in, out/out, in/in, out/out, and so on. You need much less air than that. Keep on going until you forget how to stop. Now stand up and keep panting while you get dressed and go up the stairs. A piece of advice: whenever you exert yourself, start Double Panting at the same time.

Before the patient begins Double Panting, the therapist should relax his upper lip by manipulation and show him how he can do this himself, and should do so whenever he feels he is getting out of breath. Jaw movements against light guiding resistance are also helpful.

Monitoring the movement by palpation, we can feel the clear intercostal movement of the ribs and normal activity of the diaphragm (particularly evident in the upper abdomen), relaxed lateral neck muscles and a calm pulse rate. There is plenty of saliva.

4.3 Air Gulper (Figs. 38, 39)

The name "Air Gulper" refers to a habit to be got rid of.

■ Goal of the Exercise

The goal is for the patient to learn to expel swallowed air from the intestinal tract and stomach and to learn to avoid gulping air.

▶ Functional Analysis in Therapist Language

● Conception of the Exercise

From the definition of the goal it is clear that this is a problem that will not be overcome with just one exercise. Restricting ourselves just to the three problems mentioned in the goal, we arrive at three different exercises:

– Intestinal Wind: to eliminate swallowed air in the intestines
– Belching: to eliminate swallowed air in the stomach
– Prevention of air gulping.

Intestinal Wind

Where a habit of excessive gulping of air has led to flatulence, we try functionally stimulating its discharge.

The procedure has to be simple and easy for the patient to perform at any time. It must be adaptable to any restrictions of movement, e.g. arthritis in the hip, or other pathological conditions such as cardiac insufficiency. For this reason we need to offer a variety of starting positions each of which makes for external compression of the abdominal area. Then, breathing in deeply causes the diaphragm to drop, compressing the abdominal cavity from cranially. With a little patience and overcoming of inhibitions, the excess air can now take the path of least resistance and escape through the intestines to the outside world.

Belching

It is normal to swallow air along with food and liquids as we eat and drink. The normal reaction of the body is to belch: excess air is expelled via the shortest way from the stomach, i.e. via the oesophagus and the mouth.

It is normal for an infant to burp after a meal; indeed, the mother expects it. If the baby doesn't burp, we think something is wrong and respond accordingly. In our culture, it is regarded as very bad manners for adults to belch at the table, and those who do are looked on with distaste. On the other hand, in Eastern Asia it is quite the thing for men to do. It meets the natural need to get rid of an unpleasant feeling of fullness in the stomach.

The causes of pathological air gulping are unclear. What is clear is that those who do it are swallowing air not only during mealtimes, but at other times as well, sometimes every time they breathe in.

A distinction can be made between patients with digestive disorders, in whom pathological flatulence arises in the gut or is attributable to gastrointestinal surgery, and the far more numerous nervous gulpers of air. Hyperactivity, nervousness, dissatisfaction and anxiety all lead to a particular type of stress that promotes constant air gulping.

All air gulpers exhibit signs of functional respiratory disorders in the form of pressured breathing. This occurs at first in nervous air gulpers only in stress situations, but later it becomes a habit. One could well say that these chronic air gulpers are in a habitual "mini state of stress".

Whether the chronic air gulping is of a gastric aetiology or the result of autonomic dystonia, the specific physiotherapeutic treatment should be complemented by a general relaxation exercise program.

Preventing Air Gulping
Gulping air has become a habit. The patient is aware only of the unpleasant consequences: a feeling of fullness in the stomach, difficulty in breathing, a distended abdomen. But he can't feel when he's actually gulping air, the root of the problem. How is one supposed to get rid of a habit when one can't even feel when and how one is doing it?

There is one sure way of solving this and other problems like it: we look for an activity that is incompatible with the problem. So we look for a simple activity that makes it impossible to swallow air. If we succeed in keeping the patient from gulping air for a long period of time, he'll be in a better position to unlearn his bad habit. The simple activity during which it is impossible to swallow air is whistling. But the patient must whistle without stopping not only the normal way, i.e., while exhaling, but while inhaling too. Almost any other activity can be carried out at the same time.

● **Position and Activation in the Starting Position**

Intestinal Wind (Fig. 38)
Since we must be able to adapt the starting position of sitting to the needs of the patient, we will need a stool, a box, a treatment bench or maybe even just the edge of a bed (Fig. 38 a–c). The patient can also kneel over a box or over the side of a bed, or he can stand facing a solid table without having to kneel. If the patient has good flexibility in the spinal column and unrestricted movement in the hip joints, supine is the right starting position from which to move into the end position shown in Fig. 38 e.

Belching (Fig. 39)
The best starting position is upright sitting on a stool or upright standing. The exercise can also be easily performed lying down.

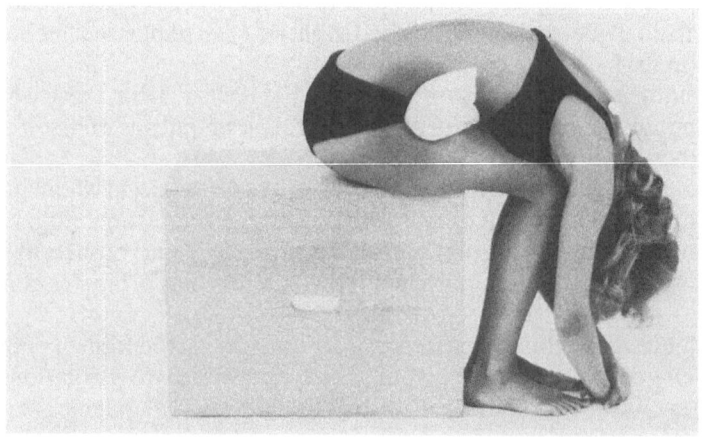

a

Fig. 38 a–e. The Air Gulper. **a** Compression of the stomach

154

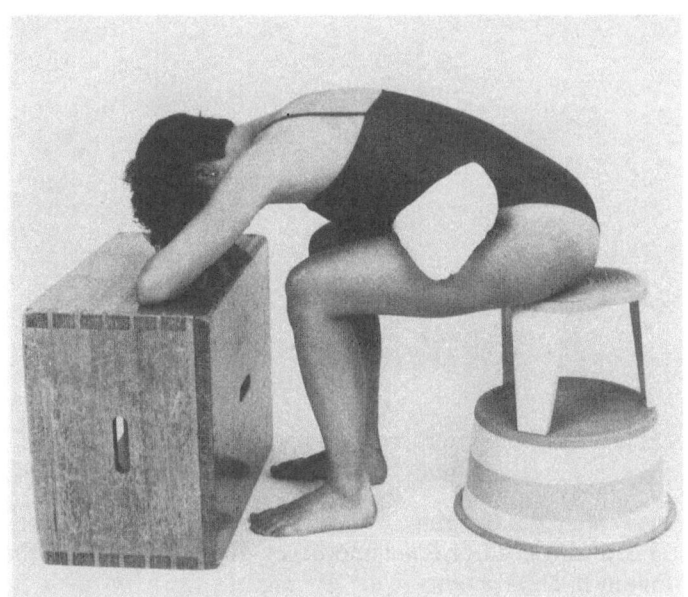

Fig. 38 b. Compression of the stomach when the upper body is disportionately long or the thighs disportionately short. The head is well supported

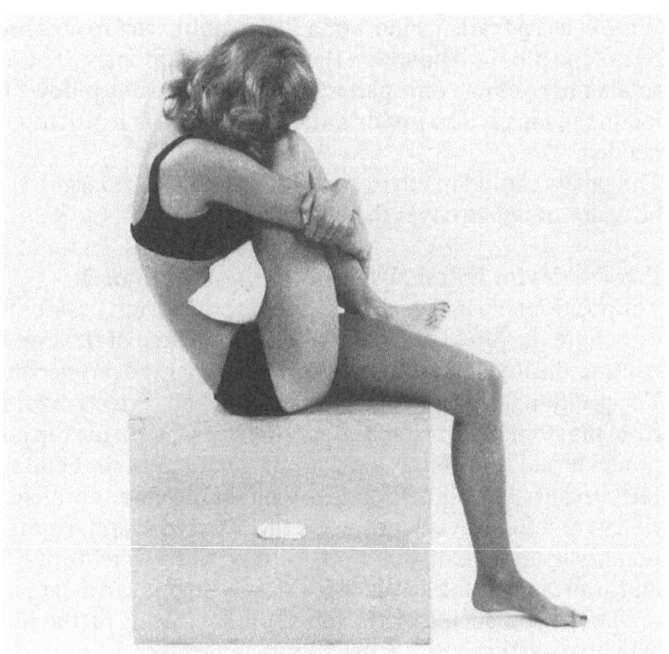

Fig. 38 c. This type of compression of the upper and lower abdomen is particularly effective

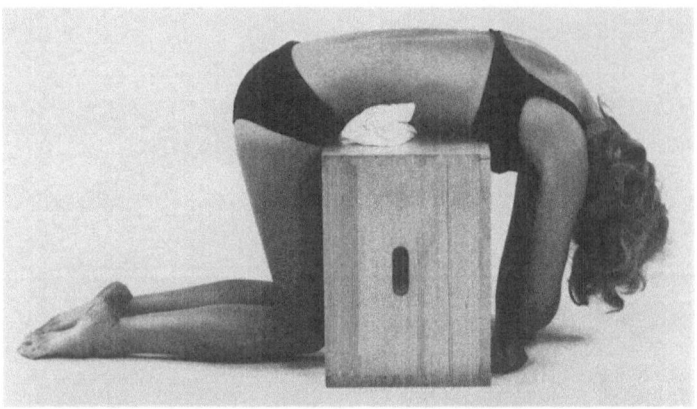

Fig. 38 d. Compression of the stomach when hip flexion is limited

Preventing Air Gulping

The starting position is not important. The best position is the accustomed posture for any familiar activity of daily living.

● Actio and Conditio of the Movement Sequence

Intestinal Wind

We will use a feather pillow or a foam rubber roll to compress the abdomen. The size of the pillow depends on the size of the abdomen. The larger the stomach, the smaller the pillow; some patients may not need any pillow at all. The range of flexion in the hips is also important; if hip flexion is restricted, a larger pillow will be needed.

The pillow should reach from the lower thoracic margin to the inguinal folds and be wide enough to cover the entire area.

Possibilities for Externally Compressing the Stomach

The positions illustrated in Fig. 38 a, b are the easiest to assume during the day. However, here the hip joints must have a good range of flexion. If lowering the head is contraindicated, the head and arms can be parked on a second stool (Fig. 38 b).

The position illustrated in Fig. 38 c is especially effective for rapidly eliminating air from the stomach, but it requires good tolerance in the hip joints for flexion/adduction/external rotation. If the patient cannot park his head on his knee without effort, because his thigh is too short, he should carry his head freely. It must be carried so that the cervical spine and the atlanto-occipital and atlanto-axial joints are potentially mobile. In addition, the combined weights of BSs pelvis, thorax, head and arms, as well as that of the leg clasped in both arms, are in unstable equilibrium on the seat, balancing on the hip of the leg resting on the floor and using this as an activated passive buttress or support as necessary.

The position illustrated in Fig. 38 d is recommended when flexion in the hip joint is restricted. Instead of a box, a normal, solid kitchen table can also be used; the patient will not have to kneel on the floor and can place his head on the table.

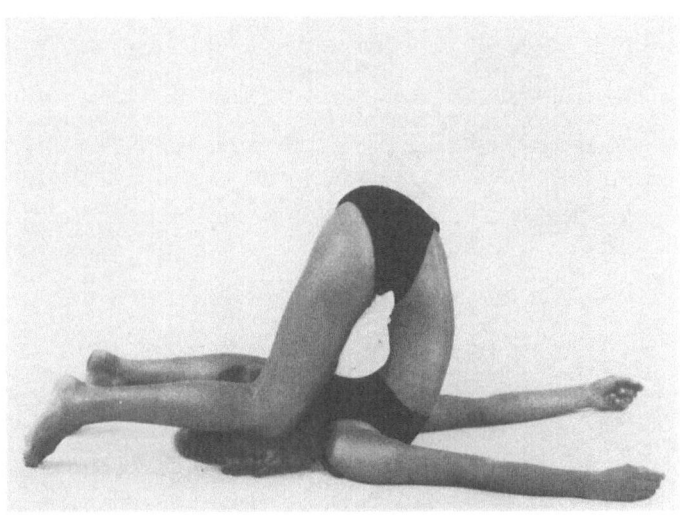

Fig. 38 e. Compression of upper and lower abdomen in patients with freely mobile vertebral and hip joints

Some very flexible and/or younger patients will find the position illustrated in Fig. 38 e very successful, especially to eliminate distending air from the intestine.

As soon as the patient has taken up one of the positions described above and the pillow has been placed properly, he patiently waits until he is breathing normally. The sensation of the pulse beating in the abdominal aorta is normal and is no cause for alarm. When normal breathing is well established, the patient makes the transition to Slow Motion Breathing. The respiratory pause at the peak of inspiration is prolonged. The patient now feels the intra-abdominal pressure building up, caused by the combination of the pillow pressing on the abdomen from the outside and the diaphragm pressing down on it from the inside. If the patient relaxes the anal sphincter and pushes down lightly as if making a bowel movement, the intestinal wind will escape.

Belching

As a word of encouragement, I'd like to say in advance that I've never had a patient who couldn't learn to belch.

To eliminate swallowed air from the stomach, the body employs the belching reflex. In professional jargon, the term is efflation or eructation. If this reflex does not act automatically, we attempt to trigger it. If the reflex is to be triggered functionally, the patient will have to learn how to "choke" the excess air out of his stomach. There are two possibilities: Swallowing Nothing and Spitting Nothing.

Swallowing Nothing: If one tries to swallow three times in the respiratory mid-position without breathing in between, one finds that this takes a great deal of effort on the part of the muscles of the pharynx and stomach. What is missing is the normal swallowing reflex triggered by the pressure of the food bolus. One therefore tries hard to produce as much saliva as possible. But the severe demand on the pha-

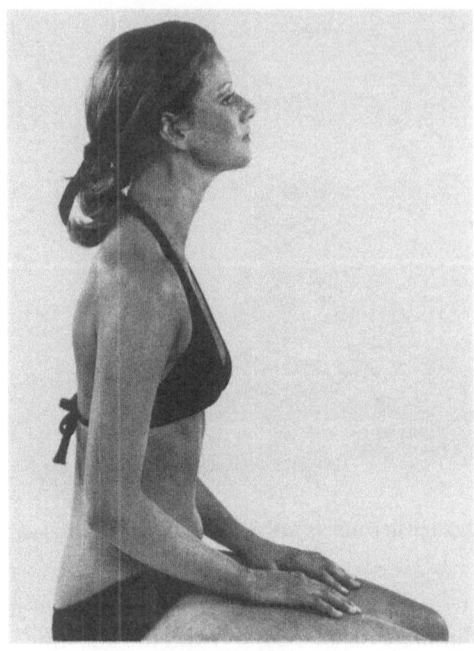

Fig. 39. Swallowing Nothing

ryngeal and abdominal muscles is still there. It is worse with the second and worse still with the third empty swallow. Associated nodding movements of the head are helpful. Similar head movements can be seen in animals, especially birds, drinking (Fig. 39).

These unusually strong, convulsive contractions of the pharyngeal muscles, augmented by the contractions of the abdominal muscles, may directly trigger the belching reflex; in any case they considerably increase any disposition to belch. The air in the stomach is radically mobilized and released, taking the path of least resistance outwards through the mouth. When the patient has learnt Swallowing Nothing properly, he can use it whenever he needs to. Sitting or standing, he attempts to swallow three times without breathing in between, pouting his mouth and with the tip of the tongue supported gently against the inside of the lower front teeth. With the tongue positioned as if it were just about to click, the flow of saliva is stimulated and swallowing is facilitated. This is initially accompanied by flexion, then, during the actual swallowing, by extension in the atlanto-occipital and atlanto-axial joints: critical DP tip of the chin moves caudally/dorsally with the flexion in these joints, then cranially/first ventrally, then dorsally with the extension, before returning to the neutral position.

The extent and intensity of economical activity of these associated head movements increase with each swallow, while the pace, due to the growing resistance, becomes more and more sluggish and slow.

If Swallowing Nothing this way does not succeed, we change the starting position. The patient sits on a chair with a backrest and armrests. He leans back so that the pelvis and the lower thorax are supported. With his forearms he exercises pressure activity on the armrests until the pressure from BS pelvis on the seat starts to let up and he feels that considerable weight is now hanging from his shoulder girdle. This is the weight of the thorax, head and, in part, the pelvis.

To begin the exercise, the patient now relaxes the abdominal and lumbar muscles, by which the pelvis hung from the thorax. The pelvis is now parked on the seat and the patient can begin to swallow.

After the third swallow, the patient gradually relaxes the remaining tension in the pharyngeal and abdominal muscles and, just as gradually, admits an inhalation. At this moment belching usually comes effortlessly, either by reflex or voluntarily.

Spitting Nothing: In normal spitting one automatically begins with an inhalation. The glottis closes and the inhaled air is compressed by the muscles of expiration until the glottis bursts open and the object being spat out is propelled in the accelerated flow of air from the body.

Example: A group of adolescents are betting who can spit cherry pits the farthest. If we discount enthusiasm and practice, the winner will be the one who can form with his tongue and mouth a good narrow nozzle pointing forwards and who has a large vital capacity and an optimal tidal volume per second.

For Spitting Nothing, the patient starts in the respiratory mid-position and fully exhales crescendo (i. e., getting louder) on a "sh" or "s", pouting out his mouth. At the end he stops for a moment and then, without breathing in between, "spits nothing" three times. The patient can feel the extreme contraction of the abdominal muscles and the tension in the glottis. Since there is no air in the respiratory space, the expiratory muscles must contract to the maximum to further narrow this area for spitting. The air in the stomach is now energetically mobilized, looks for the path of least resistance and escapes in a belch.

This easy-to-learn exercise can be performed whenever the patient feels uncomfortably full in his stomach.

The starting position for Spitting Nothing is identical to that for Swallowing Nothing. After Spitting Nothing, the patient can inhale again in different ways:

- While still in the exhalation position, the patient attempts to belch after spitting. Only thereafter does he breathe in slowly.
- After spitting, the patient pauses, but without closing the glottis. Then, simultaneously with the slow inflow of air through his nose at the end of a moderate inbreath, he belches effortlessly, whether automatically or voluntarily.
- After spitting, the patient pauses, this time with the glottis kept closed while the abdominal muscles relax. The glottis is then opened very slowly so the inhaled air doesn't flow in too quickly. After this inspiration, belching generally either happens automatically or the patient has no difficulty in doing it voluntarily. This last variation is somewhat more difficult to learn, but is also the most successful.

Preventing Air Gulping

How air is swallowed at times other than eating and drinking is an open question. My hypothesized answer is based on years of practical experience working with patients who gulp air.

Gulping air at times other than mealtimes is due to a specific functional respiratory disorder. At the end of an inhalation which began too quickly, the inhaled air is held in the respiratory space by glottal closure. The muscles of inspiration then reflexively lose tone because the air cushion trapped in the respiratory space makes their activity superfluous, for normally it is the inspiratory muscles which have to hold the respiratory space and hence also the thorax in the expanded position of inhalation in order to keep the inhaled air from escaping. The respiratory pause at the peak of inhalation is especially important for gas exchange and consequently for oxygen absorption. In the respiratory disorder just described, with glottal closure at the peak of inhalation, air can easily get into the stomach when the glottis reopens for exhalation, for, because the air has been dammed up in the respiratory space and the muscles of inspiration are not ready for performing their isotonic braking activity at the beginning of expiration, the opening of the glottis is explosive, particularly if the thoracic spine has become destabilized because it was held in the neutral position partly by the trapped cushion of air. So, first the air escapes too quickly and then, in the end phase, not enough air can be exhaled because, among other things, the oblique abdominal muscles lack active buttressing by an extensionally stabilized thoracic spine. Regulating the expiratory flow is thus left almost entirely to the vocal cords.

An experiment that one should try for oneself and which often interests patients is to reproduce the movements of inspiration voluntarily with the glottis open. The diaphragm is energetically pushed down and the ribs lifted and spread. The sucking in of the air is clearly perceptible. If, however, the glottis is closed during this process and then reopened, the air can be felt to rush in quite dramatically.

Now comes the opposite movement. The muscles of inspiration are slowly relaxed with the thoracic spine dynamically stabilized in neutral position and the glottis open. Then the ribs are dropped, the epigastric angle is narrowed and the abdominal walls are physiologically contracted. One can clearly feel the air escaping. If the glottis is closed during this process, the build-up of pressure under the vocal cords is readily perceptible.

Anyone who finds it difficult to voluntarily close the glottis has only to imagine he wishes to clear his throat. As the glottis reopens, the air is released suddenly like a cough.

A further experiment is effective in teaching awareness of the respiratory processes. One performs an exercise that stresses the circulation until one is out of breath. Now, rather than increasing the respiratory frequency, the diaphragm is pushed down and the thorax expanded to the position of inspiration and an extended respiratory pause taken with the glottis open. It will be seen that breathing quickly returns to normal. This can be repeated as often as desired.

We now intend to prevent air gulping with inspiratory and expiratory whistling during ordinary, everyday activities of daily living. We will use a song the patient knows well as the basis for melody and rhythm. Expiratory whistling causes little trouble. The patient should whistle softly, keeping a steady rhythm and being thrifty with the amount of air he uses. At first, inspiratory whistling is more difficult. It is actually a sucking whistle. Lack of skill in inspiratory movements is particularly noticeable in patients with functional respiratory disorders (the muscles of expiration are exercised in skill whenever one speaks). If sucking is a great effort, a narrow drinking straw and a glass of water are helpful. In the beginning one often sees a patient able to whistle away vigorously while breathing out but literally gasping for air when whistling on an inward breath.

The therapist must be careful that, in whistling the chosen melody, the patient makes the transition from inhalation to exhalation and from exhalation to inhalation without a break in the tune and without breathing in between.

On top of this comes the patient's self-monitoring. He must not get out of breath, but he must also not hyperventilate. Incipient hyperventilation causes a sense of discomfort which feels like lack of air, but the harder the patient breathes, the worse he feels. There is only one thing to do then: take a break and wait until breathing has returned to normal again.

The therapist must make sure that the patient is always whistling around the respiratory mid-position, i. e. he must chance frequently enough from inspiration to expiration and back again.

Whistling to prevent air gulping can be done for any amount of time – for hours, if the patient likes.

Note

In all of the exercises for functional respiration training, hyperventilation is always a possibility. This is mainly because the exercises are performed in the absence of any particular stress on the cardiovascular system. For this reason there must always be enough pauses for breath. In the event of acute hyperventilation, the therapist simply holds the patient's nose and mouth closed.

---

5 Functional Treatment of Posture-Related Syndromes of the Spinal Column

Functional treatment of syndromes of the spinal column related to postural statics offers relief or at least alleviation of pain and irradiation in the spine by normalizing posture.

Pain and irradiation may be the result of faulty stress on the passive structures. The problems may be motor, sensory, circulatory or trophic in nature and may affect the cranial nerve, the cervical plexus, the brachial plexus, the thoracic nerves, the lumbar plexus, the pudendal nerve and the autonomic nervous system.

However, pain and irradiation can also arise from inappropriate demands made on muscles due to poor posture. The problem is then ischaemic in nature. Posture-related syndromes of the spinal column may be associated with other disorders as well, e.g. rheumatic or metabolic disorders, fractures, structural deformities, discopathies, wear and tear degeneration, osteoporosis, and many others. Such secondary diagnoses do affect the guidelines of functional treatment, but the changes are only a matter of degree and are made in relation to the prognosis.

Guidelines for Functional Training for Syndromes of the Spinal Column of Postural Static or Pathological Origin

In functional kinetics, postural statics are concerned with the influence a person's posture exerts, in the form of stresses and strains, on his motor apparatus (see *Functional Kinetics*, p. 244).

Because pain and irradiation in the spinal column are caused by improper posture, we have developed a movement therapy which is carried out under conditions of the least possible stress on the motor apparatus. Since the human musculature always has to cope with the weights of the parts of the body, we pay special attention to the latter in our attempt to reduce stress.

From the functional point of view, the muscle is the effector of posture and movement. It can act as a mover or lifter of weights, a breaker of falling weights, or a preventer of weights from falling, i.e. a fall-preventer (see *Functional Kinetics*, p. 55). During these actions, the movement causing the least stress will be the one that can be performed at a suitable speed and neither positive or negative lift is necessary (see *Functional Kinetics*, pp. 57–61).

> **Note**
> With lift-free and reduced-lift mobilization of the spinal column we aim to achieve maximum fine coordination of fine deformations (changes in position of joints) and dynamic stabilization of the spinal column in posture and movement, with a minimum of stress.
> Because the spinal column is functionally an antagonistic system, its physiological segments, the lumbar, thoracic and cervical spines, can be regarded neither as a whole not as entirely independent of one another.
> If one segment of the spinal column is to be successfully mobilized lift-free or with reduced lift, the movement event aimed at must be limited either by active buttressing within the body or by physical manipulation from the therapist.

Functional treatment of the spinal column has taught us the following:

- In postural deviations within the physiological curvatures of the spinal column (lumbar lordosis, thoracic kyphosis and cervical lordosis), flattening out of the curvatures leads to instability, and exaggeration of the curvatures leads first to hypermobility and later often to stiffness.
- When these physiological curvatures have been displaced upwards or downwards, stiffness develops in some movement segments and the postural muscles are stressed inappropriately. This is the case when there is kyphosis in the lordotic region, lordosis in the kyphotic region or scoliosis overlapping with any transition between the physiological curvatures of the spine.
- A patient with partial stiffnesses in the spinal column will not be able to normalize his posture by himself. In addition to lift-free and reduced-lift mobilization of the spinal column, another possible treatment technique is mobilizing massage (see *Functional Kinetics,* p. 301). Alongside this, the patient is taught how always to neutralize the inappropriate stress on the passive structures and the muscles, including the shoulder girdle, the shoulder and hip joints, by assuming relief postures at work and at rest.

5.1 Lift-Free/Reduced-Lift Mobilization of the Spinal Column (Figs. 40–56)

"Lift-Free/Reduced-Lift Mobilization of the Spinal Column" is a functional name. Both the patient and the therapist must never forget that reducing stress is the key to success with syndromes of the spinal column. The less weight has to be lifted against gravity or prevented from falling, the lower the stress.

163

■ Goal of the Exercise

The goal is for the patient to learn, without having to work against gravity, to:
- Freely move to vertebral joints, the vertebral-intervertebral disc articulations, the costovertebral joints and the hip joints
- Coordinate fine movements and fine changes in position of particular segments of the spinal column with dynamic stabilization of the adjacent segments, in order to reactivate the economical equilibrium reactions of the spinal column
- Improve the trophic conditions of the bony and serous structures, the ligaments, cartilage, muscles and nerves in the spinal region, the shoulder girdle, the pelvis and the hip joints, by activating the autochthonous muscles of the back
- Stimulate activity of the autochthonous muscles of the back in order to increase the capacity of the spinal column to endure posture-induced stress.

▶ Functional Analysis in Therapist Language

● Conception of the Exercise

When working to bring about lift-free/reduced-lift fine movements and dynamic stabilization in the spinal region through the dominant activity of the autochthonous muscles of the back, we must remember that this activity cannot be perceived as such by the patient. All he can feel is its aftereffect, a distinct feeling of local warmth. Therefore, to learn and to be able to reproduce these fine movements, the patient needs signals that he can perceive, described according to the orientation of the individual.

BSs pelvis, thorax and head should be aligned as well as possible in the long axis of the body. Then all the vertebral joint articulations are roughly in neutral position, and there is movement tolerance for all the components of movement.

In lift-free/reduced-lift mobilization of the spinal column, no joints of the body should be at end-stop in any of the starting positions. The weights of all the body segments must be so arranged that they neither hang in an uncontrolled manner from the spinal column nor will cause sudden strain on it during the movement sequence. Frictional resistance as parts of the body are moved about on a base support must be kept as low as possible.

Criteria of Lift-Free Mobilization of the Spinal Column

The activity involved in lift-free changes of position in the spinal column is primarily alternating concentric isotonic.

The axes of the intended lift-free movements are vertical. In this way, the weight of the body parts involved is only moved to and fro and no positive or negative lift is required.

Criteria of Reduced-Lift Mobilization of the Spinal Column
The activities involved in reduced-lift changes of position in the spinal column are coordinated isometric, concentric isotonic and eccentric isotonic. Weights are lifted and let down, held and shifted, but they are reduced to a minimum. We do this by neutralizing the weights of the non-moving body segments located above the moving segment, by positioning their long axes vertically or by transferring the weight onto a base support or a supportive or suspension device, as is done in relief positions.
The axes of movement of the intended reduced-lift movements are not bound to a particular position, but they are not vertical. It is advisable to begin with the axes of movement horizontal, because this makes it easiest to combine lift-free and reduced-lift movements, but in the long run the axes can be positioned at any angle.

● **Position and Activation in the Starting Position**

Position in Space of the Critical Axes
Points of Contact Between the Body and the Environment
Components of Movement in Relation to the Neutral Position of the Joints
For lift-free mobilization of the spinal column in lateroflexion, translation to the right/to the left and cranial/caudal traction, the patient lies on his back or on his stomach, because then the critical axes of movement, the gliding planes and the planes of contact are vertical (Figs. 40–43).
For lift-free mobilization of the spinal column in flexion/extension, ventral/dorsal translation and cranial/caudal traction the patient lies on his right or left side, because then the critical axes of movement, the gliding planes and the planes of contact are vertical (Figs. 44–46).
For lift-free mobilization of the spinal column in rotation, the patient sits or stands upright, because then the critical axes of rotation are vertical. The distance between the seat and the floor must be at least as great as the distance between the knee and the floor (including the heel of the patient's shoes) (Figs. 47–51).

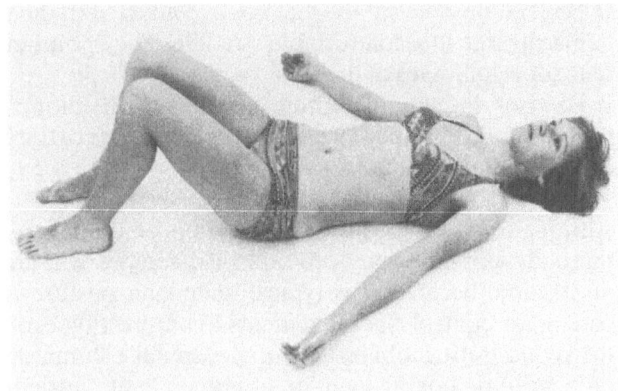

Fig. 40. Lift-Free Mobilization of the Spinal Column in Lateroflexion. Starting position

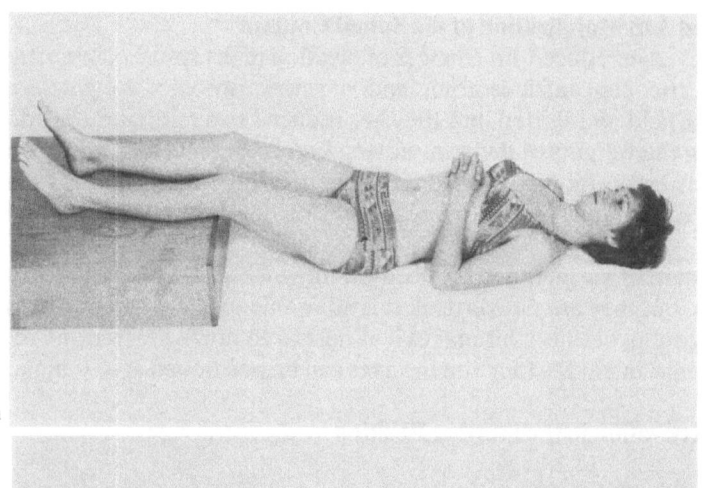

a

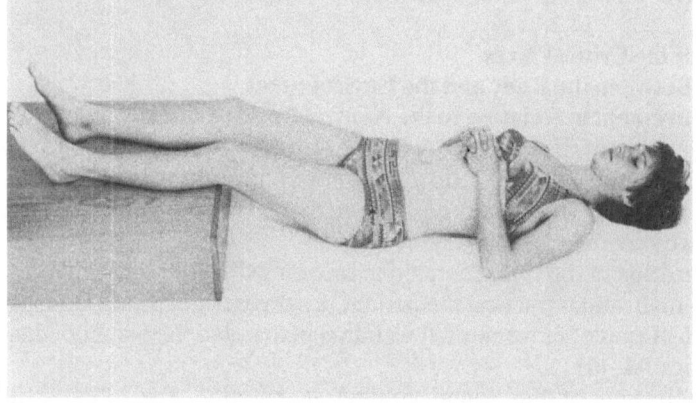

b

Fig. 41 a, b. Lift-Free Mobilization of the Thoracic and Cervical Spine in Lateroflexion. Movement tolerance for extension at the hip and flexion in the lumbar spine. **a** Thoracic spine left-concave, cervical spine right-concave lateroflexion. **b** Thoracic spine right-concave, cervical spine left-concave lateroflexion

In BS legs, the soles of the feet are in contact with the floor. The long axes of the thighs diverge in a comfortable straddle. They point in the same direction as the functional long axes of the feet.

In BS arms, the shoulder girdle is parked on the thorax and the hands rest one on top of the other on the sternum. The index finger of the hand underneath can hook onto the jugular notch.

Although for reduced-lift mobilization of the spinal column the long axis of the body can be in any position in space, we will choose upright standing for illustration, because it is typical of human posture and makes it easy for the patient to control his movements. The prototype of a good starting position for reduced-lift mobilization of the spinal column, as an alternative to sitting on a stool or box as mentioned above, is the upright two-legged stance (Figs. 52–56).

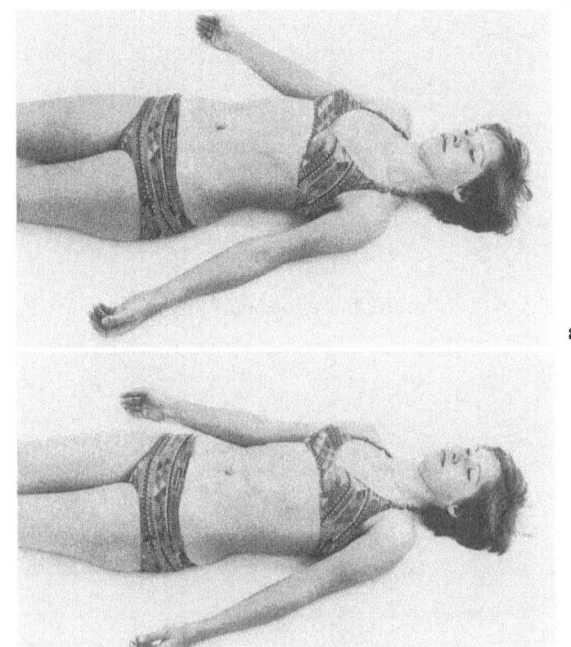

Fig. 42 a, b. Lift-Free Mobilization of the Thoracic and Cervical Spine in Lateroflexion. **a** Thoracic spine left-concave, cervical spine right concave lateroflexion. **b** Thoracic spine right-concave, cervical spine left-concave lateroflexion

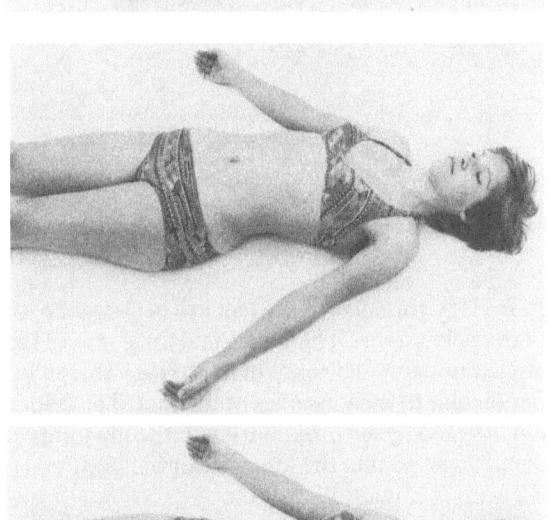

Fig. 43 a, b. Lift-Free Mobilization of the Lumbar Spine in Lateroflexion. **a** Left-concave lateroflexion, right hip in abduction, left hip in adduction. **b** Right-concave lateroflexion, right hip in adduction, left hip in abduction

167

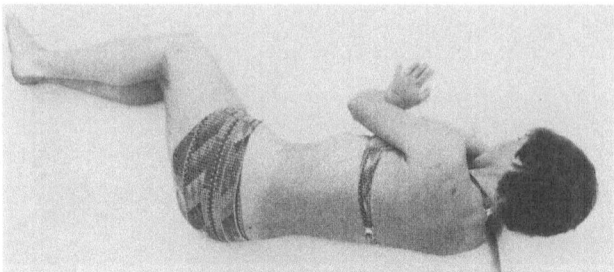

Fig. 44. Lift-Free Mobilization of the Spinal Column in Flexion/Extension. Starting position

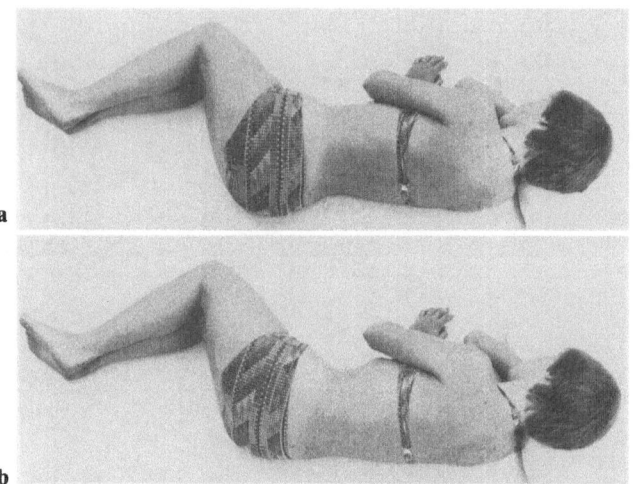

Fig. 45 a, b. Lift-Free Mobilization of the Lumbar Spine in Flexion/Extension. **a** Lumbar spine in extension, hips in flexion. **b** Lumbar spine in flexion, hips in extension

In BS legs, the soles of the feet are in contact with the floor. The feet are the width of the pelvis apart. The functional long axes of the feet point forwards or at a slight angle outwards. The axes of flexion/extension in the slightly flexed knees are perpendicular to the long axes of the feet. The talocrural joints are in slight dorsiflexion effected by the proximal lever, the hip joints are in slight flexion effected by the distal lever, so that the long axis of the body can be vertical.
BS arms is in neutral position.

**Distribution of Body Weight on a Base Support or Suspension Device,
Against a Supportive Device, or Over a Support Area,
and the Resulting Activity States of the Musculature**
In all of the positions described below – sidelying, supine, prone, or semisidelying – the alignment of BSs pelvis, thorax and head in the virtual long axis of the body should be maintained as closely as possible. Every body segment or part of a body segment must have an appropriate base support, so that the intensity of economical activity is almost the same as resting muscle tone.

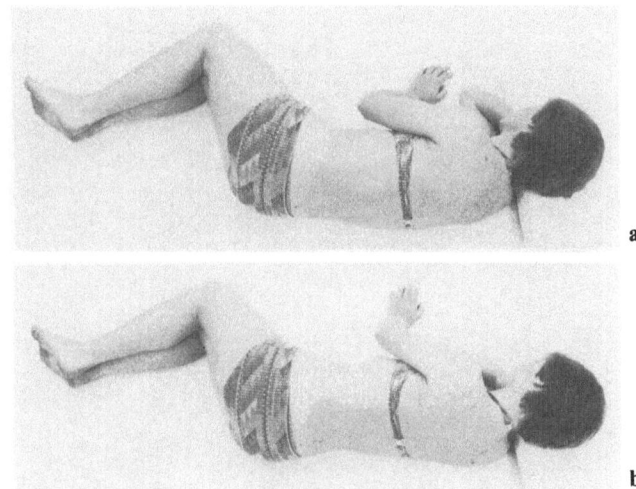

Fig. 46 a, b. Lift-Free Mobilization of the Thoracic Spine/Cervical Spine in Flexion/Extension. **a** Thoracic spine in flexion, cervical spine in extension. **b** Thoracic spine in extension, cervical spine in flexion

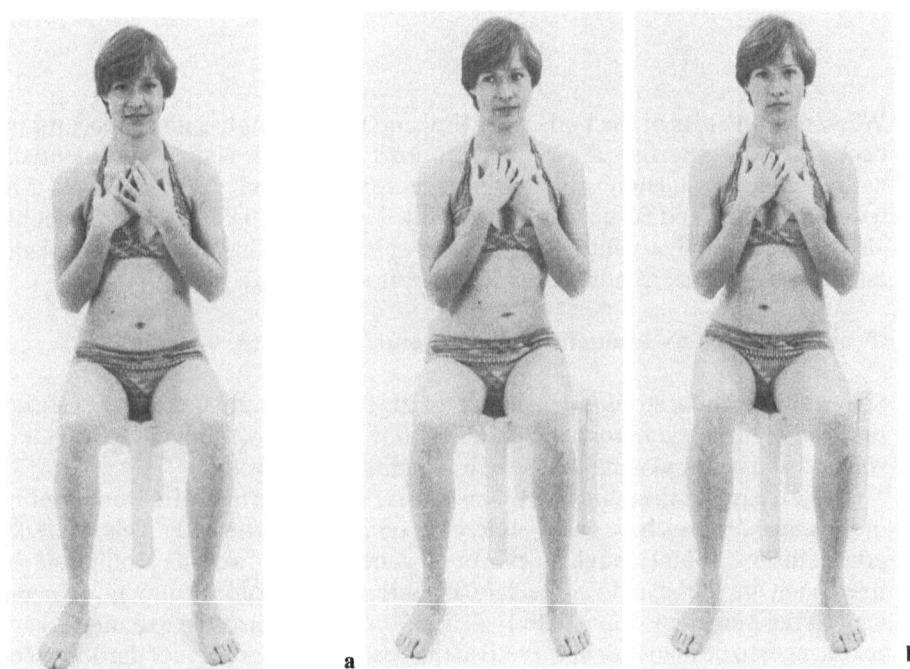

47

Fig. 47. Lift-Free Mobilization of the Spinal Column in Rotation, seated. Starting position

Fig. 48 a, b. Lift-Free Mobilization of the Thoracic Spine in Rotation. **a** Pelvis-negative rotation, right hip in horizontal abduction, left hip in horizontal adduction. **b** Pelvis-positive rotation, right hip in horizontal adduction, left hip in horizontal abduction

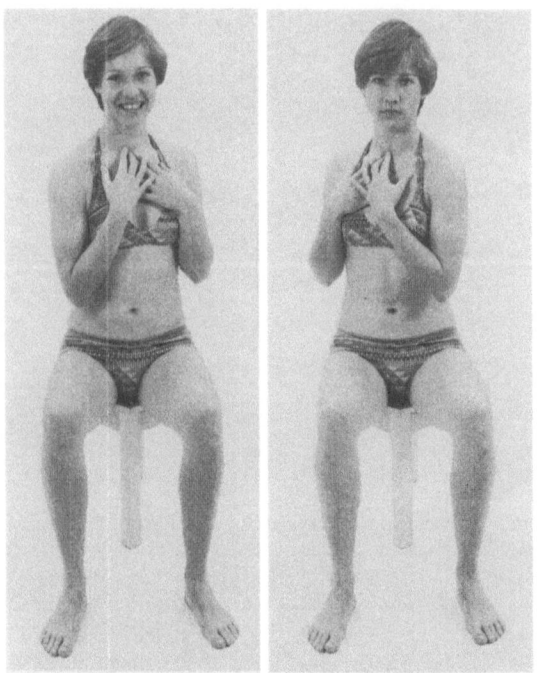

Fig. 49 a, b. Lift-Free Mobilization of the Thoracic Spine/Cervical Spine in Rotation. **a** Thoracic spine and cervical spine in thorax-negative rotation. **b** Thoracic spine and cervical spine in thorax-positive rotation

When the long axis of the body is vertical and the patient has no support for his back and no supporting devices for his arms, the pelvis should be potentially mobile in the hip and lumbar joints, the thoracic spine dynamically stabilized in its neutral position, and BS head, well-positioned in the long axis of the body, should also have potential mobility in the cervical spine and in the atlanto-occipital and atlanto-axial joints. Breathing should be normal and relaxed.

● **Actio, Conditio – Limitatio of the Movement Sequence**

Since lift-free/reduced-lift mobilization of the spinal column basically consists of simply moving a lever, pointer or gliding body to and fro, the many possibilities will be listed below as actio, followed by conditio and limitatio.

To make it easy for the patient to follow what is happening in lift-free mobilization of the spinal column, he is given a reference point on his own body. This reference point is the fixed point, and changes in the distance between a distance point and the fixed point are thus easy to appreciate. In therapist language the direction components (cranial/medial/ventral, etc.) will be given in detail, in order to define exactly the changes to be made (or observed) in the positions of the joints of the body. Too much detail in the instructions to the patient, however, would be confusing.

Example
Lift-free mobilization of the movement level lumbar spine/hip joint in lateroflexion/abduction/adduction the patient supine.

170

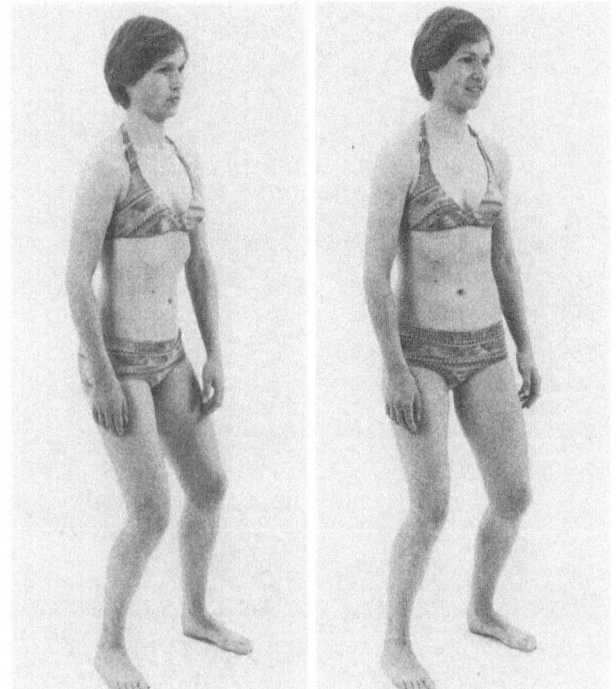

Fig. 50 a, b. Lift-Free Mobilization of the Thoracic Spine in Rotation, standing. **a** Pelvis-negative rotation, right hip in external rotation, left hip in internal rotation. **b** Pelvis-positive rotation, right hip in internal rotation, left hip in external rotation

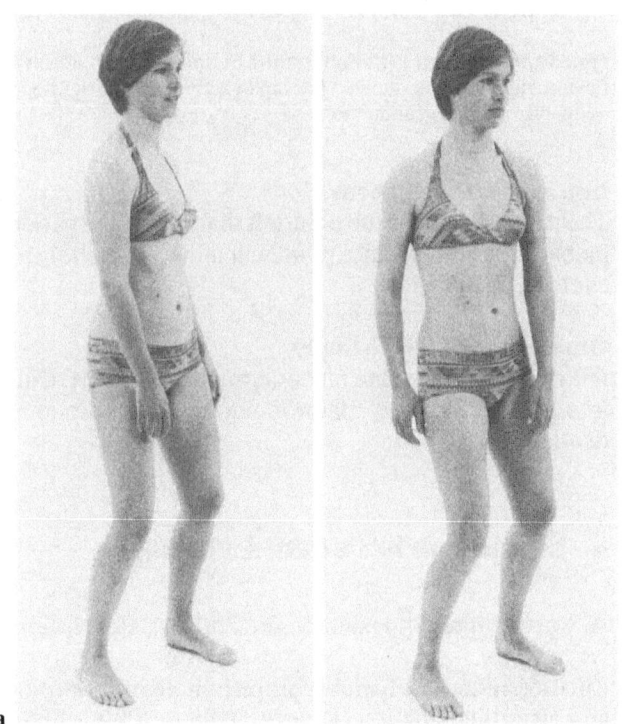

Fig. 51 a, b. Lift-Free Mobilization of the Thoracic Spine/Cervical Spine in Rotation, standing. **a** Thoracic and cervical spine in thorax-negative rotation. **b** Thoracic and cervical spine in thorax-positive rotation

171

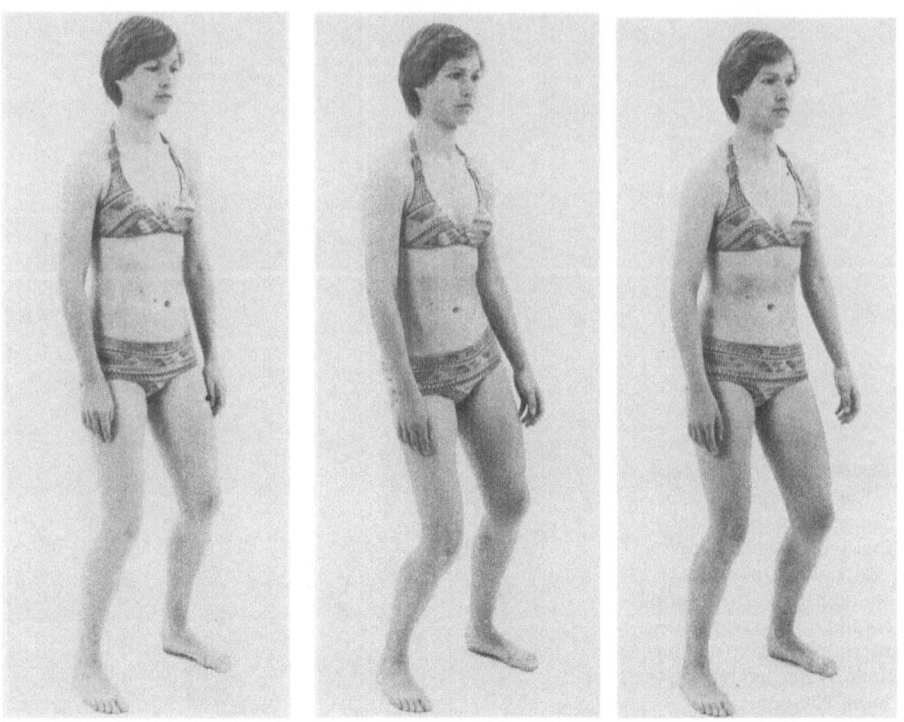

52

b

Fig. 52. Reduced-Lift Mobilization of the Spinal Column, standing. Starting position

Fig. 53 a, b. Reduced-Lift Mobilization of the Lumbar Spine in Lateroflexion. **a** Left-concave flexion, right hip in abduction, left hip in adduction. **b** Right-concave lateral flexion, right hip in adduction, left hip in abduction

Instruction to the Patient
The distance point is the right/left iliac spine (the patient learns to identify these by palpation). This distance point will move alternately towards the right and the left ear lobe (fixed point).

Observation by the Therapist
DP right/left iliac spine moves cranially/medially, causing the lumbar spine to go into right-/left-concave lateroflexion and the hip joints to go into adduction/abduction.

▶ Instruction in Patient Language

● Instructions Appealing to the Patient's Perceptions

Lift-free/reduced-lift mobilization imitates normal motor behaviour economically and gives the patient a chance to experience his body positively. Although cues

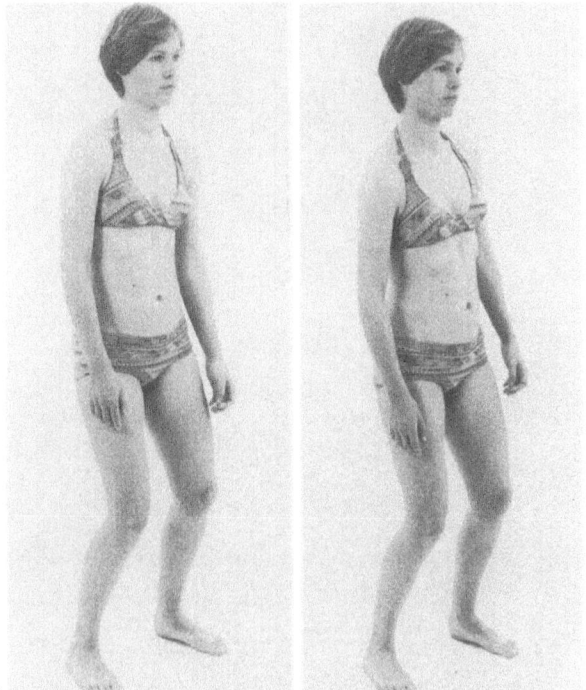

Fig. 54a, b. Reduced-Lift Mobilization of the Thoracic Spine/Cervical Spine in Lateroflexion. **a** Thoracic spine left-concave, cervical spine right-concave. **b** Thoracic spine right-concave, cervical spine left-concave

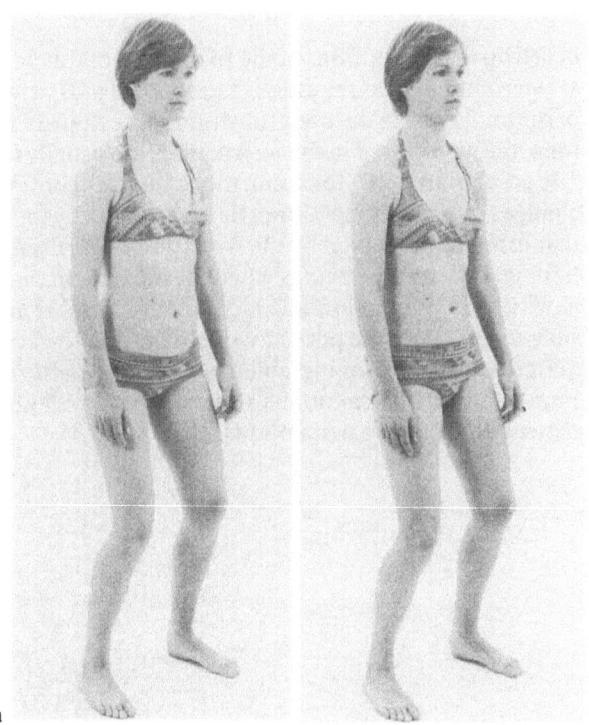

Fig. 55a, b. Reduced-Lift Mobilization of the Lumbar Spine in Flexion/Extension. **a** Lumbar spine in extension, hips in flexion. **b** Lumbar spine in flexion, hips in extension

173

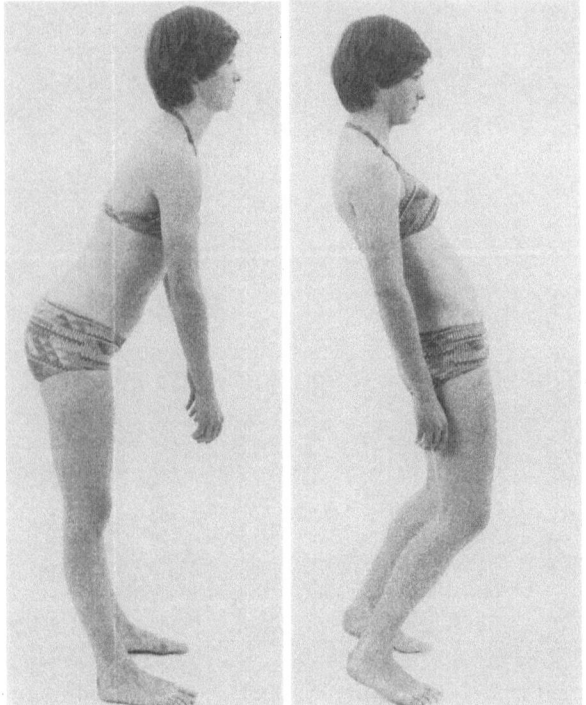

a

b

Fig. 56 a, b. Reduced-Lift
Mobilization of the Cervical
Spine in Flexion/Extension.
a Dorsal displacement of the
right/left greater trochanter,
cervical spine in extension.
b Ventral displacement of
the right/left greater trochanter, cervical spine in
flexion

based on the perceptions of the five senses of touch, taste, sight, hearing and smell
are in common general use as instructional aids, when it is changes in the position
of the joints within the body or within space that are required, or changes in muscle
tone, the words used in the instructions are usually inappropriate for the purpose.
"Bend and stretch" for joint movements, "contract and relax or release" for
changes in muscle tone cannot be understood by the body, because they cannot, in
that form, be perceived by the five senses. The uselessness of that kind of instructions is particularly obvious when the movement or change in tone required is one
in which the patient already has a disturbance. If an instruction is incomprehen-
sible to the body, the patient will not be able to carry it out on the strength of acquired conventions or ingrained behavioural patterns.

Impaired function cannot be restored to normal unless the language used to the
patient speaks to his perceptions.

Observation Criteria for the Therapist

Movement Level: Lumbar Spine/Hip Joints

Lumbar spine	*Lateroflexion*	*Translation* Caudal gliding body pelvis to the right/left	*Flexion/extension*
Hip joints	*Ab-/Adduction*	*Ab-/Adduction*	*Extension/flexion*
Position in space	Supine	Supine	Sidelying
Axes of movement	Vertical		Vertical
Gliding planes		Vertical	
Planes of movement	Horizontal	Horizontal	Horizontal
Position within the body			
Axes of movement	Sagittotransverse		Frontotransverse
Glinding planes		Transverse	
Planes of movement	Frontal	Frontal	Sagittal
Actio			
Moving lever	Line connecting right/left iliac spines		Long axis of the sacrum
Direction of the critical DPs:			
right/left iliac spines	Cranial/medial Caudal/medial	Lateral/to right Lateral/to left	Ventral/caudal Cranial/dorsal
right/left heels	Cranial/caudal	Fixed/starting position: straddle	Knee flexion
symphysis	Lateral/cranial to left/right	Lateral to right/left	Ventral/cranial, dorsal/caudal
coccyx	Lateral/cranial to right/left	Lateral to right/left	Ventral/caudal, dorsal/cranial
Conditio			
Constant distances	DP navel to DP jugular notch	DP chin to DP jugular notch	DP jugular notch to DP navel
Fixed spatial points	Frontotransverse diameter of the thorax Long axis of the sternum		Long axis of the sternum
Limitatio			
Active buttressing	TS contralateral lateroflexional	Thorax contralateral translational	TS antagonistic flexional/exten- tional

TS, thoracic spine

175

Movement Level: Lumbar Spine/Hip Joints		
Lumbar spine	*Translation* Caudal gliding body pelvis moves ventral/dorsal	*Rotation lower TS* Pelvis-positive/negative rotation
Hip joints	*Extension/flexion*	*Internal/external rotation* in standing *Transverse abduction/adduction* in sitting
Position in space Axes of movement Gliding planes Planes of movement	Sidelying Vertical Horizontal	Erect sitting/standing Vertical Horizontal
Position within the body Axes of movement Gliding planes Planes of movement	 Transverse Sagittal	 Frontosagittal Transverse
Actio Moving lever	Long axis of the sacrum	Line connecting right/left iliac spines
Direction of the critical DPs: right/left iliac spines	Ventral/dorsal	Ventral/medial, dorsal/lateral
right/left heels	Fixed	Fixed
symphysis	Ventral/dorsal	Lateral/dorsal/to the right/to the left
coccyx	Ventral/dorsal	Lateral/ventral/to the right/to the left
Conditio Constant distances		DP jugular notch to DP chin
Fixed spatial points	Long axis of the sternum	Frontotransverse diameter of the thorax
Limitatio Active buttressing	TS flexional/extensional Thorax ventral/dorsal trans- lational, antagonistic	TS antagonistic, rotational

TS, thoracic spine

Movement Level: Thoracic Spine/Cervical Spine

	Lateroflexion	Translation	Flexion/extension
Thoracic spine	*Lateroflexion*	*Translation* Cranial gliding body thorax moves to right/left	*Flexion/extension*
Cervical spine	*Contralateroflexion*	*Translation* Caudal gliding body thorax moves to right/left	*Extension/flexion*
Position in space Axes of movement Gliding planes Planes of movement	Supine Vertical Horizontal	Supine Vertical Horizontal	Sidelying Vertical Horizontal
Position within the body Axes of movement Gliding planes Planes of movement	Sagittotransverse . Frontal	Transverse Frontal	Frontotransverse Sagittal
Actio Moving lever	Frontotransverse diameter of thorax	Long axis of sternum	Long axis of sternum
Direction of critical DPs:			
C7	Lateral/caudal to right/left	To right/left	Ventral/caudal, dorsal/cranial
Jugular notch	Lateral/caudal to right/left	To right/left	Ventral/caudal, dorsal/cranial
Right/left nipple	Cranial/medial, caudal/medial		
Xiphoid process	Cranial/lateral to right/left	To right/left	Dorsal/caudal, ventral/cranial
Conditio Constant distances	DP right/left ears to DP right/left iliac spines		DP chin to DP symphysis
Fixed spatial points	Line connecting right/left iliac spines Line connecting right/left eyes		DP symphysis DP chin
Limitatio Active buttressing	Contralateroflexional in atlanto-occipital and atlanto-axial joints Abductional/adductional in right/left hip joints		Extensional/flexional in atlanto-occipital and atlanto-axial joints Flexional/extensional in hip joints and in LS

LS, lumbar spine

Movement Level: Thoracic Spine/Cervical Spine

Thoracic spine	*Translation* Cranial gliding body thorax moves ventrally/ dorsally	*Rotation lower TS* Thorax-positive/-negative rotation
Cervical spine	*Translation* Caudal gliding body thorax moves ventrally/ dorsally	*Rotation* Thorax-positive/-negative rotation
Position in space Axes of movement Gliding planes Planes of movement	Sidelying Vertical Horizontal	Erect sitting or standing Vertical Horizontal
Position within the body Axes of movement Gliding planes	 Transverse Sagittal	 Frontosagittal Transverse
Actio Moving lever	Long axis of the sternum	Frontotransverse diameter of the thorax
Direction of the critical DPs: C7	 Ventral/dorsal	 Ventral/lateral/to right/left
Jugular notch	Ventral/dorsal	Dorsal/lateral/to right/left
Right/left nipple	Ventral/dorsal	Ventral/medial, dorsal/lateral
Xiphoid process	Ventral/dorsal	Dorsal/lateral/to right/left
Conditio Constant distances	DP chin to DP symphysis	DP right/left iliac spines to DP right/left ear lobes
Fixed spatial points	DP right/left iliac spines DP chin	DP symphysis DP right/left eyes
Limitatio Active buttressing	Pelvis and head: antago- nistic, ventral/dorsal translational	Antagonistic rotational active buttressing by the pelvis in the hip joints Antagonistic rotational active buttressing by the head in the atlanto-occipital and atlanto-axial joints

5.1.1 Lift-Free Mobilization of the Spinal Column at Movement Level Lumbar Spine/Hip Joints

Lumbar Spine in Lateroflexion, Hip Joints in Abduction and Adduction (in Supine)

● **Actio**

On the moving lever, the line connecting the right and left iliac spines, critical DP right iliac spine moves cranially/medially and DP left iliac spine moves caudally/medially in relation to the plane of symmetry in the starting position. As they move, the lumbar spine goes into right-concave lateroflexion and the pelvis, as proximal lever, brings about adduction in the right hip and abduction in the left hip. (For the opposite movement, DP left iliac spine moves cranially/medially, and so on.)

● **Conditio – Limitatio**

The undesired continuing movement of right-concave lateroflexion of the thoracic spine is prevented by left-concave lateroflexional active buttressing in the thoracic spine.
The long axes of the legs move keeping parallel to each other, discreet internal rotational active buttressing in the hips keeping them in rotational neutral with the patellae facing roughly upwards/ventrally.

● **Verbal Instruction**

● **Instruction by Manipulation**

Position and Activation in the Starting Position

"Lie on your back. Together we're going to try to find the most comfortable position for you. You can lie your arms along your body on the floor with the palms facing upwards (Fig. 40) or you can fold your hands over your abdomen. Your eyes are looking straight ahead, your knees are facing slightly outwards. Breathing is quiet and easy."

The pillow should be just thick enough for the patient's head to rest on. The therapist must remember that the thicker the pillow, the further BS head is translated ventrally. Particular attention should be given to the placing of the arms. If the upper arms are short, they must be propped up off the support area by pillows, especially if the patient has a markedly deep thorax (frontosagittal diameter), otherwise the shoulder girdle will be displaced ventrally/caudally by continuing movement, bringing the cervical spine into increased extension and robbing it of its potential mobility. The decisive criterion in the placement of BS legs is that there must be movement tolerance for extension in the hip joints; this is essential for the potential mobility of the lumbar spine. A small roll placed under the knees often suffices. The therapist should not hesitate to position the lower legs so high that the lumbar spine is potentially mobile in all directions (Figs. 41).

Actio and Conditio of the Movement Sequence

"Right and left of your navel you can clearly feel your pelvic bones under the skin. If you move the one on the right towards your right shoulder, the left one moves towards your feet. And the other way around. Now move to and fro, effortlessly and at a good pace. Keep going. As you do, first one of your legs and then the other gets longer. Your rib cage lies quietly, as do your head and arms.

Let the movement slow down gradually. When you're done, have a good stretch and a big, luxurious yawn. Can you feel a little warmth in the small of your back? Good."

To learn the exercise, the patient places his hands on his iliac spines, and the therapist places her hands on top of the patient's. In this manner, the therapist can start the movement and make sure that DPs right and left iliac spines move in their frontal plane. At first, the patient won't even realize that he's doing anything himself. This is the best way to success in the fine movement of the lumbar spine. Gradually the therapist stops helping altogether and ultimately removes her hands. If the movement of the pelvis is transmitted to the thorax, no active buttressing has occurred and the mobilization is too far cranial; it has turned into an avoidance mechanism. The therapist can fix the frontotransverse diameter of the thorax with her hand, but must do so very lightly, for if it is perceived by the patient as a resistance, it will in effect reinforce the avoidance mechanism.

Lumbar Spine in Translation, Pelvis to the Right/Left, Hip Joints in Abduction and Adduction (in Supine)

● **Actio**

On the moving lever, the line connecting the iliac spines, critical DPs right and left iliac spines move right in their frontal plane. As they go, the movement of the pelvis deforms the lumbar spine by translation to the right, the right hip into adduc-

180

tion and the left hip into abduction. It is advisable for the heels to be somewhat more than the width of the pelvis apart in the starting position.

● **Conditio – Limitatio**

Any undesired deformation of the thoracic spine by right-concave lateroflexion and/or translation of the thorax to the right is prevented by thorax-left translational active buttressing (i. e. activation of the muscles that would be responsible for translating the thorax to the left). This keeps the distance between DP tip of the chin and DP jugular notch constant. DPs right and left heels remain on the base support, in slight rotation because the long axes of the legs, following the hips, have moved in their frontal planes. Discreet active buttressing in the hip joints, internal rotational in the right and external rotational in the left, holds them in rotational neutral and keeps the patellae facing roughly upwards/ventrally.

● **Verbal Instruction**

● **Instruction by Manipulation**

Position and Activation in the Starting Position

"You are lying on your back with your legs comfortably straddled and knees facing upwards. Touch those two bony projections on your pelvis with your thumbs."

The therapist checks the positioning, perfecting it with pillows. The only activity against gravity is that required to keep the patellae facing upwards.

Actio and Conditio of the Movement Sequence

"These two points are going to move a little bit to the right, and only to the right. You just have to imagine it properly first, and there it goes, you're moving without any further effort. Now come back to the centre. Repeat the process, first picturing it in your mind, then moving. When you have got used to this, practise the same thing to the left. Only then will you be ready to slide your pelvis in a leisurely kind of way, alternately right and left. Next, place one hand on your stomach and the other on your rib cage, touching the hollow of your neck with your index finger. You can feel the beat of your heart in it. Your 3rd, 4th and 5th fingers wander along down your breastbone towards your pelvis. When all your fingertips are resting on your breastbone, you can

In lateral translation of the pelvis, it is sometimes helpful for the heels to press down on the base support a little, to reduce frictional resistance. A towel can also be placed under the patient's pelvis, and the therapist can neutralize the frictional resistance by pulling on the towel in alternate directions while the patient is learning the movement. If associated movements of the thorax indicate that the lateral translational movements of the pelvis have triggered undesired continuing movements, the patient can be instructed to check for this avoidance mechanism by touching the long axis of his sternum. He must observe himself how the movement of the thorax is coordinated with the primary movement of the pelvis. He must find out for himself where the thorax

181

feel whether it is nice and straight in the middle of your rib cage or if it is slanting sideways. The little finger expecially is able to check whether the breastbone moves left or right with the pelvis. It shouldn't. The breastbone should stay still, while the pelvis moves easily right and left."

moves when the pelvis slides, for example, to the right. As soon as he understands this, he can prevent the avoidance mechanism himself. For this, the therapist must point out to him that the long axis of the sternum which he is touching must stay where it is, i.e. is a fixed spatial point. If the sternum stays in the right place, the avoidance mechanism has been checked by active buttressing.

Lumbar Spine in Flexion and Extension, Hip Joints in Extension and Flexion (in Sidelying)

● **Actio**

On the moving lever, the long axis of the sacrum, critical DP tip of the coccyx moves ventrally/caudally. The symphysis moves ventrally/cranially. As it does, the lumbar spine is brought into flexion and the pelvis, as proximal lever, brings about extension in the hip joints. If DP tip of the coccyx moves dorsally/cranially and DP symphysis moves dorsally/caudally, the lumbar spine is brought into extension and the pelvis, as proximal lever, brings about extension in the hip joints.

● **Conditio – Limitatio**

The undesired continuing movement of total flexion of the lumbar and thoracic spines is prevented by extensional active buttressing in the thoracic spine. The undesired continuing movement of total extension of the lumbar and thoracic spines is checked by flexional active buttressing in the thoracic spine. To keep the knees flexed as they were in the starting position, flexion in the hip joint effected by the pelvis as proximal lever is actively buttressed extensionally in the knee, and extension in the hip joint is actively buttressed flexionally in the knee.

● **Verbal Instruction**　　　　　● **Instruction by Manipulation**

Position and Activation in the Starting Position
"Lie on your side. You can rest your head on your lower arm or on a pillow it it's more comfortable. Your back should be long and straight. Pull your knees up a little so you can lie securely

If a pillow is needed under the head, it should be half as thick as the shoulders are wide, so as to keep BS head well-positioned in the long axis of the body.

and not roll onto your stomach. Your upper leg rests exactly on top of the lower one. If that's not comfortable, we can put a pillow between them."

If a pillow is needed under the upper leg, its thickness should correspond to the distance from the lower greater trochanter to the upper hip and it should be big enough for the medial aspect of the knee, the lower leg and the foot to lie on. Then the lower leg will be somewhat extended at the knee and hip joint.

If the weight of the upper arm threatens to compromise the vertical position of the frontotransverse diameter of the thorax, it will have to be propped up on a pillow. Ideally this pillow should be as thick as the shoulders are wide.

Actio and Conditio of the Movement Sequence

"You are lying on your right side. If you want, you can support yourself a little with your left hand in front of your navel. I am going to press down on the spot where your tail would begin if you were a dog. Imagine you have a tail. First you pull it in between your legs like a dog feeling cold, than you raise it high over your back to wag it happily. So it goes, to and fro, to and fro, quickly and easily. This makes your stomach short at first, then long. The same thing happens to the small of your back. Your back and neck stay the same length the whole time. You can keep moving like this as long as you like. When you stop, you can feel a slight warmth in the small of your back."

When giving the physical manipulative cues for this pelvic movement, the therapist places one hand on the patient's lower abdomen and the other on his sacrum. Another way to help the patient feel DP symphysis or DP tip of the coccyx is to press on them gently, while saying what changes in distance (e. g. from the navel) are to take place. In the legs the therapist observes the change in muscle activation, especially in the thighs, as the pelvis turns in flexion/extension at the hip joints. During flexion the dorsal muscles of the thighs are activated, during extension the ventral muscles are activated, but DPs right/left knees do not move in space. The therapist can clearly demonstrate the active buttressing in the thoracic spine region by applying slight resistance: during flexion of the lumbar spine (actively buttressed by extensional activity) the resistance is applied to the sternum; during extension of the lumbar spine (actively buttressed by flexional activity) the resistance is applied at the epigastric angle.

Lumbar Spine in Translation: Pelvis Ventrally/Dorsally, Hip Joints in Extension/Flexion, Knee Joints in Extension/Flexion (in Sidelying)

● **Actio**

The moving lever is the long axis of the sacrum. The critical distance points of the primary movement, DP tip of coccyx and DP symphysis, move alternately ventrally and dorsally in the plane of symmetry. When the distance points move ventrally, the lumbar spine is deformed by pelvis-ventral translation (i. e. translation brought about by the pelvis moving ventrally), the hip joints extend by ventral displacement of the fulcrum, and the thighs as proximal levers extend the knee joints. When DP tip of coccyx and DP symphysis move dorsally, the lumbar spine is deformed by pelvis-dorsal translation, the hip joints go into flexion by dorsal displacement of the fulcrum, and the thighs as proximal levers flex the knee joints.

● **Conditio – Limitatio**

The undesired continuing extensional effect on the thoracic spine as the pelvis translates ventrally is actively buttressed flexionally and dorsal-translationally, starting from the thorax. The undesired continuing flexional effect on the thoracic spine as the pelvis translates dorsally is actively buttressed extensionally and ventral-translationally, starting from the thorax. The long axis of the sternum has thus become a fixed spatial point and the distance from DP jugular notch to DP tip of the chin remains constant.

● **Verbal Instruction**   ● **Instruction by Manipulation**

Position and Activation in the Starting Position

"Lie comfortably on your side. Your legs lie on top of each other. Your knees and feet are farther forward than your stomach, so you can't roll over onto your stomach. Your upper hand can rest on the treatment bench in front of your navel or it can touch the bony spot below your navel."

In order for lift-free ventral/dorsal translation of the pelvis to take place unhindered, the flexion at the hip and knee joints should only be slight, even if, because of the patient's constitutional build, the upper leg needs to be parked ventrally to the other on a pillow. If the legs are not symmetrically placed, it is more difficult for the hip joints to move ventrally/dorsally in the displacement of the fulcrum. Placing a pillow between the patient's knees, lower legs and feet may be better. A pillow will also have to be put under the patient's waist if the distance between the greater trochanters is wide and the waist is narrow.

Actio and Conditio of the Movement Sequence

"This bony spot will move to and fro stomachwards and backwards. It will be easiest if you first just picture the movement in your mind. It must be quite effortless. You can use the other hand to help. Put your thumb in the hollow of your neck and the other fingers on your breastbone. Now you can feel if your breastbone moves when your pelvis does. It mustn't."

While the patient is learning the translation, the therapist can grasp his pelvis dorsally and ventrally between her hands and move it to and fro on the base support. As soon as the patient has felt this small movement, he will easily find the way to do it that suits him best. The therapist must realize, however, that the extent of the movement can only be about 2–3 cm.

Transition Lumbar Spine/Lower Thoracic Spine Pelvis-Positive and -Negative Rotation, Hip Joints in Transverse Abduction and Adduction (Upright Sitting on a Stool) or Internal and External Rotation (Upright Standing)

NB: With the patient sitting upright on a stool, the therapist must make sure that he doesn't shift weight from right to left as he moves his ischial tuberosities backwards and forwards. If the patient is standing, he must not shift weight from the right foot to the left. Weight shifting backwards and forwards along the functional long axes of the feet should be permitted, however, in order to allow the tolerance for rotation in the lower thoracic spine to be completely used up. This exercise can also well be performed standing on one leg.

● Actio

On the moving pointer, the line connecting the iliac spines, critical DPs right and left iliac spines move alternately ventrally/medially and dorsally/laterally in their transverse plane. If the right iliac spine moves laterally/dorsally and the left ventrally/medially, the spinal column, at the transition from the lumbar spine to the lower thoracic spine, deforms with the pelvis-positive rotation. If upright sitting is chosen as the starting position, the right hip joint moves into transverse adduction by backwards displacement of the fulcrum, and the left into abduction by forward displacement of the fulcrum.

If upright standing is chosen as the starting position, the pelvis as proximal pointer rotates internally in the right hip joint and externally in the left hip joint. By continuing movement, the weight over the right foot shifts slightly towards the heel and that over the left foot slightly towards the toes.

If upright one-legged standing is chosen as the starting position, the pelvis as proximal pointer either rotates internally in the right hip joint while the left forefoot rotates against the floor and the knee rotates inwards by continuing movement, or the pelvis rotates externally in the right hip joint while the left forefoot rotates against the floor and the left knee rotates outwards by continuing movement.

● Conditio – Limitatio

The undesired continuing movement of thorax-positive rotation in the cervical spine is actively buttressed thorax-negative rotationally in the lower thoracic spine. The frontotransverse diameter of the thorax thus becomes a fixed spatial point and the distance between DP jugular notch and DP tip of chin remains constant. If upright sitting is chosen as the starting position, the contact between the soles and the floor is kept as a fixed spatial point. When the hip joint moves into transverse abduction by forward displacement of the fulcrum, continuing movement brings the lower leg into dorsiflexion in the talocrural joint. When the hip joint moves into transverse adduction by backward displacement of the fulcrum, continuing movement brings the lower leg into plantarflexion in the talocrural joint.

● Verbal Instruction

● Instruction by Manipulation

Position and Actvation in the Starting Position

"Sit down on the stool; across the corner will be best. Your legs rest on the floor, comfortably straddled. Your hands are crossed gently on your chest. Your back is long and straight. Your head balances above your shoulders; don't let it slip down forwards. Your eyes look straight ahead. Your breathing is slow and quiet."

The patient should be sitting on his ischial tuberosities. The stool must be at least as high as the knees from the floor. The legs should be parked on the floor. BSs pelvis, thorax and head are aligned in the long axis of the body, which is vertical. The activity is economical. The weight of the arms is partly parked on BS thorax; the rest hangs via the hands from the jugular notch and facilitates stabilization of the thoracic spine in extension; in patients with – TS (flat back) this weight effective ventral to the flexion/extension axis is indispensable for the stabilization of the thoracic spine. The reduced activity of the abdominal and lumbar muscles makes normal breathing possible and facilitates readiness for rotation. It may be easier for the patient to learn the proper position of BS head if the therapist translates it dorsally by manipulation.

Actio and Conditio of the Movement Sequence

"You are sitting across the corner of the stool, hands crossed gently over each other on your chest, and looking

In this exercise, the patient will usually rotate BSs pelvis and thorax en bloc in the cervical spine instead of rotating

186

straight ahead. Estimate your distance from some object in your field of view. Now make this distance a bit longer, without looking away. Your back and neck are long and you feel no tension in your stomach or in the small of your back. Your breathing is effortless and automatic. Then push now your right, now your left knee backwards a little, alternately, without straining and at a good pace. You slip to and fro on the stool with the movement, but without transferring any weight to right or left. Your rib cage and head stay quietly where they are. With your hands resting on your rib cage, you can feel whether it is moving too. When you stop moving, you can feel a slight warmth in the small of our back and around your hip joints."

just the pelvis at the level upper lumbar/lower thoracic spine. To ensure that BS pelvis rotates below BS thorax, with transverse abduction and adduction in the hip joints (owing to the starting position on the seat of the stool), the therapist can grasp the patient's thorax in the right and left axillae and fix the frontotransverse diameter of the thorax in space. This fixation must be very gentle and must not be perceived as resistance: it is rather a perceptual aid to show the patient what it feels like when his thorax doesn't turn with the pelvis. The therapist can also help the pelvic rotation, by either grasping the pelvis itself by the iliac spines or by pushing one knee backwards and pulling the other forwards alternately.

5.1.2 Lift-Free Mobilization of the Spinal Column at Movement Level Thoracic Spine/Cervical Spine

Thoracic Spine in Right-/Left-Concave Lateroflexion, Cervical Spine in Left-/Right-Concave Lateroflexion

NB: There are two variants of lift-free mobilization of the spinal column at the movement level thoracic spine/cervical spine: either BS arms moves with the thorax or the thorax moves in the sternoclavicular joints with the right and left pincer jaws stationary. The movement of the latter variant is more complicated and finely differentiated; it is indicated for patients with uneven muscle tone in the muscles connecting the shoulder girdle to the thorax. In practice, either arm or both are brought into the relief position of the Little Shepherd Boy (see p. 290).
There are similar variants of translations of the thorax to right and left.

● **Actio**

The moving lever, the frontotransverse diameter of the thorax, rotates in the midfrontal plane. While critical DP jugular notch moves alternately caudally/laterally/right and caudally/laterally/left, and critical DPs right and left nipple move alternately cranially/medially and caudally/medially, the thoracic spine deforms in

187

lateroflexion and the cervical spine in contralateral lateroflexion. If DP jugular notch moves caudally/laterally/right, DP right nipple caudally/medially and DP left nipple cranially/medially, the thoracic spine goes into right-concave lateroflexion and the cervical spine into left-concave lateroflexion.

● **Conditio – Limitatio**

The undesired continuing movement of right-concave lateroflexion in the lumbar spine and of adduction in the right hip joint with abduction in the left by cranial and caudal displacement of the fulcra, respectively, is actively buttressed left-concave lateroflexionally in the lumbar spine, abductionally in the right hip joint and adductionally in the left hip joint (and the other way around for left-concave lateroflexion of the lumbar spine). Thus the line connecting the right and left iliac spines remains fixed in space. The undesired inclination of the head to the right due to caudal-to-cranially continuing movement is actively buttressed by the head left-concave lateroflexionally in the atlanto-occipital and atlanto-axial joints (and vice versa). Thus the line connecting the right and left eyes remains fixed.

● **Verbal Instruction**   ● **Instruction by Manipulation**

Position and Activation in the Starting Position

"Lie comfortably on your back. Place both hands on your rib cage with your index fingers touching the hollow of your neck."

The positioning of the hands on the thorax must be comfortable and also enable the patient to feel the thorax moving.

Actio and Conditio of the Movement Sequence

"When your right hand moves with your rib cage towards your head, your left hand moves with your rib cage towards your feet. Your head stays quietly where it is, your eyes looking at the ceiling. The to-and-fro movement continues easily, like a perpetual motion machine, with no exertion and at a good pace. If you want, you can place one arm over your head and with the other feel how your thorax can go on moving without disturbing the shoulder girdle lying on the bed. When you stop, you can feel a slight warmth between your shoulder blades."

Whether the shoulder girdle and the arms move with the thorax or whether the arms are placed in the Little Shepherd Boy position is decided in each case individually. If the line connecting the iliac spines remains frontotransverse, the therapist knows that the active buttressing has taken place in the lumbar spine and the hip joints. She must also watch that the patient's head stays still: that is a sign of active buttressing in the atlanto-occipital and atlanto-axial joints.

Lower Thoracic Spine in Thorax-Right/-Left Lateral Translation, Cervical Spine in Thorax-Right/-Left Lateral Translation (in Supine)

● Actio

On the moving lever, the long axis of the sternum, critical DPs jugular notch and xiphoid process move right/left, each in its frontal plane. If the two distance points move right, the lower thoracic spine is deformed by thorax-right translation performed by its cranial gliding body, and the cervical spine is deformed by thorax-right translation performed by its caudal gliding body.

● Conditio – Limitatio

The undesired continuing movement of left-concave lateroflexion in the thoracic spine is checked by right-concave lateroflexional active buttressing at that level. Pelvis-left translation of the lumbothoracic spine is prevented by pelvis-right translational active buttressing. Now the line connecting the iliac spines is fixed in space. Inclination of the head to the left is prevented by right-concave lateroflexional active buttressing in the atlanto-occipital and atlanto-axial joints. Now the line connecting the eyes is fixed in space and the distances between DP right ear and DP right iliac spine and between DP left ear and DP left iliac spine remain constant.

● Verbal Instruction

● Instruction by Manipulation

Position and Activation in the Starting Position

"Lie comfortably on your back. Link your fingers so that you can line them up (without the thumbs) along your breastbone, nicely in the middle of your rib cage, with your index fingers near the hollow of your neck."

The therapist must make absolutely sure that the virtual long axis of the body has been soundly constituted by proper alignment of BSs pelvis, thorax and head. A pillow may only be placed to raise the head if the cervical spine would otherwise lose its potential mobility. This happens especially in functional cervical kyphosis, when the head cannot be properly aligned even when the patient is standing upright. If the head is markedly raised, the lateral translation of the thorax will not be economically transmitted to the cervical spine. In such cases, one should attempt to reduce the existing stiffness by mobilizing massage.

Actio and Conditio of the Movement Sequence

"Your breathing is very quiet. Imagine that you want to move this straight piece of breastbone that you feel under

If the therapist sees any avoidance mechanisms during lift-free lateral translation of the thorax, she helps the

your fingers a little to the right, about 2 cm. It's very easy. Now come back to the middle. Now move it to the left. Think – move – think – move. As soon as your body has absorbed this movement it flows easily to and fro with no effort or haste. But you still have to pay attention. The breastbone under your fingers must not roll around or bob up and down. Just a little bit to the right, then a little to the left. Now we're going to check really closely. Your left hand stays on your breastbone, moving right and left with it. Your right thumb and index finger form pincers and grip your cheekbone. Nothing should move there; everything stays still. Now place your right hand, that's doing the monitoring on your stomach, on the footward side of your navel. There can be rumblings down there, but there mustn't be any to-and-fro movement."

patient to feel the incorrect movement of the fixed points, and the direction in which they have moved, by touching the critical distance points. Thus the patient learns how to refrain from avoidance mechanisms himself, unless existing pain or restrictions of movement make correction impossible.

Thoracic Spine in Flexion/Extension, Cervical Spine in Extension/Flexion (in Sidelying)

NB: During flexion/extension, the upper pincer jaws and the upper arm move with the thorax, while the lower pincer jaws are fixed by being lain on and do not participate in the movement. This is also the case in ventral and dorsal translations.

● **Actio**

On the moving lever, the long axis of the sternum, critical DP jugular notch moves ventrally/caudally and critical DP xiphoid process dorsally/caudally in the plane of symmetry. The thoracic spine flexes cranial-to-caudally while extension takes place in the cervical spine, effected by its caudal lever.
If DP jugular notch moves dorsally/cranially and DP xiphoid process moves ventrally/cranially in the plane of symmetry, the thoracic spine extends and the cervical spine is flexed by the caudal lever.

● **Conditio – Limitatio**

The unwanted continuing movement of a total flexion of the thoracic and lumbar spines caudally and hyperextension of the cervical spine cranially are actively buttressed caudally by the pelvis, flexionally in the hip joints and extensionally in the lumbar spine. The pelvis thus becomes a fixed spatial point. Cranially, fixed spatial point DP tip of the chin is held steady by flexional active buttressing in the atlanto-occipital and atlanto-axial joints.

● **Verbal Instruction**　　　　　　　● **Instruction by Manipulation**

Position and Activation in the Starting Position

"Lie comfortably on your right side. Your pelvis, rib cage and head are like a tower on its side. Your knees and hips are comfortably flexed."

When the therapist checks the starting position, she will almost always find that the head needs to be dorsally translated into the correct position.

Actio and Conditio of the Movement Sequence

"Put the tip of middle finger of your left hand in the hollow of your neck. Move this spot gently towards your chin, then away from it, without letting your head drop forwards. You shouldn't breathe in rhythm with the movement; the best thing would be to whistle a tune softly through your teeth, inwards and outwards. Your tail doesn't move. When the movement stops, your back feels nice and warm."

To guide the movement of the thorax, the therapist places her one hand on the patient's sternum and the other on the middle part of his thoracic spine. To flex the thoracic spine, she pulls the sternum gently caudally; to extend the thoracic spine, she pushes a little harder on the spinal processes of the thoracic spine. She watches the patient's breathing, which should be light and independent of the movement. *Caution:* Patients often hyperventilate performing this exercise.

If the therapist wants to facilitate the active buttressing in the area of the lumbar spine, she applies fine extensional resistance for the lumbar spine at the coccyx during thoracic spinal flexion and flexional resistance on the symphysis during thoracic spinal extension.

Lower Thoracic Spine in Ventral/Dorsal Translation of the Thorax, Cervical Spine in Ventral/Dorsal Translation of the Thorax (in Sidelying)

● **Actio**

On the moving lever, the long axis of the sternum, critical DPs jugular notch and xiphoid process move alternately ventrally and dorsally in the plane of symmetry.

When they move ventrally, the lower thoracic and upper lumbar spines are ventral-translationally deformed by the ventral movement of their cranial gliding body and the cervical spine is ventral-translationally deformed by the movement of its caudal gliding body. When DPs jugular notch and xiphoid process move dorsally, the dorsal movement of the thorax as cranial gliding body causes dorsal-translational deformation of the lower thoracic and upper lumbar spines, and as caudal gliding body causes dorsal-translational deformation of the cervical spine.

● **Conditio – Limitatio**

The unwanted movement continuing from a ventral translation of the thorax is, in the caudal area, a flexional movement of the pelvis in the hip joints together with extension in the lumbar spine. Dorsal-translational active buttressing of the pelvis prevents this avoidance mechanism. Dorsal translation of the thorax can cause an unwanted continuing extensional movement of the pelvis in the hip joints and flexion of the lumbar spine. Ventral-translational active buttressing of the pelvis prevents the avoidance mechanism. In the cranial area it is the head that undertakes active buttressing antagonistically to the ventral/dorsal translation of the thorax, thus actively buttressing the unwanted forward or backward inclination of the head by extensional or flexional activity at the atlanto-occipital and atlanto-axial joints and keeping the fixed spatial point DP tip of the chin in place.

● **Verbal Instruction**   ● **Instruction by Manipulation**

Position and Activation in the Starting Position

"Lie comfortably on your right side. The inside of the left leg rests on the right leg. Your knees and hips are comfortably bent to keep you from rolling onto your stomach."

The sidelying position must be adjusted individually for every patient. In addition to needing a shoulder-wide pillow under the head, we may, in patients with small frontotransverse diameter of the thorax and wide distance between the greater trochanters, need to raise the entire thorax on a thin pillow. We will also have to place pillows under a narrow waist. Patients with a wide distance between the greater trochanters will need a suitably thick pillow between the upper leg and the lower.

Actio and Conditio of the Movement Sequence

"Place your left palm on your stomach, footwards of your navel. Put your right

If the patient has trouble monitoring the thorax with his right hand, he can hand on your rib cage so that the whole underside of your thumb runs like a rail down your breastbone. Now, without turning, your whole breastbone, together with your hand, moves about 2 cm forwards. The hand on your stomach can feel that your stomach doesn't move from where it is. Your navel in particular must not move forwards even the tiniest bit. When you have repeated this slight movement several times and you can do it effortlessly, we'll turn the skewer around and let the breastbone and hand do the same parallel movement backwards, while your navel and lower abdomen stay quite still and don't allow themselves to be enticed backwards."

use his left. Because the pelvis remains stationary during ventral/dorsal translation of the thorax, the upper hip joint can be flexed up to 90°. The only important thing is that the entire lower leg, foot and of course the knee are properly positioned. If the therapist is working with trainee assistants, one person can hold the pelvis in place and another the head, while the third helps to translate the thorax. If the therapist is working alone with the patient – as is usually the case – it is advisable during the learning stage of this none-too-easy exercise to hold sometimes the pelvis, sometimes the head, and sometimes to help translate the thorax.

Lower Thoracic Spine in Thorax-Positive/Negative Rotation, Cervical Spine in Thorax-Positive/Negative Rotation (in Upright Sitting on a Stool)

● **Actio**

On the moving pointer, the frontotransverse diameter of the thorax, critical DPs right and left nipples move alternately ventrally/medially and dorsally/laterally. DP jugular notch, lying in the plane of symmetry, moves alternately dorsally/laterally/right and dorsally/laterally/left. If DP right nipple moves dorsally/laterally, DP left nipple ventrally/medially and DP jugular notch dorsally/laterally/right, the lower thoracic spine will be rotated thorax-positively by its cranial pointer and the cervical spine thorax-positively by its caudal pointer (and the other way around for rotation in the other direction). The pointer rotates and the distance points move in their transverse planes.

● **Conditio – Limitatio**

The unwanted continuing movement of the pelvis, with transverse adduction in the right hip joint and transverse abduction in the left hip joint by backward/forward displacement of the fulcrum, is actively buttressed pelvis-negative rotationally by transverse abductional activity at the right hip joint and transverse adductional activity at the left hip joint.

If upright standing is chosen as the starting position, the pelvis-negative rotational active buttressing will be by external rotational activity at the right hip and internal rotational activity at the left hip joint. In both cases, DP symphysis remains stationary as a fixed spatial point. The unwanted continuing movement in the cranial area, rotation of the head to the right, is actively buttressed negative-rotationally in the atlanto-occipital and atlanto-axial joints. The line connecting the eyes remains stationary as a fixed spatial point.

● **Verbal Instruction**

● **Instruction by Manipulation**

Position and Activation in the Starting Position

"Sit diagonally, straddling the corner of a stool, and cross your hands gently on your chest. Look straight ahead and estimate how far it is to any object in your line of vision. Make it a bit further, without changing the direction you are looking in. Keep your breathing relaxed. Although your back and neck are long, you feel no tension anywhere, neither in your stomach nor in the small of your back."

In this exercise, the observing therapist must make sure that the dorsal and ventral muscles of the waist are brought into economical activity before BS thorax rotates. Hyperactivity in these muscles will block rotation at the proper level in the thoracic spine (normal breathing). It is helpful to manually translate BS head dorsally and then apply slight compressive resistance to the long axis of the body at DP vertex. The therapist must be very careful to watch that the patient is breathing normally.

Actio and Conditio of the Movement Sequence

"Now your rib cage starts to turn smoothly and easily to and fro below your head and above your pelvis. Your hands stay on your chest, going with the movement left and right. You keep the pace brisk, like the rhythm of a hiking song. You shouldn't slide about on the chair. Your legs stay calmly on the floor and the knees don't change their distance from one another. When the movement stops, you can feel a slight warmth about your spine and in your waist and neck."

To make the active buttressing easier, the therapist can touch the left iliac spine, applying very light resistance against positive rotation of the pelvis (when the thorax has rotated negatively), but this resistance should only be enough to keep the line connecting the two iliac spines (caudal pointer of rotation) fixed in space. This activates the horizontal abductors and adductors at the hips alternately.

5.1.3 Reduced-Lift Mobilization of the Spinal Column at Movement Level Lumbar Spine/Hip Joints

> **Note**
> The position of the fulcra, axes of movement, gliding planes and planes of the body; the levers, pointers and gliding bodies moved; and the directions in which the critical distance points move, the constant distances on the patient's own body, and the definition of fixed spatial points, are all the same in reduced-lift mobilization as in lift-free mobilization. What has changed is their position in space, and with this, positive and negative lifting strain stress arise.

Example 1
A patient who can do the exercises for lift-free/reduced-lift mobilization of the spinal column wants to do economical spinal column mobilization at home in the morning lying on his back in bed.
As a base support, the bed offers more frictional resistance than the floor or treatment bench. In right/left translation he can reduce this resistance on his pelvis by pressing down slightly on the base support with his heels; for the thorax he can reduce it by pressing down slightly with his elbows and head. When he performs mobilization in flexion/extension in supine, there is lifting stress on the abdominal muscles and lifting stress in bridging activity on the muscles of the back. In rotations, it is functionally very important to lift the rotating body, the pelvis or the thorax, higher than usual, so that the rotations can be carried out without any translation.

Example 2
Reduced-lift mobilization of the lumbar spine in lateroflexion, of the hip joints in abduction/adduction (while standing on the right leg).

● **Verbal Instruction**   ● **Instruction by Manipulation**

Position and Activation in the Starting Position

"You are standing with your legs a little apart and can feel the floor pressing against the sole of your right foot – to be specific, against your heel and forefoot, especially the ball of your big toe. Your toes are relaxed and you shouldn't feel any tension in the back of your knee. Your left leg is resting on the floor,

If necessary, the therapist grasps both of the patient's greater trochanters and shifts them gently, together with everything above them, over the contact point right sole/floor. Shifting the weight towards the forefoot corrects any passive hyperextension of the right knee. If the patient does not succeed in

toes next to the arch of your right foot. To keep the left leg from being too long, the knee and hip joints bend a little. Your right hand rests on the pelvis, your left a little lower, at the spot where the hip is bent in. Your fingers point forwards, the thumbs backwards. You feel no effort and your breathing comes quietly. Your eyes look straight ahead and keep a certain distance from what they see. This makes you feel secure and as though you have a long back. Swaying slightly to and fro in rhythm with your breathing keeps you from getting tired."

shifting his weight towards the ball of the big toe, we can achieve activation of the longitudinal arch of the foot by either verbal instruction or manipulation to reduce the stress on the ball of the little toe. Resting his right hand on the right pelvic crest and grasping the left trochanter (critical DP) with his left hand, makes it easier for the patient to take in the movements of the pointer, the line connecting the greater trochanters.

The reduction of the activity of the abdominal muscles, coordinated with the tendency of BS head to translate dorsally ("eyes keeping a distance"), conditions normal breathing. Being aware of the slight swaying of the body will help the patient to find economical activity more easily. The flexion in the hip and knee joints of the parked left leg brings about the functional shortening of the leg necessary to offset the plantarflexion in the left foot.

Actio and Conditio of the Movement Sequence

"You are holding something firm in your left hand. It is your left hip. That is the spot from which the movement starts. Smoothly and easily, this spot with the hand on it starts to move up and down, but not forwards or backwards. When it goes down, your left leg bends a little more; when it goes up, your left leg straightens, but without the tip of your foot either leaving the floor or pressing against it too hard. If you look in the mirror, you can see what you can already feel: when your left hand goes down, the right one goes up and vice versa. You can do this movement fast or slow, just as you like. But everything above the waist stays still, like a picture in a frame. Watch yourself in the mirror: your reflection must not move, not to the right, not to the left, not upwards, not downwards. And be

The therapist can manually help the movement of the greater trochanter, the distance point for lateroflexion in the lumbar spine and for abduction and adduction of the right hip joint, in its midfrontal plane. She can see whether active buttressing (limitation) of the abduction/adduction in the right hip joint has taken place by whether or not the very frequent avoidance mechanism of inversion/eversion in the subtalar and talocalcaneonavicular joints of the right foot has occurred. If the fronto-transverse diameter of the thorax remains in its horizontal resting position, she knows that active buttressing of the lateroflexion of the lumbar spine has taken place. In the functional shortening of the leg the left knee must move forwards, otherwise BS pelvis cannot move in the frontal plane. When the leg

careful of your right foot. Don't tip from the inner to the outer edge as you move."

is functionally relengthened, the left knee moves back again. The therapist must make sure that the left leg doesn't go into free play by becoming suspended from the body. On the other hand, the parking function of this leg may be compromised by a little judicious pressure activity during the lifting of the weight of the pelvis and a little braking negative lift during the lowering, thus achieving the desired reduced lifting stress on the lumbar spine.

Conditio of Movement Speed
Limitatio of Economical Activity by Finding the Optimal Speed

The first thing we aim for in lift-free/reduced-lift mobilization of the spinal column is low intensity of economical activity. This is the only way in which potential mobility of the lordotic segments of the spinal column can be achieved and more or less maintained even when the position of the spinal column in space changes: for example, the potential mobility of the atlanto-occipital and atlanto-axial joints when the long axis of the body is inclined forwards. Then we stimulate the activity of the autochthonous muscles of the spinal column called for in the goal of the exercise. For a good speed, the speed of normal gait suggests itself, i.e. around 120 movement excursions per minute, for this rate, the rhythm of human locomotion, is likely to be as economical as we can find. A speed nearly double that, however, may be more suitable for some work units, particularly those that are lift-free. A very slow speed is only indicated in the learning stage.
It is essential that breathing remain normal throughout.

▶ Adapting the Exercises to the Patient's Constitution and Condition

● Adaptation to Constitution: Role of Lengths, Widths, Depths and Distribution of Weights

In lift-free/reduced-lift mobilization of the spinal column, any constitutional deviations from the norm are only significant when the body is placed with its long axis horizontal, because in all starting positions BSs thorax and head must be aligned as well as possible in the long axis of the body.

● **Adaptation to Condition**

Restricted Movement and/or Hypermobility
In lift-free/reduced-lift mobilization of the spinal column it is primarily movement restrictions in the spinal column and the hip joint that will prevent optimal alignment of the body segments in the long axis of the body. It is therefore always the first goal of treatment to overcome these restrictions. If there are muscle contractures, intensive stretching exercises are performed. If the cause lies in the passive structures and radiography indicates no irreversible ankylosis, therapy must work towards remobilization. This is a lengthy process, but is usually successful, and in the interim the patient should be taught relief postures to be used in all activities of daily living.

5.2 Building Blocks: Basic Exercise for Posture-Related Problems in the Spinal Column and in the Hip Joints (Fig. 57)

"Building Blocks" is an invented name. The demand in lift-free/reduced-lift mobilization of the spinal column for alignment of BSs pelvis, thorax and head in the long axis of the body makes it natural to imagine the body segments as building blocks. Like children with their wooden blocks, we can build the body segments up on top of each other, and if we want to tilt the turret we have built out of the vertical, we must hold the blocks together so that none of them slips out of line.

■ Goal of the Exercise

A good block builder should be able to:
– Produce the best possible vertical virtual long axis of the body by building up BSs pelvis, thorax and head on top of each other
– Bring the body segments thus aligned into economical activity: BSs pelvis and head are then in the activity state of potential mobility and the thoracic spine is in extensional dynamic stabilization in the neutral position
– Keep the virtual long axis of the body intact by keeping BSs pelvis, thorax and head aligned even when the axis inclines forwards out of the vertical
– Keep the stabilization of the thoracic spine in its neutral position even when the long axis of the body inclines backwards or to the side out of the vertical and, for reasons of economy, the lordotic segments of the spinal column slightly deform.

▶ Functional Analysis in Therapist Language

● Conception of the Exercise (Fig. 57 a–c)

In order to align BSs pelvis, thorax and head vertically in the long axis of the body, we take upright sitting on a stool as the starting position. The knees are as far off the floor as the hips, or perhaps a little closer, so that it is no effort to place the building block "pelvis" vertically on the stool. Now blocks "thorax" and "head" can be built on top, and BS legs exerts no more than its own weight on the contact points soles/floor. To avoid the possible confusing factor of an inappropriate height of the seat, the patient should sit on his ischial tuberosities, preferably straddling the corner of the seat, so that the dorsal aspects of the thighs have no contact with the seat. This is the only way to attain potential mobility of the pelvis in the hip joints and joints of the lumbar spine and of the head in the atlanto-occipital and atlanto-axial joints and cervical spine, and dynamic stabilization of the thoracic spine in its neutral position. The classic Building Blocks exercise consists of swaying the long axis of the body backwards and forwards by flexion and extension in the hips. The changing of the position in space causes changes in the demands on the fall-preventing muscles, although in forward inclination there is no joint movement in the spinal column and in backward inclination there are slight movements only in the atlanto-occipital and atlanto-axial joints, to keep the gaze directed forwards, and in the lumbosacral articulation, to prevent shearing stress in this area.

● Position and Activation in the Starting Position

Position in Space of the Critical Axes
Points of Contact Between the Body and the Environment
Components of Movement in Relation to the Neutral Position of the Joints
The long axis of the body is vertical. With the patient sitting upright on a stool and the soles touching the floor a comfortable distance apart, the hip joints are in a maximum of 90° flexion/transverse abduction, the knee joints in a maximum of 90° flexion/0° rotation. If the heels are below and somewhat behind the knee joints, the talocrural joints are slightly dorsiflexed by their proximal lever (Fig. 57 a).

Movement Tolerances at the Critical Joints in Relation
to the Intended Primary Movement
The intended primary movement is to incline the long axis of the body forwards and backwards. We assume sufficient tolerance for flexion/extension in the hip joints, to be effected by the proximal lever.

Distribution of Weight on a Base Support or Suspension Device,
Against a Supportive Device, or Over a Support Area,
and the Resulting Activity States of the Musculature
The weights of BSs pelvis, thorax, head and arms press down on the seat. The smallest area encompassing the contact point between the pelvis and the seat and those

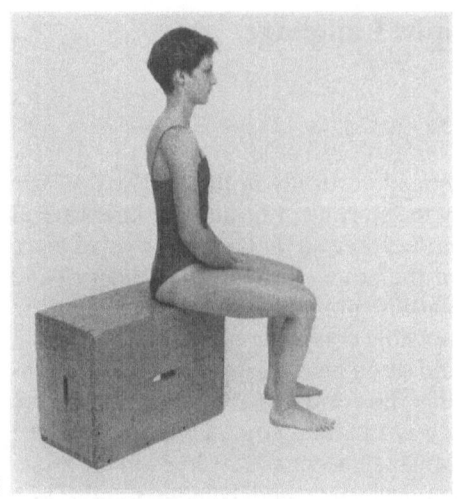

a

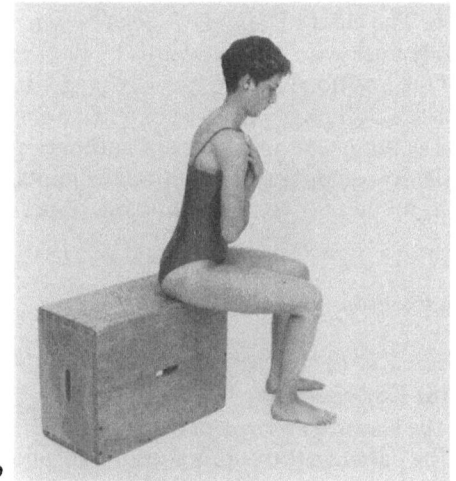

b

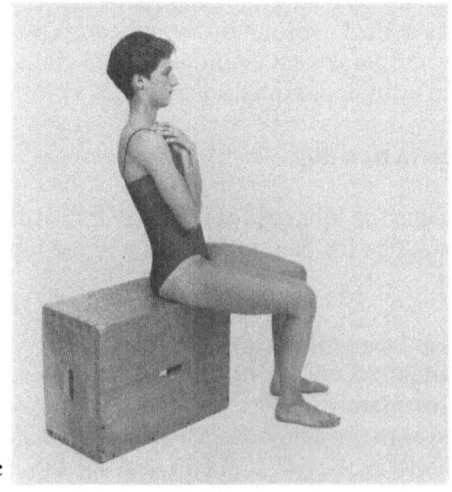

c

Fig. 57 a–c. Building Blocks. **a** Starting position, **b** turret inclines forwards, **c** turret inclines backwards

between the soles and the floor is the support area, or rather, it will be as soon as the long axis of the body inclines forwards.

BS legs is parked. BS pelvis has potential mobility in the hip joints and the joints of the lumbar spine. In BS thorax, the thoracic spine is stabilized in neutral position. BS head balances in free play and potential mobility above the thorax. In BS arms, the shoulder girdle is parked on the thorax and the arms are parked on the thighs. These activity states provide the right conditions for automatic normal breathing.

Intensity of Muscle Activity Required with Economical Activity
Respiration
The intensity of economical activity in the starting position of Building Blocks is very low.

● Actio – Reactio of the Movement Sequence

Actio: The Primary Movement
The actio of Building Blocks is the to-and-fro movement of forward and backward inclination of the long axis of the body as the patient leans forwards and backwards. Because of the horizontal direction components, we can expect a clear reactio.

Leaning Forwards: The critical distance point of the primary movement, DP jugular notch, moves forwards/downwards by flexion in the hip joints. Thus, DPs right and left iliac spines move towards the long axes of the thighs; DP vertex and DPs left and right eyes have also moved forwards/downwards (Fig. 57 b).

Return to Upright Sitting and Leaning Backwards: The critical distance joint of the primary movement, DP jugular notch, moves backwards/first upwards, then downwards by extension in the hip joints. DPs right and left iliac spines thus move away from the long axes of the thighs; DP vertex and DPs right and left eyes have also moved backwards/first upwards, then downwards (Fig. 57 c).

Reactio: Activated Passive Buttressing
As long as the body is touching the seat, there is no activated passive buttressing when *leaning forwards.*

Because in the starting position, BS legs is in parking function, the weight of the legs will become suspended from the pelvis by flexional activity at the hip joints when the long axis of the body *leans backwards* and thus becomes an activated passive buttress even though the soles remain in contact with the floor.

Reactio: Change in the Support Area
When the patient *leans forwards,* the potential support area of the starting position becomes actual, because BS legs is now exerting more pressure on the contact point soles/floor than just that of its own weight.

When the patient *leans backwards,* the support area becomes smaller because there is less contact between the soles and the floor. Instead the point of contact between the body and the seat enlarges backwards slightly.

Actio: Accelerating Weights
Reactio: Braking Weights
Because the horizontal direction components in Building Blocks go backwards and forwards, the bisecting plane in the starting position is identical to the midfrontal plane of BSs pelvis, thorax and head aligned vertically in the long axis of the body. The bisecting plane therefore shifts forwards when the patient *leans forwards;* if the body lost contact with the seat, this plane would pass through the point of contact soles/floor. All of the weights in front of the bisecting plane have an accelerating effect on the movement sequence, and those behind it have a braking effect. When the patient *leans backwards,* the bisecting plane displaces backwards only slightly; if the soles lost contact with the floor, it would pass approximately through the caudal pole of the iliosacral joints. All weights in front of the bisecting plane have a braking effect on the movement sequence, while all of those behind it have an accelerating effect.

● **Conditio – Limitatio of the Movement Sequence**

Conditio: Constant Distances Between Body Distance Points
Limitatio: Active Buttressing and Stabilization
Conditio: The distance between DP navel and DP jugular notch remains constant during forward and backward leaning.
Limitatio: To keep this distance constant, the thoracic spine must be dynamically stabilized in its neutral position, extensionally in forward leaning, flexionally in backward leaning, with increasing intensity of economical activity.

Conditio: During forward leaning, the distances between DP symphysis pubis and DP navel and between DP jugular notch and DP tip of the chin remain constant.
Limitatio: To keep these distances constant, the lumbar spine, the cervical spine and the atlanto-occipital and atlanto-axial joints must stabilize extensionally in their neutral positions with increasing intensity of economical activity, and the frontotransverse diameters of BSs pelvis, thorax and head must remain parallel to each other.

Conditio: The distance between DPs right and left patellae remains constant during forward and backward leaning.
Limitatio: For this distance to remain constant it must be held by alternate transverse-abductional/-adductional activity in the hip joints, plantarflexional/dorsiflexional in the talocrural joints, and inversional/eversional in the talocalcaneonavicular joints.

Conditio of Absolute and/or Relative Fixed Spatial Points
Limitatio by Limiting the Primary Movement, Activated Passive Buttressing and/or Change in the Support Area
In Building Blocks, there are absolute and relative fixed spatial points.

Conditio: The contact between the right and left soles and the floor is an absolute fixed spatial point.

Limitatio: This fixed point checks the backward inclination of the long axis of the body. Because BS legs is already parked in the starting position, only a small amount of extension may take place at the hip joints. The smallest bit too much would bring BS legs into free play, losing the contact of the soles with the floor.

Conditio: The continuous contact between the body and the seat is an absolute fixed spatial point.
Limitatio: This fixed point checks forward inclination of the long axis of the body. Although BS legs goes into supporting function, the major portion of the weight of BSs pelvis, thorax, head and arms is borne by the seat as long as the patient continues to sit on it.

Conditio: During backward leaning, the gaze remains directed forwards.
Limitatio: This relative fixed point makes the atlanto-occipital and atlanto-axial joints flex adaptively. DP tip of the chin moves closer to DP jugular notch.

Conditio: During backward leaning, the symphysis moves away from the seat.
Limitatio: This relative fixed spatial point causes the lower abdomen to shorten slightly as DP symphysis comes a little closer to DP navel. This loosens the extensional lumbosacral anchoring, causing the lowest motion segments in the lumbar spine to flex slightly, which improves the motive components of the abdominal muscles. This prevents shearing stress in the lumbar area.

Conditio of Movement Speed
Limitatio of Economical Activity by Finding the Optimal Speed
The patient should take about 2 seconds to lean forwards and backwards. This tempo allows him enough time to become aware of everything necessary for Building Blocks to work perfectly. While working up into the rhythm, it is best if the patient crosses his hands on top of each other on his sternum. That way he can feel the jugular notch. Next he will need his hands to monitor the continual movement of the right and left iliac spines towards and away from the supporting thighs. He must also feel the activity of the fall-preventing muscles coming and going: as he leans forwards, he can feel by palpation the activation of the lumbar and cervical extensors; as he leans backwards, he can palpate the ventral muscles of the abdomen and neck. He will then be able to find the middle position (analogous to the starting position), where neither ventral or dorsal muscles are activated against gravity in the lumbar and cervical areas. Now BSs pelvis and head have optimum potential mobility.

▶ Instruction in Patient Language

● Instruction Appealing to the Patient's Perception

In Building Blocks, it is above all by palpating his muscles himself that the patient rediscovers a feeling for good upright posture with economical activity and breathing.

Position and Activation in the Starting Position

"Sit down across the corner of a box, or you could take a stool. Your knees are a comfortable distance apart, facing forwards and outwards, as do the tips of your feet. The soles of your feet feel the floor. To do this, your feet must be below your knees. Now place one hand on your abdomen and the back of the other against the small of your back, not too high up. Now you are holding the building block 'pelvis' between your hands. Place this block on the stool such that your stomach won't spill out forwards and your pelvis won't tip backwards. Let the pelvis block stay there, nice and upright, and grasp your head from both sides in your hands. If you hold your ears between your index and middle fingers, you can rest your chin on the balls of your palms. Now we have to shift the head block backwards a little so that it's well over the pelvis block, being careful not to move the pelvis backwards as well, of course. Keep looking straight ahead. Now let your stomach go flop, but without allowing the turret you have just built up of the pelvis, rib cage and head blocks to fall down anywhere or require too much effort to keep up. Now that your stomach has gone flop, the pelvis block is automatically in the right position. You feel that your breathing is easy, you're not strained or cramping up anywhere. You can check with your hands on the thorax block that your upper abdomen is nice and long, but soft. After you've finished your work, you can place your hands, not in your lap, but one over the other on the middle of your rib cage. One of your index fingers has found the hollow of your neck. Now feel how warm your hands are, or your rib cage.

In this exercise, the correct starting position is really the main goal of the exercise. As the patient takes up the starting position, the therapist is particularly careful that he learns to feel the difference between hyper- and hypoactivity and economical activity. The first way for the patient to monitor himself for this is self-palpation; other ways are to check where he is looking (direction of gaze) and to become aware of the sense of well-being that comes from normal breathing at rest (p. 131). When the patient palpates his BSs pelvis and head, the therapist can also touch them if, in the continual dialogue between patient and therapist, it emerges that the patient is still unclear about what he can and should be feeling.

In Building Blocks, as anywhere else, it is impossible to align the body segments in the long axis of the body if there is any stiffness in the spinal column that cannot be overcome spontaneously. If the patient is unable to relax his abdomen, the therapist can hold his thorax and the exercise be done without extensional stabilization of the thoracic spine (see. Fig. 80).

You can also feel the beating of your heart distinctly, and how your rib cage widens and narrows with your breathing."

Actio and Conditio of the Movement Sequence

"Now this solid little turret starts to sway to and fro, first forwards and then backwards. These are little movements, the one forwards is a little bigger than the one backwards. The to-and-fro movement continues at a comfortable speed like a perpetual

During the rhythmic alteration by extension and flexion in the hips of forward and backward inclination of BSs pelvis, thorax and head stabilized in the long axis of the body, it is good training in perception for the patient to become aware of the changes in the

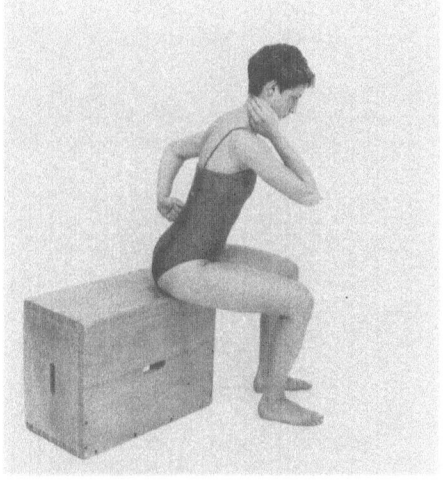

d

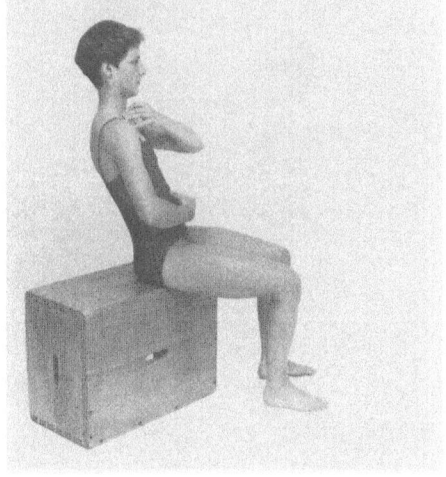

Fig. 57 d, e. Building Blocks. **d** As the turret inclines forwards, the patient can feel by palpation the fall-preventing activity automatically arising in the extensor muscles in the lumbar and cervical region. **e** As the turret inclines backwards, the patient can feel by palpation the fall-preventing activity automatically arising in the flexor muscles of the lumbar and cervical region

e

motion machine, while your sensory system registers it.

First you feel the pressure of your feet on the floor changing. Every time it increases you say 'Now'. Your thumbs touch those bony projections you know on your pelvis and your middle fingers are on your thighs. You feel how the pressure under your feet increases when the spot your thumbs are touching comes closer to your thighs and decreases when it moves away.

You have learned how the pressure of your feet on the floor increases when the turret leans forwards and decreases pressure of his feet on the floor and relate them to his leaning forwards and backwards. He should then feel the activation of the fall-preventing dorsal and ventral muscles around the lordotic segments of the spinal column by palpating these muscles himself and relating their activity to the leaning to-and-fro rhythm of the "turret" (Fig. 57 d, e). When the turret leans forwards, the entire spinal column remains in neutral position and the patient no longer looks "forwards" but "down forwards". The angle of forward inclina-

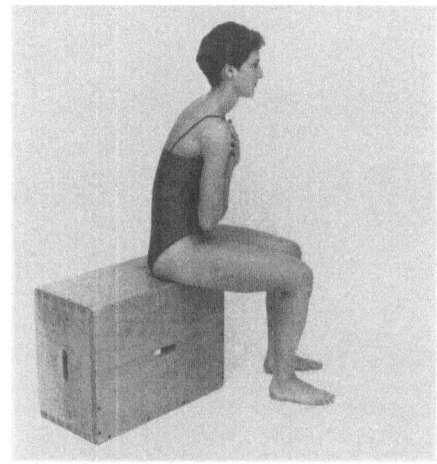

f

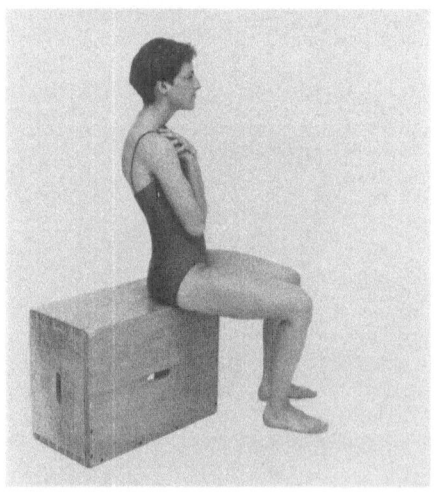

g

Fig. 57 f, g. Building Blocks. **f** Avoidance mechanism in forward leaning. **g** Avoidance mechanism in backward leaning

when it leans backwards. Now you're going to find out how your muscles have to work to keep the tower together. This is how you're going to do it: one hand is on your abdomen and the fingers of the other are up in the hollow of your neck. When you feel your muscles spring into action you say 'Snap!' and notice that you have started to lean backwards. Now move the hand on your abdomen to the small of your back, just at the top of your pelvis, and the hand at your neck to the back of your neck. Say 'Snip!' when the muscles spring into action and see how you are leaning forwards. Now you know how the turret is kept together. Now for the last experiment. One hand on your abdomen or your neck, the other on the small of your back or the back of your neck. You can feel the muscles spring into action and you say 'Snip, snap!' in double time. Between the 'snip' and 'snap' there's a gap when all the muscles are soft. That means that the turret is upright."

tion should be small enough – about 30°–40° – to keep the forward component predominant.

If total flexion of the lumbar/thoracic spine and hyperlordosis of the cervical spine occurs when the patient leans forwards, the cause may be restricted flexion in the hips and/or restricted extension in the lumbar spine (Fig. 57 f).

In backward inclination, slight flexion in the atlanto-occipital and atlanto-axial joints is desirable. This keeps the gaze directed forwards. Very slight flexion in the lumbosacral articulation is also to be expected if lumbar lordosis is normal. The therapist should know that this accommodating flexional movement will not take place if there is even the slightest lumbar kyphosis, because the lumbar spine is then unable even to achieve its optimal neutral position.

One avoidance mechanism seen frequently is when the extensional movement of the pelvis in the hip joints as the patient leans backwards is blocked; instead there is dorsal translation in the upper lumbar/lower thoracic spine while the head translates ventrally in the cervical spine. The first suspect for the cause of this is abdominal muscle insufficiency (Fig. 57 g).

By introducing free movement of the hands freely or combining Building Blocks with Short and Sharp (see Sect. 5.6.4), a transition to normal movement patterns is made (Fig. 57 h, i).

▶ Adapting the Exercise to the Patient's Constitution and Condition

● Adaptation to Constitution: Role of Lengths, Widths, Depths and Distribution of Weights

In Building Blocks, the constitutional measurements will only affect how far forwards and backwards the patient leans. The smallest amount of flexion/extension of the stabilized long axis of the body in the hip joints will be seen in patients with + + + topheavy upper body length, short thighs and light legs.

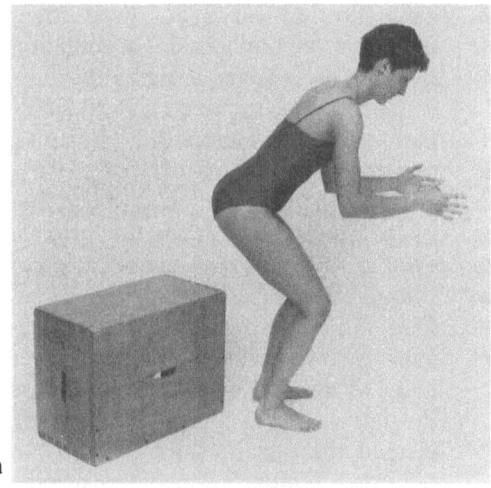

h

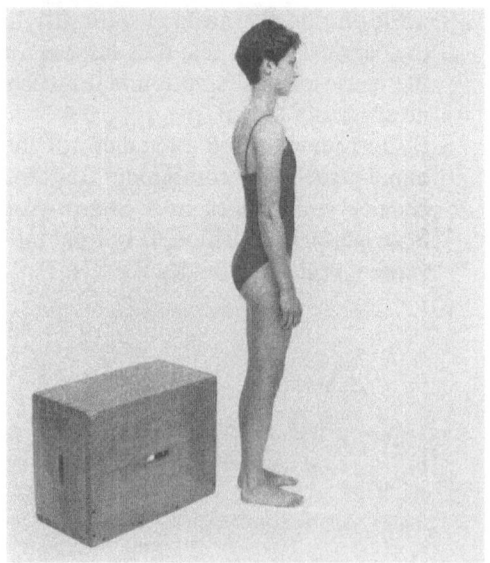

i

Fig. 57 h, i. Building Blocks. **h, i** Continuing the movement into upright standing

● **Adaptation to Condition**

Poor Physical Fitness or Wish to Increase Performance

For a patient with spinal instability or hypermobility, an increase in the speed of the exercise and the addition of arm activities can be very helpful in improving physical condition. If the movement is expanded so that in backward leaning the feet leave the floor and in forward leaning the pelvis leaves the seat, the movement of the "turret" stops at the hip joints. There can then be a smooth transition into functional training for stressing the long axes of the legs (Fig. 57 h, i).

Pain Arising During the Exercise a Contraindication

Ischaemic pain resulting from inappropriate demands on the muscles of the spinal column, shoulder and hip joints can be relieved completely with this exercise. Radicular pain may worsen because unstable motion segments may be stressed. In such cases, the exercise should be stopped and specific treatment in a relief posture begun with mobilizing massage, etc.

Restricted Movement and/or Hypermobility

Up to a certain extent, restricted hip flexion can be overcome by raising the seat. It is advisable to seat the patient on the treatment bench. As soon as the seat is higher and the thighs no longer horizontal, care must be taken that they do not touch the seat dorsally.

If the axes of flexion/extension in the hip joints cannot be brought parallel, performing the exercise is impossible.

As mentioned above, movement restrictions and asymmetry in the spinal column prevent the optimal alignment of the "building blocks". Nevertheless, the movement sequence can still be performed, indeed with great benefit, only reactive hypertonicity in the muscles must first be neutralized by adapting the starting position as a relief posture for these muscles.

Movement Disorders Originating in the Central Nervous System

In these cases, too, Building Blocks can often be helpful, as the legs are parked and the arms "taken care of" on the thorax. By changing the position in space, the adaptive change of the muscle tone acts as a productive influence to normalize muscle activity.

5.2.1 Relief Postures for the Entire Spinal Column (Figs. 58, 59)

The name "Relief Postures for the Entire Spinal Column" refers to the functional problem to be solved.

■ Goal of the Exercise

A relief posture for the entire spinal column must relieve the physiological axial stress of the spine without allowing shearing stress on the passive structures of the motion segments to arise.

▶ Functional Analysis in Therapist Language

● Conception of the Exercise

Relief Posture in Suspension (Fig. 58)

To relieve the axial stress on the spinal column without shearing stress on the passive structures arising, traction is exerted on the spinal column in the direction taken by the long axis of the body. The easiest way to do this is to keep the long axis of the body vertical but turn the arrangement of the blocks through 180°, i. e. head at the bottom, pelvis at the top. Traction using the patient's own body weight can be performed in a position of suspension; this requires more than 90° flexion at the hips. To attain this position, the patient lies on his stomach on a raised treatment bench – the distance between the surface on which the patient is lying and the floor must be a little more than the patient's upper body length – and he must slide headwards until only the ventral aspects of his outspread legs touch the surface of the bench. The patient grips the long sides of the treatment bench with his feet if no one is available to hold on to his legs and keep them down. The patient's hands and perhaps also forearms touch the floor; the vertex of his head may also touch the floor a little. For the long axis of the body to hang vertical, the vertex must be under the lumbosacral articulation. In this starting position, the frontotransverse diameter of the thorax as cranial pointer of the thoracic spine and caudal pointer of the cervical spine can rotate lift-free about the long axis of the body at both rotation levels.

During traction, the individual motion segments in which extension or flexion is restricted can be manually mobilized under conditions of reduced lift. Reduced-lift mobilization of all of the other movement components of the spinal column is also possible during traction.

To stand up, the patient is pulled footwards along the treatment bench by the therapist, the patient helping with his hands.

Relief Posture in Supine (Fig. 59)

For patients with normal mobility in the shoulder and hip joints, this relief posture for the entire spinal column is an excellent and very quick way to achieve relaxation of the whole body.

The patient lies on his back on a treatment bench.

BSs pelvis, thorax and head form the long axis of the body, which is horizontal. Thoracic kyphosis and cervical lordosis are somewhat less than normal.

BS arms is in the Little Shepherd Boy position (see p. 290). The arms are supported on cushions only if shoulder flexion is restricted. The position of the arms makes the cervical spine potentially mobile.

In BS legs, the hip joints are in neutral position (Fig. 59 a). The dorsal aspects of the thighs are in contact with the treatment bench, the narrow end of which is level with the flexion/extension axes of the knee joints. The soles of the feet are in contact with the floor or are supported on a pillow, depending on the height of the bench and the length of the lower legs. The functional long axes of the feet are in the sagittal plane of the hip joints, which is vertical. The lower legs are flexed at the knee joints to about 90°. In this position, it is easy to keep the hips in neutral as to rotation as well.

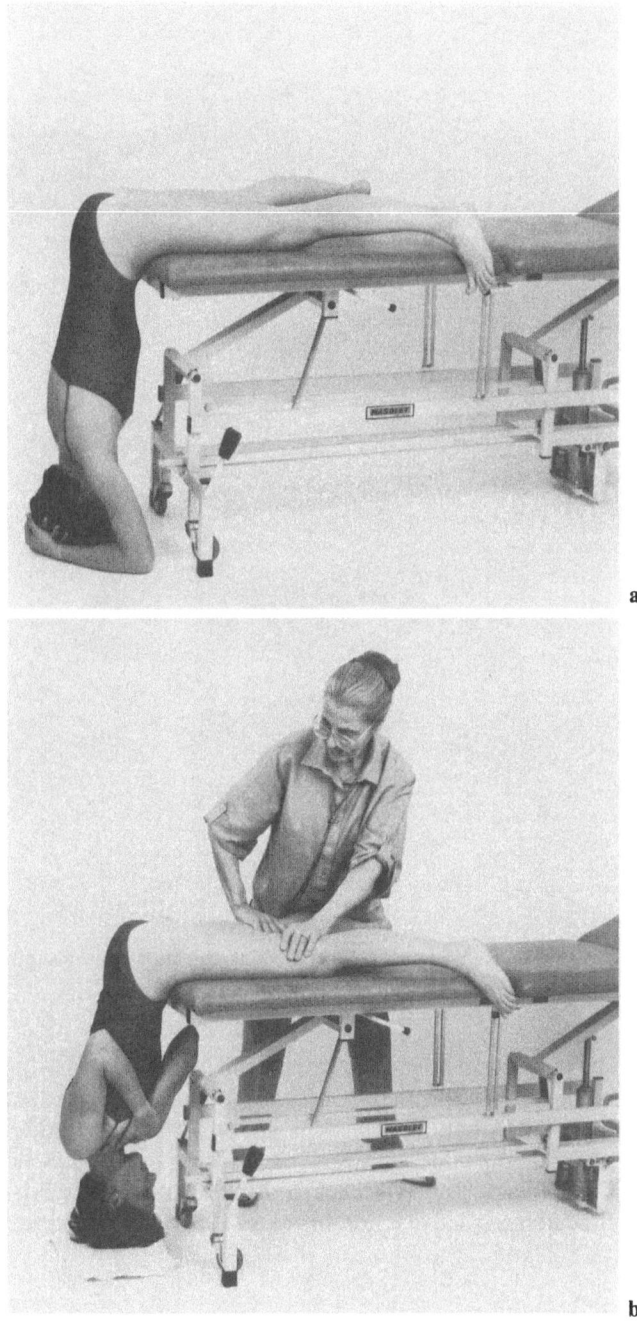

Fig. 58 a, b. Relief posture for the entire spinal column in suspension. **a** The patient hangs by her feet from the long sides of the therapy bench. BSs arms and head touch the floor and are parked. **b** The therapist makes the hanging activity of the legs redundant. The patient's hands are joined and are placed ventrocranially at mid-thorax. The thorax rotates as the cranial pointer of the thoracic spine and as caudal pointer of the cervical spine

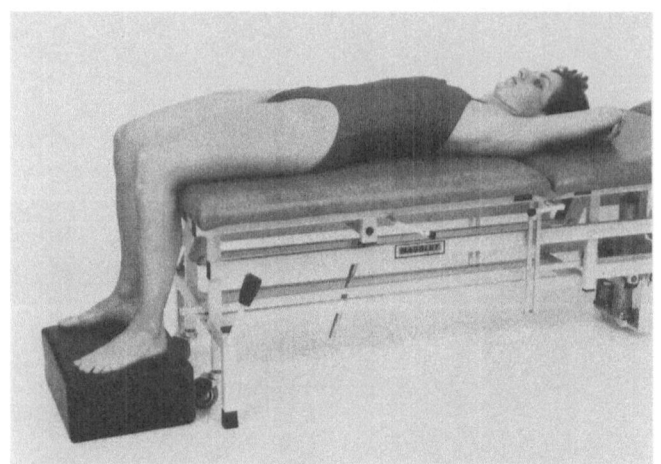

a

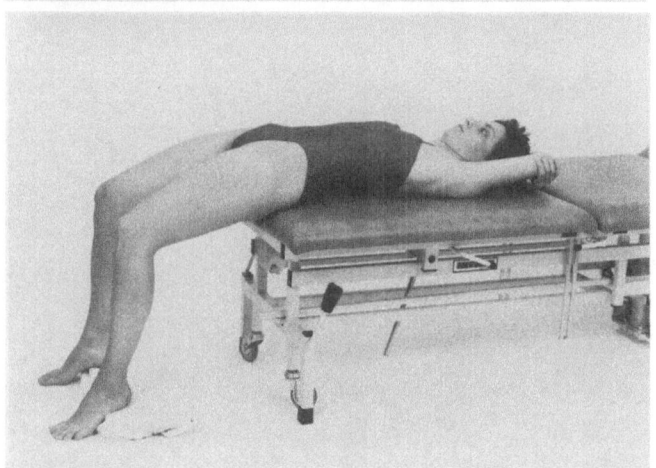

b

Fig. 59 a, b. Relief posture for the entire spinal column in supine. **a** Hips in neutral position, **b** hips in extension

In Fig. 59 b, the edge of the treatment bench is level with the flexion/extension axes of the hip joints, which are extended. The lower legs are flexed at the knee joints to slightly less than 90°. The heels are on a thin pillow and the forefeet touch the floor such that the talocrural joints are in moderate plantarflexion.

This relief posture stretches the hip flexors. If the pelvis flexes in the hip joints and the lumbar spine extends, hip extension must be abandoned and the feet raised.

5.2.2 The Snake (Figs. 60, 61)

"The Snake" is an invented name. In this exercise the spinal column has to be writhed like a snake.

212

■ Goal of the Exercise

The goal is for the patient to learn to mobilize the entire spinal column extensionally/flexionally in the plane of symmetry by a continuing caudal-to-cranial movement and lateroflexionally in the midfrontal plane by a continuing caudal-to-cranial movement.

► Functional Analysis in Therapist Language

● Conception of the Exercise

To mobilize the entire spinal column using caudal-to-cranial continuing movements of extension/flexion or lateroflexion, the best starting position is sitting upright in a chair without a backrest. This does mean that the movement sequence is not lift-free, but the patient gains the advantage of having BSs pelvis, thorax and head moving freely in space, unhindered by a base support. To make the direction of the flexion/extension movement caudal-to-cranial, we choose alternating extensional and flexional movement impulses of the pelvis in the hip joints. A flexional impulse which deforms the lumbar spine extensionally continues on cranially, but before it reaches the cervical spine the extensional impulse – rather less strong – sets in in the hip joints and, continuing, deforms the spinal column flexionally.
Lateroflexional snaking starts with internal rotation of the pelvis, e. g. in the right hip joint, and left-concave lateroflexion of the lumbar spine, which continues on cranially. Before it reaches the cervical spine, the weaker impulse of external rotation in the right hip takes over, deforming the spinal column to the other side. By keeping one hand on his back, the patient can palpate the sites that require special mobilization and even manipulate them himself with some skill.

● Position and Activation of the Starting Position

See Building Blocks (p. 199).

● Actio – Reactio of the Movement Sequence

The Snake is a constant-location movement sequence with a change in the distribution of pressure within the support area of the starting position.
The actio is characterized by a primary impulse that continues cranially unchecked, followed by a weaker secondary impulse, precisely timed to the first, in the opposite direction. In continuing precise coordination in time, the primary impulse is repeated, followed by the secondary impulse, etc.
If the direction of the primary impulse is forwards, the secondary impulse will be backwards. If the direction of the primary impulse is to the right, the secondary impulse will be to the left.
Both impulses should be allowed to continue on cranially unchecked.

Extensional/Flexional Continuing Mobilization of the Spinal Column (Fig. 60)

Actio: The Primary Movement

The critical distance point of the primary impulse, DP lumbosacral articulation, moves energetically forwards/downwards. This displacement of their fulcrum causes the hip joints to flex and the lumbar spine goes into extension effected by the pelvis. By cranially continuing movement, first the thoracic spine, then the cervical spine and finally the atlanto-occipital and atlanto-axial joints extend so that DP vertex moves backwards/downwards. By now the secondary impulse has already set in.

The critical distance point of the secondary impulse, DP lumbosacral articulation, moves gently backwards, first a little upwards, then downwards. This displacement of their fulcrum causes the hip joints to extend and the lumbar spine goes into flexion effected by the pelvis. By cranially continuing movement, first the thoracic spine, beginning at its caudal end, then the cervical spine and finally the atlanto-occipital and atlanto-axial joints flex, so that DP vertex now moves forwards/first upwards, then downwards. By now the second primary impulse has already set in.

Reactio: Activated Passive Buttressing

There is no activated passive buttressing in the classical sense. Nevertheless, the snakelike movement with its forward and backward impulses results in a harmonious interplay of the weights of BSs pelvis, thorax, head and arms swaying to and fro. Exact timing of the movement impulses is essential.

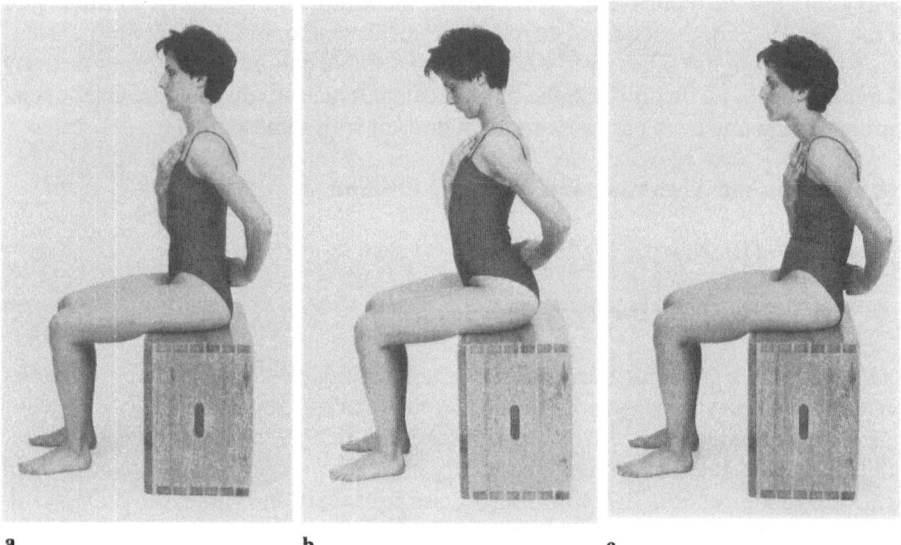

a   b   c

Fig. 60 a–c. The Snake. **a** Starting position for extensional/flexional mobilization continuing of the spinal column. **b** Pelvic impulse (flexional in the hips) to extensional continuing mobilization of the spinal column. **c** Pelvic impulse (extensional in the hips) to flexional mobilization of the spinal column

Reactio: Change in the Support Area

When the movement impulse is forwards, the pressure on the soles of the feet reactively increases; when the impulse is backwards, the pressure on the soles decreases and is transferred backwards onto the seat.

Lateroflexional Continuing Mobilization of the Spinal Column (Fig. 61)

Actio: The Primary Movement

The critical distance point of the primary impulse, DP left iliac spine, moves energetically upwards/to the right by internal rotation in the right hip joint effected by the pelvis and left-concave lateroflexion in the lumbar spine arising caudally. This primary impulse is intensified by simultaneous pushing off of the left sole from the floor downwards/to the left. By cranially continuing movement, the thoracic spine, then the cervical spine and finally the atlanto-occipital and atlanto-axial joints are deformed in left-concave lateroflexion arising caudally, so that DP vertex moves downwards/laterally to the left in the midfrontal plane, which is vertical. By now the secondary impulse has already set in.

The critical distance point of the secondary impulse, DP left iliac spine, gently moves downwards/to the left by external rotation in the right hip joint effected by the pelvis, then by internal rotation in the left hip joint effected by the pelvis, and the lumbar spine deforms in right-concave lateroflexion. By cranially continuing movement, the thoracic spine, then the cervical spine and finally the atlanto-oc-

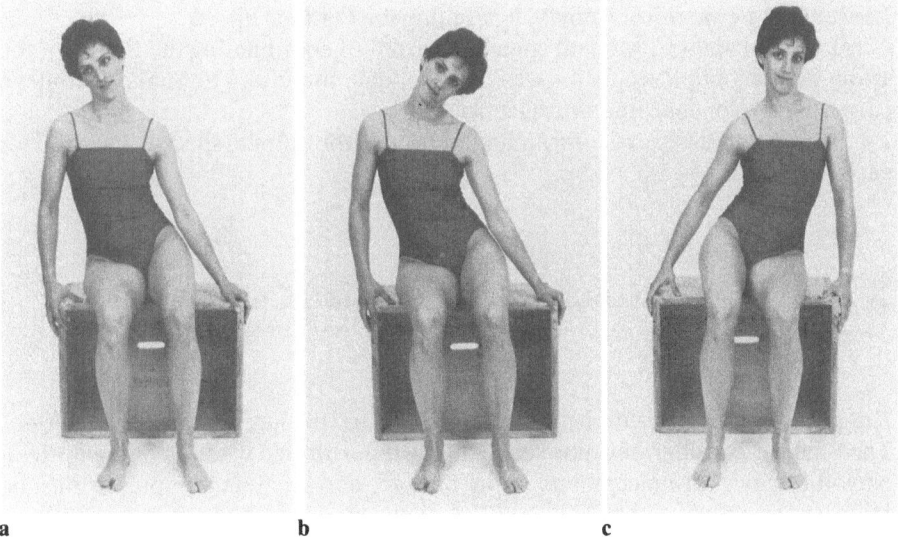

a   b   c

Fig. 61 a–c. The Snake. **a** Pelvic impulse (internal rotation in the right hip) to left-concave lateroflexional mobilization in the spinal column. **b** End position of left-concave lateroflexional mobilization of the spinal column. **c** Pelvic impulse (internal rotation in the hip) to right-concave lateroflexional mobilization of the spinal column

cipital and atlanto-axial joints are deformed in right-concave lateroflexion arising caudally, so that DP vertex moves downwards/laterally to the right in the mid-frontal plane, which is vertical. By now, the second primary impulse has already set in.

Reactio: Activated Passive Buttressing
There is no activated passive buttressing in the classical sense. Nevertheless, the snakelike movement with its impulses to the right and the left results in a harmonious interplay of the weights of BSs pelvis, thorax, head and arms swaying right and left. Exact timing of the movement impulses is essential.

Reactio: Change in the Support Area
Through the pushing off of the left foot downwards/to the left from the floor, co-ordinated with the primary impulse upwards/to the right of the left iliac spine, DP left ischial tuberosity loses contact with the seat completely, pressure on the right tuberosity is reduced, and the patient is more or less sitting on his right trochanter. The primary impulse has thus caused the support area to expand reactively somewhat to the right. The expansion to the left after the secondary impulse is much less pronounced.

● **Conditio – Limitatio of the Movement Sequence**

The only part the conditio and limitatio play in the Snake is to prevent the movement impulses from driving the undulating movement sequence out of control.

Conditio of Movement Speed
Limitatio of Economical Activity by Finding the Optimal Speed
Conditio: The right movement speed arises out of coordinating the timing of the strong primary impulse and the weaker secondary impulse. The Snake becomes a perpetual motion machine with accents.
Limitatio: Once the exercise is running smoothly, the optimal speed is 1 second for each impulse.

▶ **Adapting the Exercise to the Patient's Constitution and Condition**

Adaptations for constitution are limited to altering the intensity of the impulses. The Snake is considerably more challenging if performed when standing upright. Now the critical distance points of the primary and secondary impulses must be relocated one movement level down, i.e. to the hip joints. For extensional/flexional snaking of the spinal column, the primary impulse comes from forward movement of the flexion/extension axes of the hip joints. Through displacement of their fulcra, the hip joints go into extension. In the secondary impulse backwards, the hip joints move into flexion.

For lateroflexional snaking of the spinal column, the primary impulse comes from moving the abduction/adduction axes of the hip joints to the right. The right hip joint goes into adduction by displacement of its fulcrum. During the secondary impulse to the left, the left hip joint goes into adduction.

The pattern of movement that the axes of the legs describe in this Snake variant will be analysed in detail in the volume on gait training (Klein-Vogelbach 1991).

5.3 Adapting Lift-Free/Reduced-Lift Mobilization of the Spinal Column to Special Problems of the Lumbar Spine

Functionally speaking, the lumbar spine is regarded as part of BS pelvis. In upright, economical posture, the pelvis should be potentially mobile both in the hip joints and in the lumbar spine. This also applies to typical human locomotion, walking. This means that the lumbar part of the spine must always be ready for fine deformation by flexion, extension or lateroflexion and, at the lumbothoracic transition, rotation and translation. At the same time, this readiness to flex, extend, lateroflex, rotate or translate means that, even when the vertebral and intervertebral joints remain still, the muscles are constantly subjected to changes in tone in order to prevent falling. This motor behaviour protects the lumbar spine from premature degeneration and increases its readiness to provide fall-preventing stabilization whenever the long axis of the body inclines out of the vertical. Whether effective deformation of the lumbar spine takes place when a person is walking or engaged in manual activities or whether there are merely changes in muscle tone are questions that depend on individual condition, constitution, kinaesthetic skill and postural statics as well as, of course, most importantly, on the movement – sequence itself.

The lumbar spine is particularly sensitive to repetitive postural stress and uncontrolled rotational strain. It is particularly exposed to these because, in addition to external weight that shifts the body's centre of gravity away from the centre of the body, as in carrying and putting down small children, suitcases, boxes, etc., the weight of parts of one's own upper body, which are above and mostly in front of the lumbar spine, such as the thorax, shoulder girdle, head, arms and stomach, severely stress or overstress it. This is why, in bending and lifting, the possibilities for shortening or lengthening the weighted lever must be critically evaluated (this will be dealt with in the volume on gait training, Klein-Vogelbach 1991).

Strain caused by transient changes in position within a movement sequence is easily coped with. This is why patients with syndromes of the lumbar spine but more or less normal postural statics usually find walking a relief, as long as there are no acute radicular symptoms that make even the slightest strain unbearable.

If, for pathological reasons or merely due to poor postural statics, the position of the lumbar spine in relation to the other body segments or to gravity is not economical even when the patient is standing upright, the process of degeneration speeds up rapidly. We must therefore attempt to track down the functional relationships that underlie these disturbances and have an additional negative effect on pathological processes already existing in this area.

Common Causes of Faulty Postural Stress

Faulty postural stress can frequently be traced to:
- Instability in the vertebral–intervertebral disc articulations of the lumbar spine in intervertebral osteochondrosis, spondylolysis, spondylolisthesis and hypermobility.
- Structural kyphosis at the lumbosacral transition resulting in altered distribution of body weight in front of and behind the flexion/extension axes of the lumbar spine.
- Functional lumbar kyphosis associated with ischiocrural contracture, frequently seen where the angles of antetorsion of the femoral neck are relatively large or asymmetrical, causing the lordosis of the adjacent lumbar spine to flatten out.
- Hyperlordosis, often accompanied by restricted extension in the hip joints, making it difficult or impossible for the hips to achieve neutral the position, and by restricted flexion in the lumbar spine.
- Muscle contractures in the hip joints, often primarily in the biarticular muscles. The muscles acting upon the lumbar spine and the hip joints are iliopsoas, psoas major and minor; those affecting the hip and knee joints are the ischiocrural muscles, rectus femoris, sartorius, and gracilis. In the monarticular muscles, contracture may affect the fan of muscles stretching from the tensor fasciae latae to the adductor magnus that anchors the pelvis to the thigh when the leg is in the supporting phase of walking. Contracture can also occur in the fan of muscles that stretches from the adductor longus to the iliacus, suspending the thigh from the pelvis when the leg is in the free-play phase of walking. Contracture in any of these muscles has an immediate effect on the lumbar spine.
- Any blockage in the iliosacral joints.
- Any arthritic or arthrotic processes in the hip, iliosacral and lumbar joints.
- Poor postural statics in the axes of the legs and the arches of the feet.
- Muscular insufficiencies in the legs, the hip joints and the lumbar spine. Serious insufficiencies are those of the triceps surae, the quadriceps, the fan of extensor muscles at the hip joints and the abdominal muscles.

With the exception of inflammatory processes all the above causes of faulty stressing in the postural statics respond to functional treatment. Careful differential diagnosis is an important part of determining functional status (see *Functional Kinetics*, p. 213).

5.3.1 Relief Postures for the Lumbar Spine

The name "Relief Postures for the Lumbar Spine" refers to the functional problem to be resolved.

■ Goal of the Exercise

The goal is for the patient to learn to:
- Find positions for rest and for work in which all fall-preventing activity directed against gravity in the hip joints and the joints of the lumbar spine can automatically switch off, thereby creating the activity state of potential mobility in the pelvis
- Position the axes of the feet and the legs in such a way that the pelvis has potential mobility in the hip joints
- Arrange the weights of BSs thorax, head and arms in such a way that the lumbar spine, which is in its neutral position, is potentially mobile and will be able to undergo lift-free/reduced-lift deformation when the pelvis moves in the hip joints.

▶ Functional Analysis in Therapist Language

● Conception of the Exercise

We need positions for sleep and rest, i. e. the most completely comfortable positions possible. But we also need positions for sitting, standing and working. Relief postures for working when the long axis of the body has to be inclined out of the vertical are the most difficult because the hands are needed for work and cannot be used for support.

● Position and Activation in the Starting Position

These relief postures also apply to the thoracic and cervical spines; here we will emphasize aspects of specific relevance to the lumbar spine.

Relief Postures for the Lumbar Spine in Supine or Prone Lying (Figs. 62, 63)
To satisfy the basic principle of good resting and sleeping positions, the inherently mobile systems of the body segments must not be suspended from each other by muscular activity directed against gravity. In addition, BSs pelvis, thorax and head must be aligned in the best possible way in the long axis of the body, as in Figs. 62 and 63.
To ensure that, in supine, the lumbar spine when roughly in neutral is potentially mobile, the hip joints are flexed by their distal lever, i. e. the lower legs are placed on a raised base support, as in Fig. 62. In this manner, the pelvis, as proximal lever of the hip joints, has tolerance for extension, thus preventing flexional suspension of the legs from the pelvis or the pelvis from the legs at the hip joints, and giving the lumbar spine tolerance for flexion and extension and thus potential mobility. In patients with a hollow back, placing cushions beneath the lumbar spine is advised (Fig. 64). Patients with constitutional flat backs and increased flexion of the pelvis in the hip joints, on the other hand, should have the lumbar spine, thorax, shoulder girdle, arms and head raised by a suitable large pillow. Since these patients often have re-

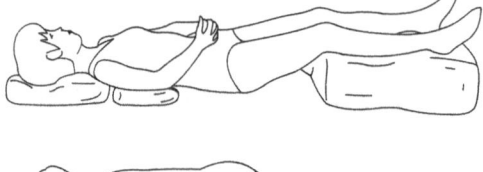

Fig. 62. Relief posture for the lumbar spine (also thoracic and cervical spine) in supine

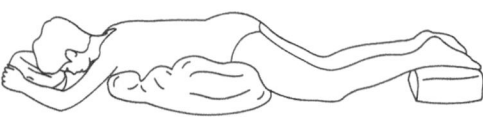

Fig. 63. Relief posture for the lumbar spine (also thoracic and cervical spine) in prone

stricted hip extension, flexion of the pelvis in the hip joints will be supported proximally with cushions. This gives the hip joints tolerance for extension, preventing flexional suspension of the pelvis from the thighs. The lumbar spine is potentially mobile.

In the prone position (Fig. 63), cushions are placed under the abdomen and under the thorax if necessary to bring about a position of flexion at the hips joints effectd by the distal lever. This positioning prevents the lumbar spine from sagging into end-stop extension.

A pillow under the ankles keeps the hips in rotational neutral.

Semisidelying Supported by Pillows (Fig. 65)

This position will be described in more detail under "Relief Postures for the Thoracic Spine." To relieve strain on the lumbar spine, plenty of cushioning under the abdomen and upper thighs is particularly important. The abdomen must be able to lean against the pillows and be compressed by them. This compression of the abdomen in turn prevents the lumbar spine from sagging into end-stop extension and creates a buttress to the lowering of the diaphragm on inspiration.

It is a substitute for good resting muscle tone in the abdominal walls. In patients with a bloated stomach, it can also stimulate the elimination of air from the intestines.

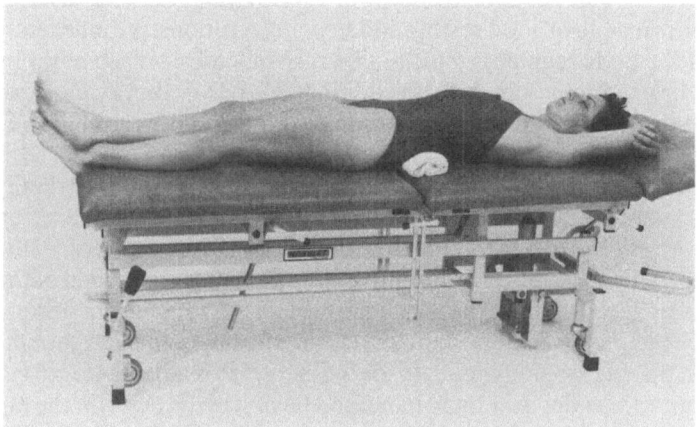

Fig. 64. Relief posture for the lumbar spine in supine for patients with hyperkypholordosis

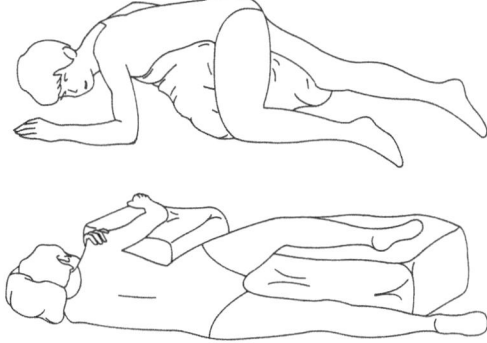

Fig. 65. Relief posture for the lumbar spine (also thoracic spine) in right semi-sidelying

Fig. 66. Relief posture for the lumbar spine (also thoracic and cervical spine) in left sidelying

Relief Posture for the Lumbar Spine in Sidelying (Fig. 66)

In sidelying as a relief posture for the lumbar spine, it is especially important to elevate the upper leg on a raised base support to prevent it from becoming suspended from the pelvis by transverse abduction in the hip joint and exerting shearing stress on the lumbar spine. The head and the upper arms also need to be propped up; if these body parts hang from the thorax and pull it forwards or backwards out of sidelying, the thorax will hang in rotation from the pelvis and stress the lumbar spine with undesired activation. In sidelying too, a pillow in front of the abdomen is indispensable. If the distance between greater trochanters is wide and the frontotransverse diameter of the thorax narrow, the thorax will have to be elevated by a large flat pillow. If only the waist is narrow, a pillow under it will suffice to prevent the lumbar spine from sagging in lateroflexion.

Relief Posture for the Lumbar Spine in Sitting (Work Posture) (Fig. 67)

For reading, writing or typing, the abdominal support shown in Fig. 67 is an ideal relief posture for the lumbar spine. BSs pelvis, thorax and head, aligned in the long axis of the body, incline forwards by flexion in the hip joints and the lumbar spine stays roughly in neutral position. By the provision of ventral support, preferably all the

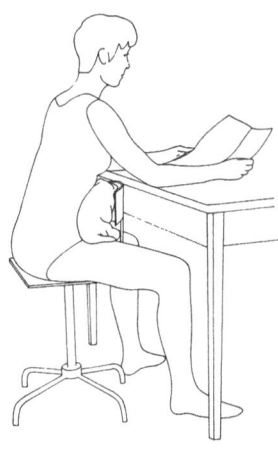

Fig. 67. Relief posture for the lumbar spine in sitting: work posture

way to the caudal portion of the thorax, the weights of the thorax, head and arms can to a large extent be transferred to the abdominal support. The arms can be parked on the desk. The fall-preventing activity holding the head in the long axis of the body stimulates stabilization of the thoracic spine in neutral. Stress on the lumbar spine, especially on the lumbosacral transition, is dramatically reduced and the fall-preventing activity in the extensor muscles can switch off completely.

Relief Posture for the Lumbar Spine in Standing (Figs. 68–70)

In standing, stress on the lumbar spine is automatically relieved by leaning the long axes of BSs pelvis and thorax backwards by extension in the supporting hip joint and the body is leant against a dorsal support at the level of the shoulder girdle (Fig. 68). The long axis of the body above the site of the support remains vertical. The extensional supported leaning occurs only in the portion of the thoracic spine below the support site, leaving the lumbar spine potentially mobile.

Figures 69 and 70 show how to relieve the lumbar spine when the long axis of the body is inclined forwards by flexion in the hip joints. The patient places one foot on a stool high enough for him to be able, depending on the length of his arm and the activity he is engaged in, to lean on his thigh with the ipsilateral hand or elbow. The spinal column is thus in flexional/extensional neutral. The weights of the forwards-leaning BSs pelvis and thorax are supported on the raised leg by the arm and can therefore neither cause shearing stress on the passive structures of the lumbar spine nor overload the fall-preventing extensors of the lumbar spine by requiring their constant activation.

Relief Posture for the Iliosacral Joints and for the Lumbar Spine in Standing (Fig. 71)

To relieve stress on the iliosacral joints we use the position illustrated in Fig. 71: standing one-legged on the right foot, a footlength away from a wall. The dorsal aspects of BSs pelvis, thorax and head, aligned in the long axis of the body, are leant against the wall. The long axis of the body remains vertical when the right hand

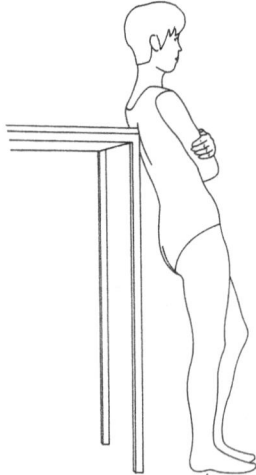

Fig. 68. Relief posture for the lumbar spine (also cervical spine) in standing

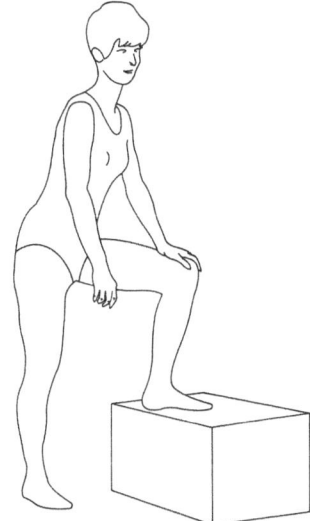

Fig. 69. Relief posture for the lumbar spine in standing: work posture

grasps the left knee from ventrally/laterally, so that the weight of the leg hangs from the hand. A horizontal tug to the right/dorsally relieves stress on the iliosacral joints and on the lumbosacral articulation.

Relief Posture for the Lumbar Spine in Sitting (Fig. 72)
In Fig. 72, the arms form a suspension device for the thorax and for the head enthroned atop it. Through the muscle activity by which the thorax is hung from the shoulder girdle, the arms go into supporting function. BS pelvis remains in contact with the seat. With the relaxation of the lumbar and abdominal muscles, BS pelvis goes into parking function. If the pressure activity of the hands is increased, the weight of the pelvis can be used to exert traction on the lumbar spine.

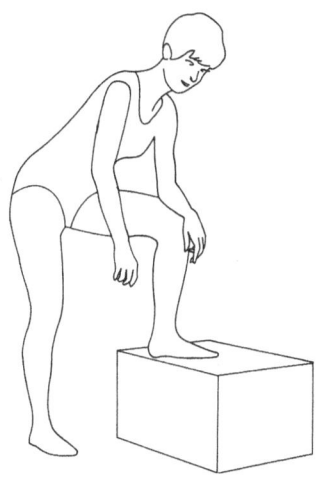

Fig. 70. Relief posture for the lumbar spine in bending: work posture

223

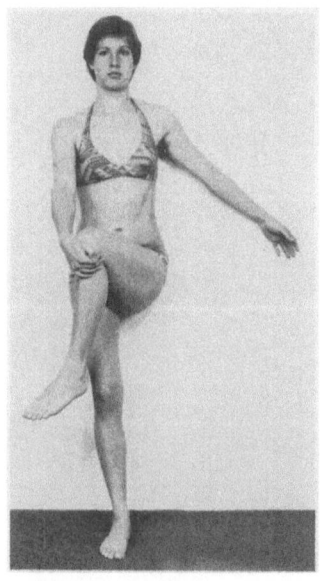

Fig. 71. Relief posture for the lumbar spine (iliosacral joints) in standing

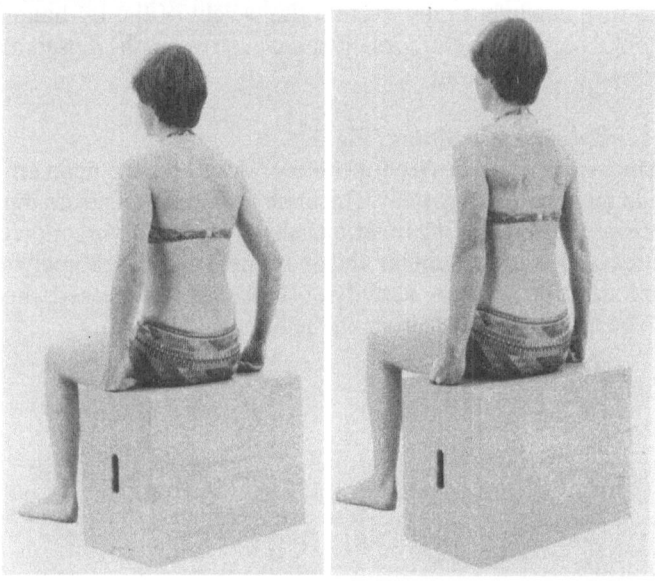

a

b

Fig. 72 a, b. Relief posture for the lumbar spine in sitting. **a** Starting position. **b** BSs thorax and pelvis are suspended from the shoulder girdle by muscle activity

Relief Posture for the Lumbar Spine in Sitting with the Arms Supported on the Thighs (Fig. 73)

In this relief posture, BSs pelvis, thorax and head are aligned in the long axis of the body, which is inclined forwards. Initially an extensional lumbosacral anchor forms while, at the same time, stress on the lumbosacral area is relieved by the arms' being supported on the thighs.

224

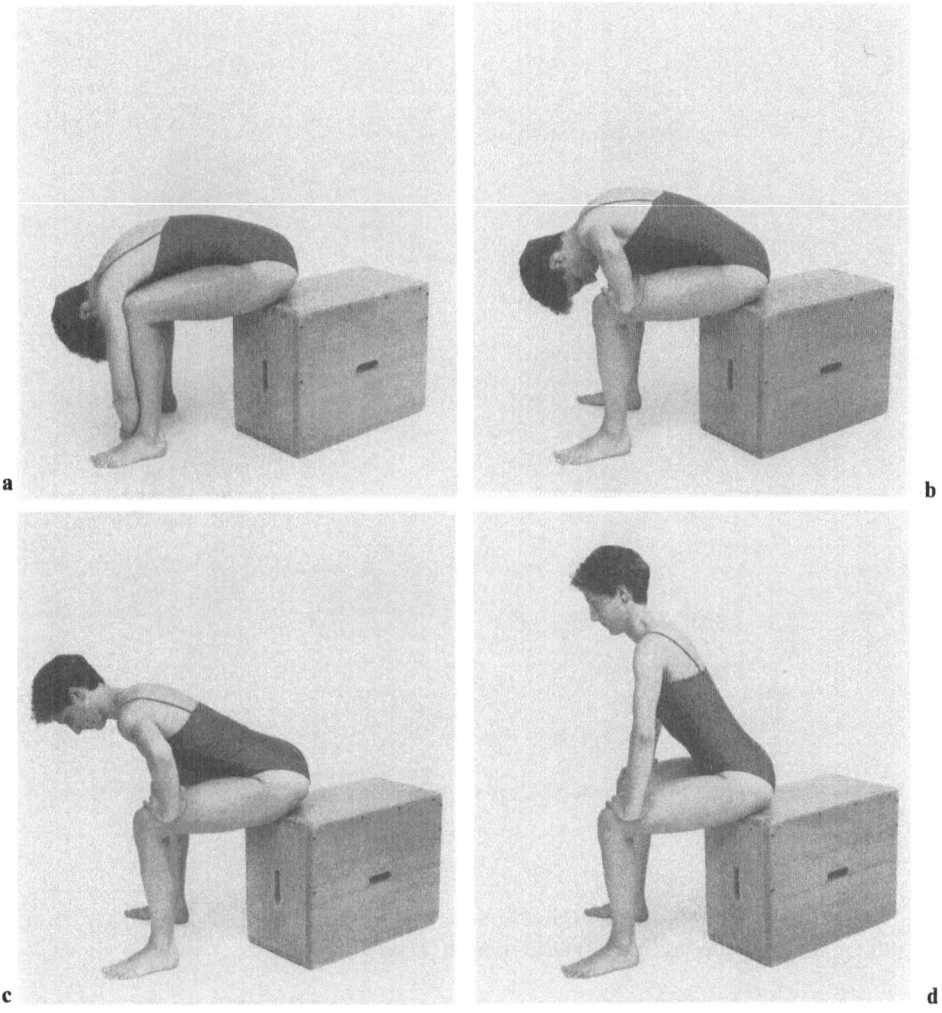

a

b

c

d

Fig. 73 a–d. Relief posture for the lumbar spine in sitting with arms supported on the thighs

Starting Position: Sitting across a corner of a box; BSs pelvis and thorax are parked on the thighs (on top of a pillow if necessary). BSs arms and head hang from the thorax (Fig. 73 a).

Actio: The hands find a place to support themselves on the thighs, close to the knees (Fig. 73 b). Through an increase in the flexion of the pelvis in the hip joints, the lumbosacral transition becomes extensionally activated. Not until then is the thoracic spine brought by extension into its neutral position, by both the pushing-off activity upwards/backwards of the hands on the thighs and the dorsal translation of the head into the virtual long axis of the body (Fig. 73 c, d).

Conditio: The distance from acromion to earlobe must not get smaller and the patient must not hold his breath. The pushing-off activity of the hands brings the arms into supporting function and must on no account bring them into free play.

225

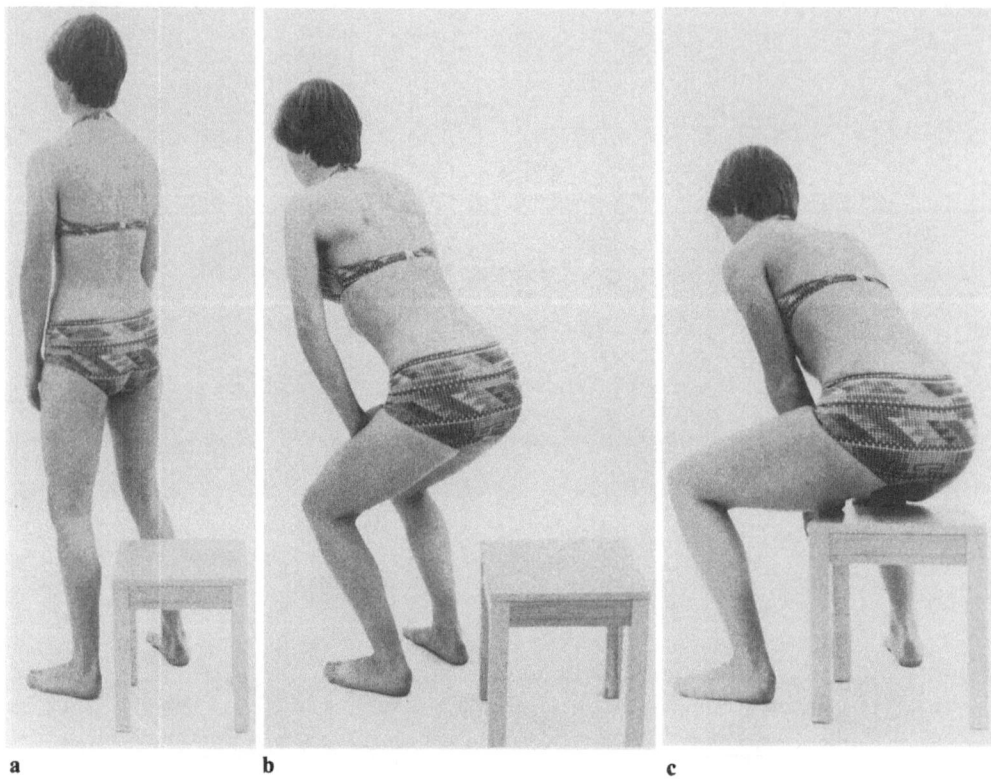

a   b   c

Fig. 74 a–c. Relief posture for the lumbar spine. **a** Standing, prior to sitting or after standing up. **b** Sitting down and **c** getting up

The intensity of economical activity in the abdominal muscles is low and the lumbar spine is extensionally activated in neutral position.

Relief Posture for the Lumbar Spine While Standing Up and Sitting Down (Fig. 74)

Standing upright (Fig. 74 a), the patient aligns BS pelvis so well under BSs thorax and head in the long axis of the body that the extensors of the lumbar spine and lumbosacral transition do not need to work against gravity at all, i.e. are not activated to prevent falling. The pelvis is potentially mobile in the hip joints and in the joints of the lumbar spine. If there is pain, the hands can be rested on the right and left pelvic crests and can then press down hard enough to suspend the weight of the thorax and the head enthroned on top of it from the muscles of the shoulder girdle. When sitting down or standing up, the long axis of the body, which has been inclined forward by hip flexion, is supported by via the arms leaning on the thighs close to the hip joints (Fig. 74 b). Immediately before sitting down or when just beginning to stand up, the arms can find support on the seat of the chair, as shown in Fig. 74 c, or, if the seat is wider, to the right and left of the hip joints.

226

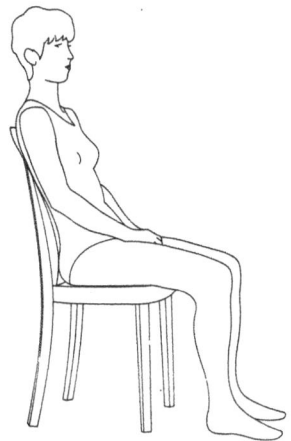

Fig. 75. Relief posture for the lumbar spine in sitting with a backrest

Relief Posture for the Lumbar Spine in Sitting with a Backrest (Fig. 75)

Figure 75 shows a person sitting with the Swedish backrest "Abo back". It is light and very useful in any standard chair, carseat or bed, and fits easily into a suitcase. To truly eliminate stress on the lumbar spine by leaning against a backrest, the entire dorsal aspects of BSs pelvis and thorax must be in contact with the backrest. The long axis of the head sticking up beyond the backrest should be vertically above the cranial end of the thoracic spine. The soles are in contact with the floor and the dorsal aspects of the thighs should be firmly in contact with the seat.

5.3.2 Movement Levels for Mobilizing Massage Around the Lumbar Spine

The name "Movement Levels for Mobilizing Massage of the Lumbar Spine" refers to the area in which the technique of mobilizing massage (see *Functional Kinetics,* pp. 301–311) is to be applied.

■ Goal of the Exercise

The goal is for the therapist to:
- Improve circulation, elasticity and contractility and normalize tone in the muscles around the lumbar spine through mobilizing massage
- Facilitate the interaction between the pelvis, potentially mobile in the hip joints and joints of the lumbar spine, and the thoracic spine, dynamically stabilized in neutral position, and explain to the patient how they work together
- Facilitate the interaction of fine deformation and/or fluctuations in tone of the surrounding muscles when the legs are involved in locomotion and explain the way it works to the patient

▶ Functional Analysis in Therapist Language

As described in the goal, Mobilizing Massage of the Lumbar Spine treats BS pelvis and the adjacent BSs thorax and legs. The levels of movement are:
- Lumbar spine in lateroflexion – hip joints
- Lumbar spine in flexion/extension – hip joints
- Transition between lumbar and thoracic spine in rotation – hip joints

Lumbar Spine in Lateroflexion, Hip Joints in Rotation (Fig. 76)

Since lateroflexion in the lumbar spine, particularly the caudal lumbar spine, is very important, we want to mobilize the effector muscles by massage. To do this we will use extensive pelvic movement in the midfrontal plane to alternately shift the lumbar spine into right- and left-convex/-concave lateroflexion and the hip joints, in a starting position of 90° flexion effected by the distal lever, into internal and external rotation. The muscles will be massaged on the concave side when the lumbar spine is in lateroflexion.

Unit 1
Displacement of the pelvis with the thighs flexed to 90° in the hip joints (Fig. 76 a). DP intersection of the left pelvic crest and the midfrontal plane moves cranially/medially, DP intersection of the right pelvic crest and the midfrontal plane moves caudally/medially. As these points move, the *lumbar spine* goes into *left-*

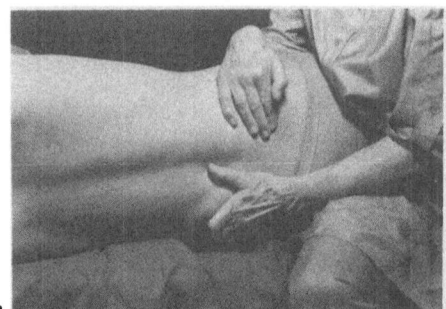

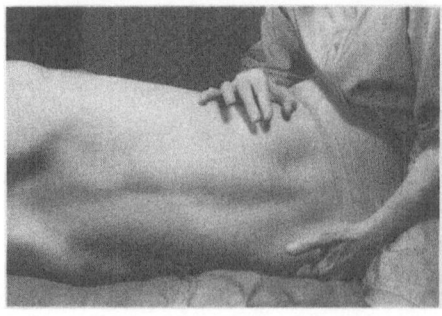

Fig. 76 a, b. Mobilizing Massage at Movement Level lumbar spine. **a** Left-concave lateroflexion. **b** Right-concave lateroflexion

concave lateroflexion, the left hip joint into *external rotation*, and the *right hip joint* into *internal rotation.*

Muscles Relaxed:
Right hip joint: obturatorius internus, piriformis, gemellus inferior and superior, gluteus medius and minimus, lateral portion of the gluteus maximus.
Left hip joint: adductor magnus, adductor longus and adductor brevis, pectineus, quadratus femoris, obturatorius externus.
Lumbar spine: quadratus lumborum, psoas major and minor, transverse abdominis, obliquus externus and internus, multifidus, intertransversarius, transversospinalis, *left* longissimus and iliocostalis.

Muscles Stretched:
Right hip joint: adductor magnus, adductor longus and adductor brevis, pectineus, quadratus femoris, obturatorius externus.
Left hip joint: obturatorius internus, piriformis, gemellus inferior and superior, gluteus medius and minimus, lateral portion of the gluteus maximus, tensor fasciae latae.
Lumbar spine: quadratus lumborum, psoas major and minor, transversus abdominis, obliquus externus and internus, multifidus, intertransversarius, transversospinalis, *right* longissimus and iliocostalis.

Unit 2
Displacement of the pelvis with the thighs flexed to 90° in the hip joints (Fig. 76 b). DP intersection of the left pelvic crest and the midfrontal plane moves caudally/medially, DP intersection of the right pelvic crest and the midfrontal plane moves cranially/medially. As these points move, the *lumbar spine* goes into *right-concave lateroflexion,* the *left hip joint* into *internal rotation,* and the *right hip joint* into *external rotation.*

Muscles Relaxed:
Right hip joint: adductor magnus, adductor longus and adductor brevis, pectineus, quadratus femoris, obturatorius externus.
Left hip joint: obturatorius internus, piriformis, gemellus inferior and superior, gluteus medius and minimus, lateral portion of the gluteus maximus, tensor fasciae latae.
Lumbar spine: quadratus lumborum, psoas major and minor, transversus abdominis, obliquus externus and internus, multifidus, intertransversarius, transversospinalis, *right* longissimus and iliocostalis.

Muscles Stretched:
Right hip joint: obturatorius internus, piriformis, gemellus inferior and superior, gluteus medius and minimus, lateral portion of gluteus maximus.
Left hip joint: adductor magnus, adductor longus and adductor brevis, pectineus, quadratus femoris, obturatorius externus.
Lumbar spine: quadratus lumborum, psoas major and minor, transversus abdominis, obliquus externus and internus, multifidus, intertransversarius, transversospinalis, *left* longissimus and iliocostalis.

Procedure for Units 1 and 2

The patient is positioned on his right or left side. For the long axis of the body to be more or less in the neutral position horizontally, the head will need a raised base support, and, depending on the patient's constitution, the thorax, waist or pelvis may require one as well. The long axes of the thighs are positioned in the transverse plane of the hip joints, the knees are flexed somewhat more than 90°. The dorsal aspects of BSs pelvis, thorax and head are vertical along the long edge of the treatment bench; this gives even long thighs enough room. If the patient is lying on his right side, the therapist sits down in the angle formed by the thighs and lower legs such that the left side of her pelvis touches the patient's tuberosities. This way she can grasp the patient's left pelvic crest from above with her left forearm and his right pelvic crest from below with her right hand. She can also push the patient's left tuberosity cranially with her body. In order for the therapist to be able to hang well from the patient's pelvis and pull it caudally or lean against his pelvis and push it cranially, she must position her legs in a stride, firmly in contact with the floor at the metatarsophalangeal joint of her right large toe, with her hip extended and knee flexed. Now she can either hang by her left arm from the patient's left pelvic crest, if necessary pushing the patient's right tuberosity cranially with her right hand, or she can push off with her right foot so that she pushes the patient's left tuberosity cranially with her pelvis, hanging if necessary from the patient's right pelvic crest by her right hand.

When pulling on the upper pelvic crest brings about right-/downwards facing concavity in the lumbar spine, the therapist lifts the relaxed lumbar muscles with her right hand while the fingers of her left hand pull the stretched lumbar muscles on the convex left side away from the spinal processes. When, by pushing the upper ischial tuberosity cranially, the lateroflexion changes so that the concavity faces to the left/upwards, the therapist kneads the relaxed lumbar muscles downwards with her left hand while the fingertips of the right hand pull the stretched lumbar muscles on the right side downwards and away from the spinal processes.

To mobilize the monarticular muscles of the hip joints by massage, the therapist can use her right hand to work the relaxed lumbar muscles on the right side when the lumbar spine is right-concave lateroflexed and manipulates the relaxed abductors of the left hip joint with her left.

One can also massage the hip abductors and adductors alternately. For this the patient is best positioned supine. One leg is placed with the sole near and caudal to the ischial tuberosity on the treatment bench, and the leg to be massaged is positioned in neutral. If the right leg is raised up, the therapist sits on the patient's left side and with her left hand on his right pelvic crest moves his pelvis in the midfrontal plane, causing lateroflexion in the lumbar spine, rotation in the right hip joint and alternating abduction/adduction in the left hip joint. The therapist massages the abductors and adductors of the left hip joint with her right hand.

Another good position for mobilizing massage at this movement level is prone. For this variation, the abdomen must be positioned high enough for there to be movement tolerance for extension in the hip joints. The head should for preference be positioned low enough that the patient can rest his forehead on his hands and the cervical spine remain in neutral.

The therapist stands at the head end of the treatment bench and leans with her hands on the right and left side of the patient's pelvis, making it turn in slight extension in the hip joints and exerting light traction on the lumbar spine. By alternating pressure on the right and left pelvic crest, the therapist starts lift-free lateroflexional mobilization of the lumbar spine and tells the patient to follow what is happening by feeling how his knees are pushed away alternately. Now the therapist can massage each side of the lumbar spine when it is concave with the ball of thumb.

If the therapist stands on the patient's right side, she can push the patient's thorax with her right elbow, push his pelvis into left-concave lateroflexion of the lumbar spine with her left elbow, and simultaneously mobilize the relaxed lumbar muscles on the left side by massage.

Lumbar Spine in Extension/Flexion, Hip Joints in Flexion/Extension

Since extension and flexion in the caudal motion segments of the lumbar spine are extremely important to good postural statics, we want to give the effector muscles, particularly the concentric-isotonic extensors and the eccentric-isotonic flexors, mobilizing massage. To do this, we alternately extend and flex the lumbar spine, particularly the caudal portion, and alternately flex and extend the hip joints within the flexion zone, out of a starting position at about 40° flexion of the thighs, by moving the pelvis in the plane of symmetry.

Unit 3
Displacement of the pelvis with the thighs in 40° flexion in the hip joints. DPs right and left iliac spines move ventrally/caudally in their sagittal plane and DP tip of the coccyx moves dorsally/cranially in the plane of symmetry. As these distance points move, the *lumbar spine* goes into *extension* and the *pelvis* moves in *flexion in the hip joints.*

Muscles Relaxed:
Hip joints: iliopsoas, tensor fasciae latae, sartorius, rectus femoris, gluteus medius and minimus (ventral portion).
Lumbar spine: iliocostalis lumborum, longissimus lumborum, intertransversarii lumborum, interspinales lumborum, multifidus lumborum, rotatores lumborum.

Muscles Stretched:
Hip joints: gluteus medius and minimus (dorsal fibres), piriformis, obturatorius externus, quadratus femoris, adductor brevis and magnus, gluteus maximus, semimembranosus, biceps femoris, semitendinosus, gracilis.
Lumbar spine: rectus abdominis, obliquus internus and externus bilaterally.

Unit 4
Displacement of the pelvis with the thighs in 40° flexion in the hip joints. DPs right and left iliac spines move dorsally/cranially in their sagittal plane, DP symphysis moves ventrally/cranially in the plane of symmetry. As these distance points move, the *lumbar spine* goes into *flexion,* the *pelvis* moves in *extension in the hip joints.*

Muscles Relaxed:
Hip joints: gluteus medius and minimus (dorsal fibres), piriformis, obturatorius externus, quadratus femoris, adductur brevis and magnus, gluteus maximus, semi-membranosus, biceps femoris, semitendinosus, gracilis.
Lumbar spine: rectus abdominis, obliquus internus and externus bilaterally.

Muscles Stretched:
Hip joints: iliopsoas, tensor fasciae latae, sartorius, rectus femoris, gluteus medius and minimus (ventral portion).
Lumbar spine: iliocostalis lumborum, longissimus lumborum, intertransversarii lumborum, interspinalis lumborum, multifidus lumborum, rotatores lumborum.

Procedure for Units 3 and 4
The patient is positioned on his right or left side. For the long axis of the body to be horizontal and roughly in the neutral position, the head will need to a raised base support, and, depending on the patient's constitution, the thorax, waist or pelvis may require one as well. The legs are comfortably positioned with about 40° flexion in the hip joints effected by the distal lever and about 90° flexion in the knee and ankle joints. If there is too much adduction in the upper hip joint, this can be rectified by placing a thin pillow between the legs. The hand of the upper arm can use the treatment bench ventrally at about the level of the navel as a supportive or suspension device; this helps control the tendency to roll on to the back or the stomach. The lower arm lies on the bench, its hand rests on the thumb side, about level with the patient's face. The shoulder is flexed to about 45° and externally rotated, the elbow flexed more than 90° and the forearm supinated.
The therapist sits behind the patient, high enough that she can lean her elbows either on her own thighs or on the treatment bench. She is careful to keep her spinal column roughly in neutral position as she leans forwards by flexion in the hip joints. By applying axial pressure with one hand (see Fig. 86 a) at motion segment S1/L5 and having the patient push back against this pressure, she causes him to flex his lumbar spine, and the pelvis moves causing extension in the hip joints. Then the patient yields to the pressure of the therapist's hand, the lumbar spine extends, and the pelvis moves back causing flexion in the hip joints. During this to-and-fro movement, the lumbosacral transition remains the critical distance point. The patient is instructed to keep this little movement going.
The muscles around the lumbar spine can either be pushed together from either side of the spinal processes when they are relaxed during the extension phase of the movement, and then stretched again when the spine flexes, or first the lower region then the upper can be kneaded. When the muscles on the lower side are relaxed the thumbs knead them, moving them towards the spinal processes; when they are stretched, they are pulled downwards, away from the spinal processes. When the muscles on the upper side are relaxed the thumbs knead them, lifting them up and away from the spinal processes; when they are stretched, the fingers knead the muscles downwards and stretch them longways.

In the upper hip joint, the flexor and extensor muscles can be massaged in alternation in the relaxed phase. This works particularly well because the fan of muscles that anchors the pelvis to the thigh in the supporting leg during walking is antagonistic within itself.

Lumbothoracic Transition in Rotation, Hip Joints in Transverse Abduction/Adduction

Well-functioning rotation at the transition from the lumbar to the thoracic spine being essential to protect the lumbar discs, we will use up the movement tolerances for rotation to end-stop by turning the pelvis in transverse abduction/adduction in the hip joints, and give the rotation area mobilizing massage.

Unit 5
Displacement of the pelvis with the thighs flexed to 90° in the hip joints. With the patient lying on his right side, DP left patella moves ventrally while DP right patella strives tendentially slightly dorsally. This causes the *spinal column* to be deformed in *pelvis-positive rotation* at the lumbothoracic transition, the *left hip joint* goes into *transverse abduction* and the *right hip joint* goes into *transverse adduction*.

Muscles Relaxed:
Left hip joint: tensor fasciae latae, ventral portions of the gluteus medius and minimus, sartorius, rectus femoris.
Right hip joint: adductor brevis, obturatorius internus and externus, pectineus, iliopsoas.
Lumbothoracic transition: obliquus abdominis internus on the *left,* obliquus abdominis externus on the *right,* the autochthonous rotators that effect pelvis-positive rotation in this area.

Muscles Stretched:
Left hip joint: adductor brevis, obturatorius internus and externus, pectineus, iliopsoas.
Right hip: tensor fasciae latae, ventral portion of gluteus medius and minimus, sartorius, rectus femoris.
Lumbothoracic transition: obliquus abdominis internus on the *right,* obliquus abdominis externus on the *left,* the autochthonous rotators that effect pelvis-negative rotation in this area.

Unit 6
Displacement of the pelvis with the thighs flexed to 90° in the hip joints. With the patient lying on his right side, DP left patella moves dorsally while DP right patella strives tendentially slightly ventrally. This causes the *spinal column* to be deformed in *pelvis-negative rotation* at the lumbothoracic transition, the *left hip joint* goes into *transverse adduction* and the *right hip joint* goes into *transverse abduction*.

Muscles Relaxed:
Left hip joint: adductor brevis, obturatorius internus and externus, pectineus, iliopsoas.
Right hip joint: tensor fasciae latae, ventral portion of the gluteus medius and minimus, sartorius, rectus femoris.
Lumbothoracic transition: obliquus abdominis internus on the *right,* obliquus abdominis externus on the *left,* the autochthonous rotators responsible for pelvis-negative rotation in this area.

Muscles Stretched:
Left hip joint: tensor fasciae latae, ventral portion of gluteus medius and minimus, sartorius, rectus femoris.
Right hip joint: adductor brevis, obturatorius internus and externus, pectineus, iliopsoas.
Lumbothoracic transition: obliquus abdominis internus on the *left,* obliquus abdominis externus on the *right,* the autochthonous rotators responsible for pelvis-positive rotation in this area.

Procedure for Units 5 and 6
The patient is positioned as for units 3 and 4.
For unit 5, the therapist sits behind the patient, who is lying on his right side, about at the level of the treatment bench. With her left hand she grasps the patient's left patella from above/ventrally, applying slight compressive resistance in a dorsal direction towards the left hip joint. At the same time, she encircles the patient's thorax from above/left-laterally with her right hand. For the time being, this hand controls the thorax and keeps it from leaning over ventrally when the left patella moves ventrally and the right patella strives dorsally.
For the transition into unit 6, the therapist grips the patient's left lower leg close to the popliteal fossa, coming from dorsally with her left hand. This allows the patient to begin the countermovement, gliding the left patella dorsally against gentle guiding resistance while the right patella strives ventrally. The therapist's right hand ensures that the thorax does not lean over backwards. As soon as this alternating movement sequence is running smoothly, the patient is instructed to keep it going in an effortless manner.
Now the therapist can modify her hand-hold and begin with the mobilizing massage. She moves the patient's pelvis and thorax counter-rotationally with the movement described above. She does this with her forearms, which she positions frontotransversely. Now her hands are free to massage. The art of therapy is the ability to find the patient's actual present level of rotation and if necessary expand it caudally or cranially (i. e. making more motion segments available for rotation) by kneading the muscles of the back while the thorax and pelvis continue to rotate. If one particular motion segment is to be mobilized, the hand-hold is modified. The therapist holds the two spinal processes between thumb, index and middle fingers. Whether she then holds the cranial spinal process still with the thorax and moves the caudal one with the pelvis, or holds the caudal process still with the pelvis and rotates the cranial process with the thorax, or twists the two segments against each other counter-rotationally, is something to be decided individually for each case.

234

5.3.3 Stretch, Little Hip (Fig. 77)

"Stretch, Little Hip" is an invented name. It refers to extension of the hip, which is of great importance for economical motor behaviour.
Any restriction of hip extension disturbs economical upright posture decisively. The potential mobility of the pelvis in the lumbar joints and in the hip joints is bound to be lost. The only way lift-free/reduced-lift mobilization can then be performed is when the hips are flexed so far that the pelvis has extensional tolerance of at least 15° in the hip joints. Stretch, Little Hip aims to achieve full tolerance for extension in the hip joint.

■ Goal of the Exercise

The goal is for the patient to be able to:
- Extend the hips easily, both actively and passively, until end-stopped by the iliofemoral ligament
- Fully extend one hip by the distal lever, the thigh, without deforming the lumbar spine in extension or lateroflexion.

▶ Functional Analysis in Therapists Language

● Conception of the Exercise

This exercise subjects the hip extensors to extreme stress, in order to trigger reflexive relaxation of their antagonists and thus eliminate or at least improve a flexion contracture of muscular origin. To this end, the starting position must meet the following conditions:
- In the hip joint with a muscle flexion contracture, there must be ample tolerance for extension.
- The extensional components of the affected hip should be subjected to unambiguous positive lifting stress.
- Natural avoidance mechanisms in the form of unwanted continuing movements in the spinal column – extension, lateroflexion or rotation of the lumbar spine – must be made impossible.

All these conditions are basically met when the patient, at the narrow end of a well-padded treatment bench, sets his right or left lower leg on the bench and parks his pelvis and abdomen on his thigh and his head on the bench, while his other leg hangs down with the foot touching the floor.
If the flexion/extension axis of the hip of the hanging leg is horizontal and the long axis of this leg is in the sagittal plane of this hip, which is vertical, the extensors of this hip will be subjected to full positive lifting stress when the leg is raised, while

235

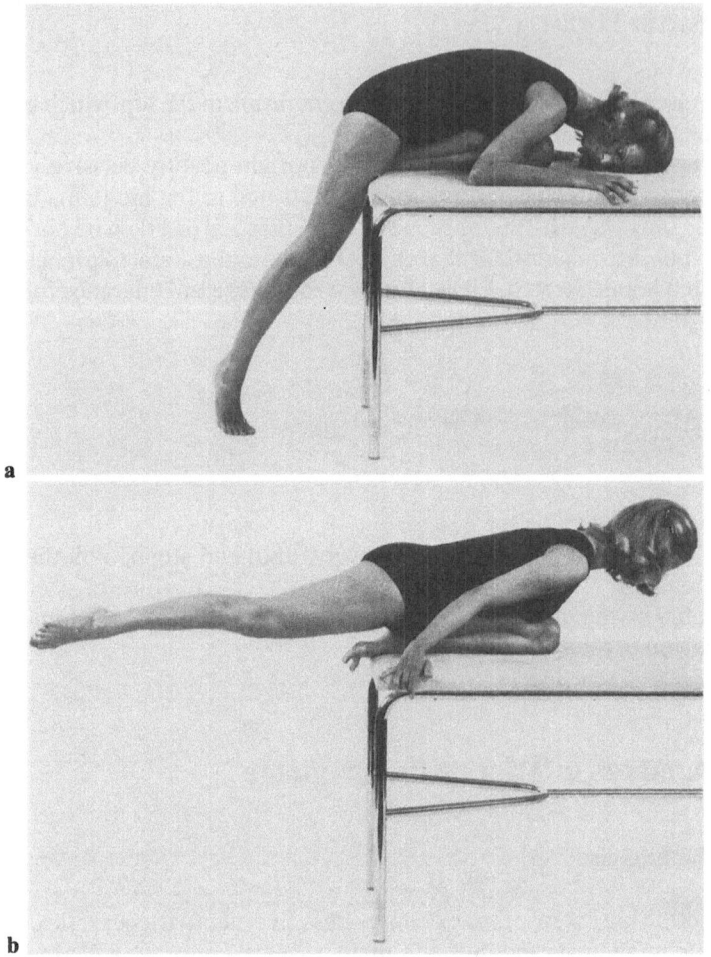

a

b

Fig. 77 a, b. Stretch, Little Hip. **a** Starting position, **b** end position

the body resting on top of the lower thigh prevents unwanted continuing movements. The patient can if necessary use the long sides of the treatment bench as a suspension device for his hands in order to keep his balance.

● **Position and Activation in the Starting Position**

Position in Space of the Critical Axes
Points of Contact Between the Body and the Environment
Components of Movement in Relation to the Neutral Positions of the Joints
The starting position is with the body sitting on the left lower leg at the narrow end of a well-padded treatment bench. The left lower leg is tucked under the left thigh, BSs pelvis and thorax rest on the left thigh, BS head is parked on the bench. The point of contact between the head and the base support is the forehead. The

forearms rest to the right and left of the left knee on the treatment bench, touching it with their flexor sides and palms. The right leg touches the floor in the sagittal plane of the right hip joint. The point of contact between the right foot and the floor is the flexor side of the toes; in the large, second and third toes floor contact is extended as far as the metatarsophalangeal joints. How far this point is from the right hip horizontally will depend on the length of the leg and the height of the treatment bench.

The joints which are not in neutral position are as follows: In BSs pelvis, thorax and head, the pelvis is maximally flexed in the left hip, the lumbar, thoracic and cervical spines are moderately flexed. We aim to make sure that as far as possible the position of the pelvis in the left hip causes no unwanted continuing movements of lateroflexion and/or rotation in the spinal column.

In BS arms, DP acromion is ventral to the body because of the protraction of the shoulder girdle in the sternoclavicular joint, the shoulder joint is in flexion/abduction/external rotation effected by the distal lever, the elbow joint is in flexion due to displacement of its fulcrum, the forearm is in pronation effected by the distal pointer, the wrist is in slight ulnar abduction and the phalangeal joints in so much flexion that if necessary they can use the long edge of the treatment table as a suspension device.

Movement Tolerances at the Critical Joints in Relation
to the Intended Primary Movement

As the name Stretch, Little Hip implies, we need the full tolerance for extension in the hip joint concerned. In the starting position we analysed above, this is the right hip joint, flexed to about 45°. The spinal column is in slight flexion. The cervical and thoracic spines have sufficient tolerance for cranial-to-caudal extension to form an activated passive buttress. Although the lumbar spine is extensionally activated by the buttressing effect between the primary movement of the right leg and the activated passive buttress, the fact that the pelvis remains in contact with the ventral aspect of the left thigh keeps it from deforming into cranial-to-caudal extension.

Distribution of Body Weight on a Base Support or Suspension Device,
Against a Supportive Device, or Over a Support Area,
and the Resulting Activity States of the Musculature

The support area is the smallest area encompassing the contact area between the ventral aspect of the left lower leg and the treatment bench and the contact point between the ventral aspect of the right thigh and the edge of the bench. The potential extension of this area, which will become effective when the patient holds on to keep his balance, will take in the points of contact between the forearms, palms and forehead and the treatment bench.

BSs pelvis and thorax are parked on the left thigh, BSs head and arms on the treatment bench and the right leg is parked on the floor.

Intensity of Muscular Activity Required with Economical Activity
Respiration

The intensity of economical activity is low. The patient should try to breathe normally.

● **Actio – Reactio of the Movement Sequence**

First of all, the palms are placed to the right and left of the left foot, resting on the corners of the treatment bench with the fingers pointing caudally/laterally. The bench can be used as either a supportive or a suspension device, as required; in the latter case the hands will need to move cranially.

Actio: The Primary Movement
The right leg performs the primary movement. The dominant direction component is vertically upwards, the horizontal component goes caudally.
The critical distance point of the primary movement of the right leg, DP tips of the toes, moves caudally/upwards/dorsally. Continuing co-rotationally, the toes are flexed by their distal levers, the subtalar and talocalcaneonavicular joints evert, the talocrural joint plantarflexes; the thigh brings the hip joint into extension and slight rotation (critical fulcrum).

Reactio: Activated Passive Buttressing
Because the vertical direction component in the primary movement is predominant, the restricted tolerance for extension acts as resistance to the primary movement at the critical fulcrum, and the potential counterweight parked on the bench, although large, can only be activated by being lifted up off the base support, activated passive buttressing will not arise reactively but must if necessary be directed.
The critical distance points of the activated passive buttressing are DP vertex and DPs right and left acromions. In continuing co-rotational movement, DP vertex moves cranially/upwards as the atlanto-occipital and atlanto-axial joints and cervical and thoracic spine extend. DPs right and left acromions move dorsally/upwards as the medial margins of the scapulae move towards the spinal processes of the thoracic spine and the pincer jaws open.

Reactio: Change in the Support Area
The support area becomes concentrically smaller because the right foot is lifted from the floor while the head goes into free play to become an activated passive buttress.

Actio: Accelerating Weights
Reactio: Braking Weights
In Stretch, Little Hip, the bisecting plane remains roughly upright, coinciding roughly with the transverse plane of the cranial pole of the iliosacral joint, which plane is vertical.
Because of the positive lift required and because the long axis of the body is horizontal, the weight of the primary moving leg has a braking effect on the movement sequence (see *Functional Kinetics,* p. 151). It is therefore important in this exercise that the primary weights and the counterweights balance each other even over the smaller support area, so that the goal is fulfilled and the right hip joint reaches the maximum extension possible under stress.

238

● **Conditio – Limitatio of the Movement Sequence**

Conditio: Constant Distances Between Body Distance Points
Limitatio: Active Buttressing and Stabilization
Conditio: The distance between DP left iliac spine and DP ventral aspect of the left thigh remains constant.
Limitatio: Keeping the left iliac spine in contact with the ventral aspect of the left thigh achieves two things: first, it makes an unwanted continuation of the primary movement of the right leg impossible, because the pelvis has no further tolerance for flexion in the left hip, and, secondly, it checks the buttressing movement which, extending the thoracic spine from the head cranially, provides a counterweight to the right leg. This leads to extensional stabilization but not actual extension of the lumbar spine, because the lumbar spine is actively buttressed flexionally by the pelvis, the proximal lever, in the left hip joint.

Conditio: The distance between DP right lateral malleolus and DP right greater trochanter remains constant.
Limitatio: If this distance is kept constant, the right knee joint becomes stabilized in extension and the right leg makes use of its entire length to increase the extensional positive lifting stress until it is horizontal.

Conditio of Absolute or Relative Fixed Spatial Points
Limitatio by Limiting the Primary Movement, Activated Passive Buttressing and/or Change in the Support Area
In this exercise there are absolute and relative fixed spatial points.

Conditio: The point of contact lower left leg/treatment bench is an absolute fixed spatial point.
Limitatio: This fixed point regulates the balancing of the weight of the primary movement against the weight of the activated passive buttress. If necessary, it also regulates the supported leaning or hanging activities of the hands.

Conditio: The points of contact right and left hand/treatment bench are relative fixed spatial points.
Limitatio: These relative fixed points ensure that the shoulder girdle and spinal column are kept symmetrical. Through hanging activity the counterweight can be increased; through supported leaning the primary weight can be reduced.

Conditio: The distance between the right iliac spine and the treatment bench is an absolute fixed spatial point.
Limitatio: This fixed point keeps the frontal plane of BS pelvis horizontal and ensures that the positive stress from the lifting of the right leg remains directed at the hip extensors and is not deflected onto the hip abductors.

Conditio of Movement Speed
Limitatio of Economical Activity by Finding the Optimal Speed
Conditio: The speed of the movement is about 3 seconds to lift the leg, 5 seconds to hold it in the end position.
Limitatio: Keeping the movement slow prevents the exercise from being performed with too much momentum. Holding the leg in the end position for a long time requires a high intensity of economical activity and allows the patient time to be aware of the return of normal breathing.

● **Position and Activation in the End Position**
  and Return to the Starting Position

As mentioned above, the end position should be held 5 seconds or longer.
The way back to the starting position is by slowly reducing the high intensity of the economical activity; the return, too, should be slow, controlled, and without deviations. The hands remain where they are for subsequent repetitions, returning to the starting position only at the end of the final repetition.

▶ **Instruction in Patient Language**

● **Instruction Appealing to the Patient's Perception**

Before beginning the movement sequence, the patient must check his starting position, become aware of where his right foot touches the floor, and feel whether he will be able to perform the exercise or whether, as is often the case, adaptation will be necessary before he starts.

● **Verbal Instruction**   ● **Instruction by Manipulation**

Position and Activation in the Starting Position
"Kneel on your left leg on top of the treatment bench (table, sofa). You can support yourself on your hands. Keep your right foot on the floor. Sit down on your left lower leg so that you can feel your heel under your bottom; your foot hangs over the side of the bench and your toes face inwards.
Now lie down along the top of your left thigh so that your forehead touches the treatment bench in front of your left knee and you can rest your head on it. Your hands slid forwards as your body

If kneeling down on the lower leg is uncomfortable, a pillow can be placed between the lower leg and the thigh. Stress is taken off the knee by having the patient support himself on his hands. The toes should face inwards. This keeps the lower leg in internal rotation when under stress, protecting the medial ligaments. Where the right forefoot touches the floor will depend on the height of the treatment bench. The lower the bench, the more the knee will have to flex, and the further

went down and are now resting on the bench on either side of your head. You should feel quite comfortable in this position and be able to breathe easily."

away the point of contact between the right foot and the floor will be. If the patient is unable to lay BS pelvis on his thigh because of restricted hip flexion, a pillow can also be pushed in between the pelvis and the abdomen. The therapist watches particularly that the only movement in the spinal column is flexion; no rotation or lateroflexion is allowed. BS thorax should lie with the middle of its ventral aspect on the thigh.

Actio and Conditio of the Movement Sequence

"Your hands go down next to your left foot with the palms facing downwards and the fingers pointing backwards. This gives you the security to make your right leg really long and lift it upwards, lifting your head at the same time – that's the best way to find your balance. But your lower abdomen stays down on your thigh. The back of your neck is long and your head doesn't feel stiff. Your are looking downwards. Your right buttock really has to work hard, but you keep breathing quietly and your tongue is relaxed against your front lower teeth. You remain motionless in this position." (Fig. 77 b)

Before the movement sequence starts, the therapist must estimate how the right leg and BSs pelvis and head will weigh against each other. If they are of about equal weight or if the leg is relatively light, as in Fig. 77 a, the hands find purchase on the support area to the right and left of the left foot in order to expand this area if necessary. If, however, the leg is long and heavy, the arms will either have to be brought in as activated passive buttresses in the projection of the long axis of the body or they will have to stay in the starting position and, holding onto the edge of the bench, hang the body onto the bench. If the patient at first has to struggle too much to extend the right hip joint, the therapist should help lift the right leg and hold BS pelvis in the correct position.

Return to the Starting Position

"Now you can move back into that comfortable starting position. It's all downhill from here, but it's steep, so go slowly, put on the brakes. You can rest for a bit as soon as your toes have found the floor again."

The therapist can make the exercise easier for the patient by hanging herself onto the patient's hands, so that he only needs to think about moving his leg while she provides a finely adjusted counterweight.

► Adapting the Exercise to the Patient's Constitution and Condition

● Adaptation to Constitution: Role of Lengths, Widths, Depths and Distribution of Weights

The relationship between the weight of the leg and the weight of the upper body length plays an important part in Stretch, Little Hip. Light legs combined with an upper length with increased weight in BSs thorax and head and a heavy shoulder girdle make the exercise easier, while heavy legs and an upper length with less weight in BSs thorax and head and a light shoulder girdle make the exercise more difficult.
In the latter case, we slightly modify the starting position before the primary movement begins. The palms slide headwards along the long edges of the treatment bench until the elbows are in neutral position. As the leg is raised, the upper body becomes hung onto the treatment bench. Now we must be especially careful to watch that the conditio requiring contact between DP left iliac spine and the ventral aspect of the left thigh is fulfilled.

● Adaptation to Condition

Restricted Movement and/or Hypermobility
Stretch, Little Hip can be helpful in relaxing muscle flexion contractures in the hip joint because the intense stress on the agonists causes the antagonists to relax reflexively.

5.3.4 Pliers (Fig. 78)

"Pliers" is an invented name: the therapist manipulates the patient's legs as if she were opening and closing a pair of pliers.

■ Goal of the Exercise

The goal is for the therapist to bring about the activity state of potential mobility in the lumbar spine in its neutral position by equal and simultaneous stressing of the flexors of one hip and the extensors of the other.

▶ Functional Analysis in Therapist Language

● Conception of the Exercise

Potential mobility in the lumbar spine in its neutral position is an important feature of economical motor behaviour. In upright standing or sitting this potential mobility is coordinated with that of the pelvis in the hip joints. Smooth transitions between potential mobility and stabilization are important when the long axis of the body changes its position in space. When the long axis of the body leans forwards, the lumbar motion segments should not alter their alignment; when it leans backwards, only the lumbosacral transition should accommodate with slight flexion.

To bring about potential mobility in the lumbar spine from the direction of the legs, we have the patient lying on his side with his legs positioned as if taking a large step. The upper hip joint should be flexed, the lower hip joint extended, and the lumbar spine should be in neutral.

If the therapist now applies flexional resistance (resistance to hinder flexion) to one hip joint, the ventral muscles that flex the lumbar spine will be activated by continuing movement. If she applies extensional resistance to the other hip joint, the dorsal muscles that extend the lumbar spine will be activated in a similar way. For the lumbar spine to remain in its neutral position there must be active buttressing: the flexors and extensors in this area contract.

If the therapist applies the flexional and extensional resistance to the hip joints simultaneously and with equal force, the two continuing activations offset each other and no buttressing is needed. There is the potential mobility we wanted. This only works because the pelvis is a stable bony ring and the springy resilience of the iliosacral joints can be used therapeutically (see Klein-Vogelbach 1991). The therapist can now move the movement system legs/pelvis, stabilized within itself, to and fro in the lumbar spine in flexion/extension (fine mobilization).

● Position and Activation in the Starting Position

Position in Space of the Critical Axes
Points of Contact Between the Body and the Environment
Components of Movement in Relation to the Neutral Position of the Joints
The starting position in the exercise example shown here is left sidelying (Fig. 78a).

BSs pelvis, thorax and head are aligned in the long axis of the body, which is horizontal. To keep the spinal column in its neutral position, the head will be placed on a suitably thick pillow.

In BS arms, the left arm rests on the base support in front of the thorax and the right arm on a pillow.

In BS legs, the left leg rests on the base support, its long axis roughly parallel to the long axis of the body. The right leg is supported on a pillow.

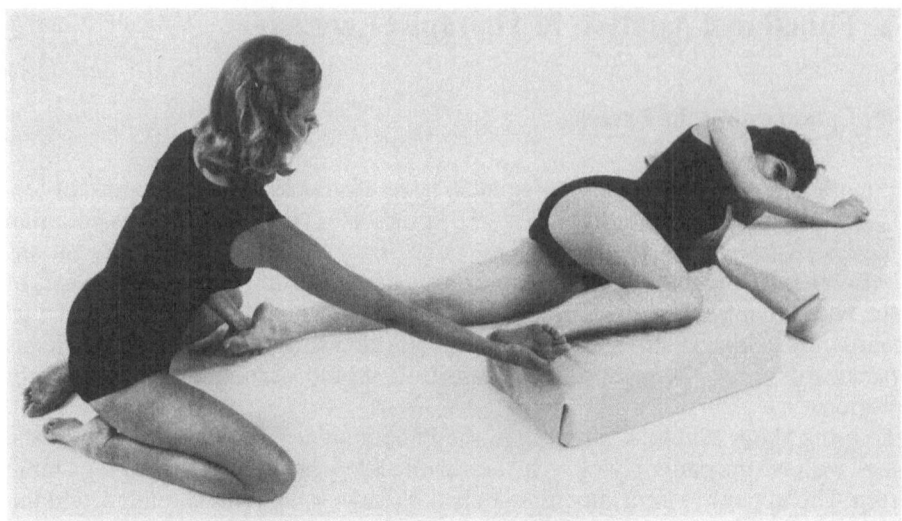

Fig. 78 a. Hip joint resistance in Pliers. **a** Right flexion, left extension

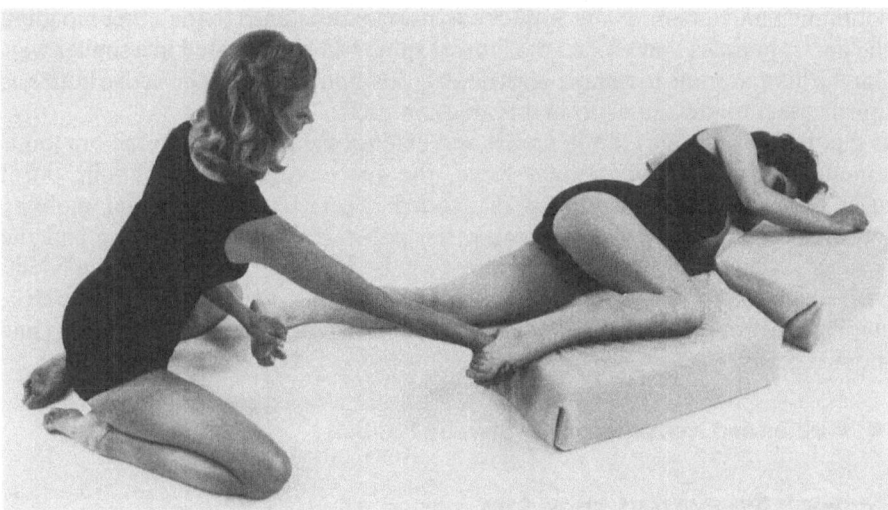

Fig. 78 b. Hip joint resistance in Pliers. **b** Right extension, left flexion

The critical joint positions in BS legs are:
- Left leg: hip joint in extension, knee joint in neutral position, joints of the foot in plantarflexion and eversion and the toes in flexion. If extension in the hip joint is unrestricted, the knee and foot of the left leg are dorsal to the midfrontal plane.
- Right leg: hip joint in so much flexion that the lumbar spine can easily remain in its neutral position, knee joint in 90° flexion, joints of the foot in dorsiflexion and inversion and the toes in extension. If flexion in the hip joint is unrestricted,

the knee is ventral to the hip joint. The knee, lower leg and foot are clearly ventral to the midfrontal plane.

Movement Tolerances at the Critical Joints in Relation to the Intended Primary Movement

The only movement excursions occur in the joints of the feet and toes. Full movement tolerance at these joints is desirable but not absolutely necessary for the exercise.

Distribution of Body Weight on a Base Support or Suspension Device, Against a Supportive Device, or Over a Support Area, and the Resulting Activity States of the Musculature

In the starting position, all the body segments are parked on their base supports.

● Actio – Reactio of the Movement Sequence

In Pliers, one cannot really speak of an actio of the movement sequence – unless one analyses instead the movements of the therapist, applying resistance. The patient pulls or pushes against this resistance without changing the position of his joints. He moves only his feet as the therapist changes the resistance to open and close the pliers.

Closing the Pliers (Fig. 78 a)

With her right hand the therapist grasps the patient's dorsiflexed foot from underneath/medially and uses it as a hook. The resistance is a tug directed caudally/ventrally. It activates the
– Extensors, invertors and dorsiflexors of the joints of the toes and foot
– Flexors of the knee joint
– Flexors of the hip joint

With her left hand the therapist grasps the patient's plantarflexed left foot from underneath/laterally and uses it as a shock absorber. The resistance is compression to the long axis of the leg coupled with a levering in a ventral direction. This activates the
– Flexors, evertors and plantarflexors of the joints of the toes and foot
– Extensors of the knee joint
– Extensors of the hip joint

If the therapist wants to mobilize the lumbar spine, particularly the lumbosacral articulation, in flexion and extension, she must tug more dorsally with her right hand without allowing the activation of the knee flexors to stop.

Opening the Pliers (Fig. 78 b)

With her right hand the therapist grasps the patient's plantarflexed right foot and uses it as a shock absorber. The pressure is directed cranially/ventrally, its course running in front of the flexion/extension axis of the ankle, behind the flexion/extension axis of the knee joint and in front of the flexion/extension axis of the hip joint, thus activating the plantarflexors of the ankle and the extensors of the knee and hip joints. With her left hand the therapist grasps the patient's dorsiflexed left foot medially/cranially and uses it as a suspension device. The resistance is a tug directed caudally/dorsally, its course running in front of the flexion/extension axis of the ankle, behind the flexion/extension axis of the knee joint and in front of the flexion/extension axis of the hip joint, thus activating the dorsiflexors of the ankle and the flexors of the knee and hip joints.

If the therapist wants to mobilize the lumbar spine, particularly the lumbosacral transition, in flexion/extension she must properly coordinate the opening of the pliers, the compressive resistance and the tugging resistance.

● **Conditio – Limitatio of the Movement Sequence**

Conditio: Constant Distances Between Body Distance Points
Limitatio: Active Buttressing and Stabilization
In Pliers, all the distances over the entire body remain constant except those at the feet and toes. Here, only those will be mentioned that are of direct relevance to the goal of the exercise.

Conditio: The distances between DP symphysis and DP navel and between DP lumbosacral transition and DP lumbothoracic transition remain constant, except if the lumbar spine is to be subjected to fine mobilization (see p. 243).
Limitatio: The lumbar spine is thus in neutral position and the resistances the therapist applies to the legs simultaneously are equally intense.

Conditio: The distance between DP navel and DP xiphoid process remains constant.
Limitatio: This keeps the thoracic spine in neutral position as well. This is especially important if the lumbar spine is to be subjected to fine mobilization.

Conditio of Absolute and/or Relative Fixed Spatial Points
Limitatio by Limiting the Primary Movement, Activated Passive Buttressing and/or Change in the Support Area
Conditio: The entire spinal column in neutral position is an absolute fixed spatial point.
Limitatio: This fixed point ensures that the resistance applied to the legs simultaneously will be of equal intensity.

▶ **Adapting the Exercise to the Patient's Constitution and Condition**

● **Adaptation to Constitution: Role of Lengths, Widths, Depths and Distribution of Weights**

Constitutional variations and weight distribution have no relevance in this exercise, except possibly when positioning the patient at the start.

246

- **Adaptation to Condition**

Restricted Movement
If restriction of movement at the hips prevents the patient from assuming the starting position shown in our example, the stride position of the legs can be adapted. Great care should still be taken that the lumbar spine stays in its neutral position if at all possible.

5.3.5 Open and Shut (Fig. 79)

"Open and Shut" is an invented name. In reference to the hip joints, "open" means flexion and "shut" means extension to end-stop.

■ Goal of the Exercise

The goal is for the patient to learn to achieve full hip extension while standing upright without disturbing the postural statics.

▶ Functional Analysis in Therapist Language

- **Conception of the Exercise**

Tilting the pelvis and righting it, or, in functional terms, flexing and extending the pelvis in the hip joints while standing upright, disturbs the statics of posture considerably. When the pelvis extends in the hip joints, all the weight above it is brought backwards with it; as it flexes, all this weight is brought forwards. This is impossible without displacing a counterweight. When we are sitting, however, flexing and extending the pelvis in the hip joints cause no problems because the support area can be extended as far forwards or backwards as we need.

Open and Shut was therefore so conceived that the horizontal displacements of weight cancel each other out. The "shut" happens when, in displacing the fulcrum (the flexion/extension axes of the hip joints) forwards, we push distal DP patella and proximal DP iliac spine backwards, thereby effecting active buttressing movement of the hip joints in extension. Unwanted continuing movements at the adjacent caudal and cranial movement levels are prevented by active buttressing; for example, no change is permitted in the distribution of weight within the support area. For the starting position we choose the "open" position, i. e. hip flexion by displacement of the fulcrum backwards and of the distance points forwards.

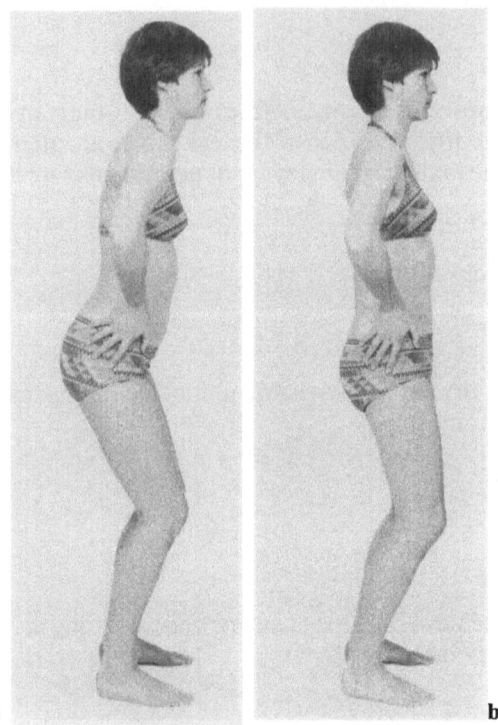

Fig. 79 a, b. Open and Shut.
a Starting position of preliminary movement. **b** End position of preliminary movement (knees remain flexed)

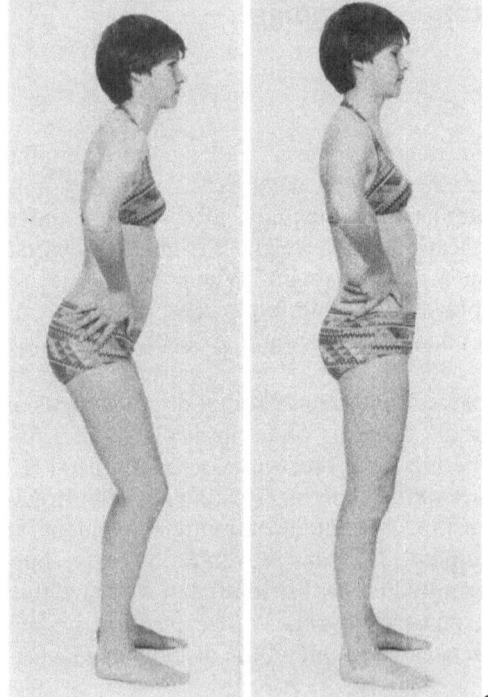

Fig. 79 c, d. Open and Shut.
c Starting position of primary movement. **d** End position of primary movement

● **Position and Activation in the Starting Position**

Position in Space of the Critical Axes
Points of Contact Between the Body and the Environment
Components of Movement in Relation to the Neutral Position of the Joints
For the "open" starting position in two-legged standing, we aim to have the flexion/extension axes of the spinal column, hips, knees and large toes horizontal and parallel.

In BS legs, the soles of the feet are in contact with the floor and the functional long axes of the feet point forwards. In relation to the midfrontal plane the knee joints are flexed forwards/slightly downwards and the hip joints are flexed backwards/slightly downwards. The long axes of the lower legs incline forwards and those of the thighs backwards.

In BS pelvis, the abdomen faces forwards/downwards. The lower abdomen is long and the lumbar spine is in extension. The long axis of the pelvis is tilted further forwards.

In BS thorax, the long axis of the sternum is roughly vertical. The upper abdomen is slightly shortened, the thoracic spine is slightly flexed.

In BS head, the sagittotransverse diameter of the head is over the feet. The neck is long at the front, the cervical spine is in extension and the atlanto-occipital and atlanto-axial joints flexed to keep the patient's gaze directed forwards.

In BS arms, the hands are holding the pelvis with the thumbs feeling the iliac spines. The shoulder joints are in front of the midfrontal plane.

Movement Tolerances at the Critical Joints in Relation
to the Intended Primary Movement
The intended movement sequence in Open and Shut requires the following movement tolerances:
– Plantarflexion into the neutral position in the talocrural joints, effected by the proximal lever
– Knee extension by displacement of the fulcrum backwards into the neutral position
– Hip extension by displacement of the fulcrum forwards into full extension
– Flexion in the lumbar spine
– Extension in the thoracic spine into the neutral position
– Flexion in the cervical spine into the neutral position
– Extension in the atlanto-occipital and atlanto-axial joints into the neutral position

Distribution of Body Weight on a Base Support or Suspension Device,
Against a Supportive Device, or Over a Support Area,
and the Resulting Activity States of the Musculature
The support area in Open and Shut is the smallest area encompassing the contact points soles of feet/floor.

BS legs is in supporting function. The flexion of the pelvis in the hip joints has activated the hip joints and the joints of the lumbar spine extensionally. BS arms is in supported leaning with the contact point palms/pelvis blades.

Intensity of Muscle Activity Required with Economical Activity
Respiration
The intensity of economical activity is only a little greater than that required for normal upright standing. Normal breathing is not disturbed.

Potential Accelerating and Braking Weights in Relation to the Bisecting Plane of the Intended Primary Movement
The bisecting plane of the intended primary movement goes through the flexion/extension axis of the talocrural joints and the vertical midfrontal plane of the head. The weights in front of and behind this bisecting plane should always be in balance, so any displacement of weight forwards is compensated by a corresponding displacement of weight backwards and the bisecting plane remains where it is.

● **Actio – Reactio of the Movement Sequence**

Actio: The Primary Movement
The critical distance points of the primary movement, DPs right and left greater trochanters, move forwards/slightly upwards by extension in the hip joints.

Reactio: Activated Passive Buttressing
Reactio: Change in the Support Area
The reactio and the lack of change in the support area are governed by the conditio, ensuring that despite the straight horizontal direction component, the primary movement does not give rise to any major equilibrium reactions.

● **Conditio – Limitatio of the Movement Sequence**

Conditio: Constant Distances Between Body Distance Points
Limitatio: Active Buttressing and Stabilization
In Open and Shut there are no constant distances.

Conditio of Absolute and/or Relative Fixed Spatial Points
Limitatio by Limiting the Primary Movement, Activated Passive Buttressing and/or Change in the Support Area
In Open and Shut there are only absolute fixed spatial points.

Conditio: Contact point right and left sole/floor is an absolute fixed spatial point.
Limitatio: This point remains fixed if, during the primary movement, the caudal and cranial distance points of the hip joints, DPs right and left patella and DPs right and left iliac spines, move backwards/slightly upwards. In this way, although the primary movement causes weight to be brought forwards, buttressing movement of the hip joint brings enough weight backwards to offset it so that this fixed point can be maintained.

Conditio: The pressure exerted by the soles of the floor does not shift within the support area.

250

Limitatio: This absolute fixed spatial point ensures that during the buttressing extension of the pelvis in the hip joints the thorax is not taken backwards as well, causing an increase in the weight on the heels. For the weight of the thorax to be distributed as neutrally as possible in front of and behind the bisecting plane, the long axis of the thoracic spine is drawn up vertical. This makes the upper abdomen somewhat longer and brings the cervical and thoracic spine into neutral position, and the dynamic stabilization of the thoracic spine functions as active buttressing to the flexion of the lumbar spine that took place with the extension of the pelvis in the hip joints.

Conditio of Movement Speed
Limitatio of Economical Activity by Finding the Optimal Speed
Conditio: Open and Shut should be performed slowly to allow time to properly coordinate the actio and its conditio. The end position should be held for a few seconds, at least until the patient – despite the high intensity of economical activity – can feel that he is breathing normally again.
Limitatio: A good speed is 4 seconds for the movement sequence, 4 seconds to hold the end position and 4 seconds to return to the starting position.

- **Position and Activation in the End Position
  and Return to the Starting Position**

The return to the starting position is by way of steadily reducing the intensity of economical activity. Now as before, no weight may be shifted within the support area. The knees are allowed to sink forwards/downwards in flexion, the hip joints backwards/downwards, and the thorax sinks down with a little flexion coming from cranially in the thoracic spine.

▶ Instruction in Patient Language

- **Instruction Aids Appealing to Perception**

Although the movement sequence of Open and Shut should be performed with low intensity of economical activity, the intensity will increase on the way into the end position. To keep the breathing normal and avoid pressured respiration, the patient can breathe with inspiratory and expiratory whistling. Having DP vertex "pull upwards" makes it easy to coordinate the two consecutively activated sets of buttressing that help to hold all the "blocks" together in the hyperactive end position.

- **Verbal Instruction**
- **Instruction by Manipulation**

Position and Activation in the Starting Position
"Stand up straight and easy. Don't pull your shoulders back. Touch the sides of your thighs and you'll feel a bone under

The therapist must watch that the activity in upright standing is economical. The positioning of the greater trochan-

the skin. That's the spot that should be over the middle of your feet. Forefeet and heels exert the same amount of pressure on the floor; your toes are completely relaxed. Now, let your knees and bottom drop down together. Your knees sag forwards, your bottom backwards, and even your rib cage caves in a little."

ters over the long arches of the feet is important for the dropping away of the knees and hips. If, when the hip joints flex, the pelvis does not also move in the direction of flexion, the therapist should guide its movement manually. To provide assistance, the therapist sits on a stool to the patient's right or left and places one hand on his knee and the other hand under his bottom. She can also take the patient's lower legs between her knees to help him into the starting position.

Actio and Conditio of the Movement Sequence

"This starting position has made you a rather sorry figure. You took off the muscle brakes in your bottom and your knees, opened them up, so to speak, as in the name of the exercise. Now it's time to shut them back on. Without haste, and without any effort, your knees move backwards and your bottom forwards, your eyes draw back, the back of your neck becomes long, and all the time you feel the pressure of your forefeet and heels on the floor. Your breathing is easy, even when you've finished moving and everything is 'shut'. Now let's see how strong you are. Your knees are trying to move backwards, your bottom wants to go forwards, your head wants to go upwards and your feet downwards. They are all equally strong, so nothing moves until you let go of all your strength, 'opening' everything up again, and you're back where you started from. Your knees have bent forwards, your bottom backwards, and your chest has collapsed a little. Now you can start up the movement again. 'Open' and 'shut' as often as you like."

Before the movement sequence starts, the therapist taps on the patient's knees and tells him that these have to move backwards while his bottom, on which she also taps, is simultaneously to move forwards, until the patient feels the stretching of the iliofemoral ligaments ventral to the hip joints as a pleasant pulling. Usually, several manipulative hand-holds are needed before the therapist can palpate the femoral artery:

1. With one hand on the patient's lower abdomen, the therapist supports extension in the hip joints by the proximal lever, while with her other hand she pushes the greater trochanter forwards, pressing the head of the femur against the iliofemoral ligament. As soon as the patient has learned the displacements in space, he will be able to repeat them without help because they will take place as equilibrium reactions.

2. The therapist provides the appropriate physical cues to ensure that BSs thorax and head are aligned in the long axis of the body.

▶ Adapting the Exercise to the Patient's Constitution and Condition

● Adaptation to Constitution: Role of Lengths, Widths, Depths and Distribution of Weights

Constitutional variations are of no relevance in Open and Shut.

● Adaptation to Condition

Restricted Movement

If extension is restricted or the neutral position cannot even be reached in either or both hip joints, the exercise will have to be adapted.

The starting position remains the same.

The knee joints become fixed spatial points. The primary movement will be very small and the direction component of the right/left greater trochanters is more forwards/upwards. Simultaneously, the right and left iliac spines make a bigger movement excursion backwards/upwards, emphasizing the extension of the pelvis in the hip joints. The flexion in the lumbar spine which necessarily follows is actively buttressed extensionally by the thoracic spine, which is stabilized in neutral. With time the fixed point patella is abandoned and the patient tries to perform the exercise as prescribed (Fig. 79).

5.4 Adapting Lift-free/Reduced-Lift Mobilization of the Spinal Column to Special Problems of the Thoracic Spine

In functional terms, the thoracic spine is part of BS thorax. The activity state of dynamic stabilization in the neutral position which is typical of the thoracic spine gives it the function of a "stabile". The thoracic spine should be dynamically stabilized in the neutral position, not only during locomotion and upright posture, but also during many activities requiring use of the hands (see *Functional Kinetics*, pp. 75–76, 86), in order to ensure that (a) the spinal column has potential rotational ability about the long axis of the body and (b) the thorax can provide a solid substructure for the shoulder girdle. This dynamic stabilization of the thoracic spine is a normal postural reflex. If for any reason it fails, severe functional disturbances result. First of all, the adjacent lordotic parts of the spine lose their potential mobility. Secondly, functional disorders of respiration occur (*Functional Kinetics*, p. 285). Thirdly, motor impulses coming from peripheral nerves encounter an a destabilized centre which is able neither to absorb them by active buttressing nor economically to transmit them further. This leads to premature degeneration of the passive structures involved and also explains the inability of the patient to make swift, powerful and precise movements.

Common Causes of Faulty Static Stressing of the Thoracic Spine

- Hypoactivity of the extensors due to deficient stabilization in patients with normal thoracic kyphosis. This important postural reflex can be lost as a result of fatigue, static overstress, sitting too long, poor postural habits, apathy or depression.
- All forms of respiratory disorder.
- Thoracic flat back. Patients with a thoracic flat back (– TS) lack the stimulus to extensional stabilization provided by the pull of gravity on clearly dominant frontal weights in combination with the available tolerance for flexion in the thoracic spine. Lumbar kyphosis is often seen in patients with – TS. If the thoracic spine is destabilized to this extent, there can be no adequate muscular anchoring of the shoulder girdle to the thorax and no economical suspension of the arms.
- Thoracic round back (+ TS). A thoracic round back is often characterized by stiffness and an extension deficit. In such cases, arm activity represents an additional stress that is difficult to offset. Hypermobile thoracic round backs often turn out to be collapsed flat backs.
- Common deformities such as scoliosis, scoliotic postures and thoracic asymmetries, which make it difficult or even impossible to stabilize the thoracic spine in its neutral position. Especially problematic are deformities at the rotation level of the lower thoracic spine, where they block rotation and thus considerably increase stress on the lordotic segments of the spine. Such problems also cause the thoracic kyphosis to extend caudally into the upper lumbar spine.
- Neck kyphosis, also called the functional C7 syndrome. Coupled with – TS in the midthoracic spine, this destroys the virtual long axis of the body, because pseudostiffness in the upper thoracic and lower cervical spine makes it impossible to align the head properly. The consequent abnormal tone in the muscles of the cervical spine and shoulder girdle should be regarded as malfunction of healthy musculature carrying out an equilibrium reaction in response to poor head posture.

5.4.1 Relief Postures for the Thoracic Spine (Figs. 80–85)

The name "Relief Postures for the Thoracic Spine" refers to the functional problem to be solved.

■ Goal of the Exercise

The goal is for the patient to:
- Find resting positions and work postures that will neutralize the weight of the thorax such that the thoracic spine in neutral position need not be held by muscle activity

– Find resting positions and work postures in which the thoracic spine and adjacent BSs pelvis and head are roughly in neutral position without the weights of the head, pelvis, arms and shoulder girdle stressing the passive and active structures of the thoracic spine.

▶ Functional Analysis in Therapist Language

Most of the following relief postures apply in part to the lumbar and cervical as well. We will limit our remarks here to the aspects that are of specific relevance to the thoracic spine.

Learning to Sit with the Thoracic Spine Dynamically Stabilized in Neutral Position and Achieve Economical Distribution of Tone in the Fall-Preventing Muscles (Figs. 80, 81)

Starting Position
Sitting upright across the corner of a stool that is at least the height of the patient's lower legs, including heels if he is wearing shoes. The shoulder girdle is parked on the thorax and the arms on the thighs.

Actio, Conditio – Limitatio
The therapist sits behind the patient: She puts one arm around the patient from behind/laterally between the thorax and the arm hanging down. With her hand she holds the patient's thorax at the epigastric angle and lifts the weight of the thorax somewhat, thereby extending the thoracic spine but not beyond its neutral position. At the same time, with her other hand she applies a counterstay against the patient's spinal column, about at the level of the lumbothoracic transition, to prevent flexion of the pelvis in the hip joints and total extension of the lumbar and thoracic spine (Fig. 80a).
Figure 80b shows a variant hand-hold that the therapist can use if the patient finds being held at the epigastric angle unpleasant.
Figure 80c shows another variant. This one is good for patients with extreme total flat back.
As soon as the therapist, using one of the hand-holds described, has assumed some of the weight of the patient's thorax and head, the patient is requested to relax his abdominal and waist muscles until he begins to breathe normally again (see p. 135, the Lion).
Figure 81 shows how patients with thoracic flat back can carry the arms in the horizontal transverse plane of the shoulder joints in front of the vertical midfrontal plane to stimulate extensional stabilization of the thoracic spine. The arms increase the amount of weight carried in front of the flexion/extension axis of the thoracic spine, thereby stimulating its extensional stabilization in neutral position.

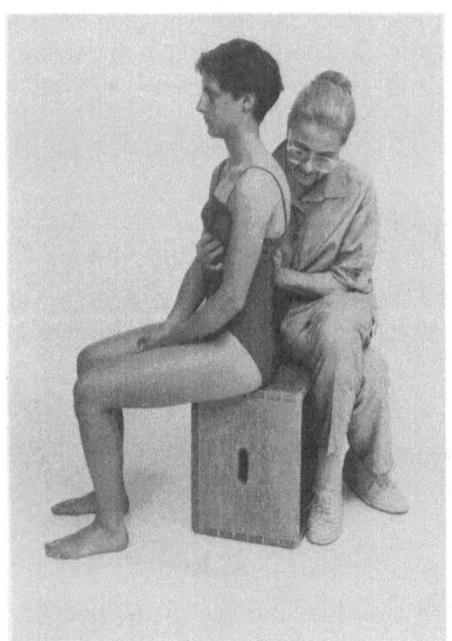

a

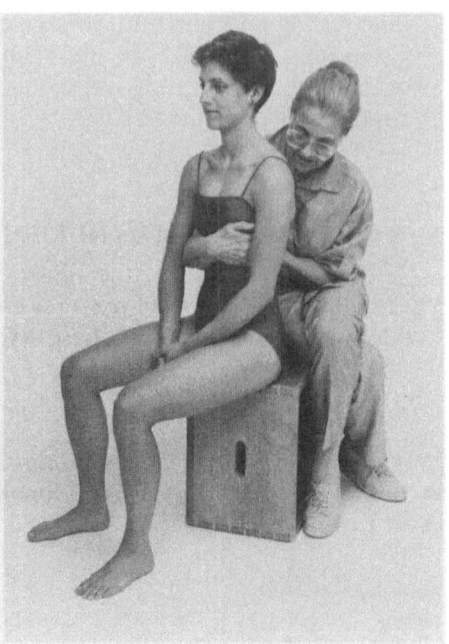

b

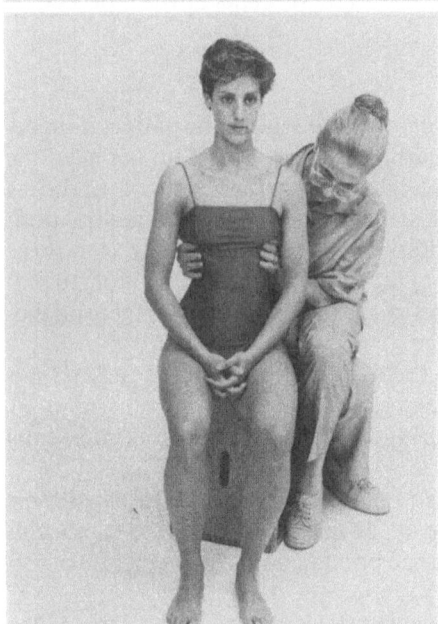

c

Fig. 80 a–c. Adaptation for thoracic spine problems in cases of functional respiratory disorders. This adaptation is for an unstable thoracic spine. The therapist supports the weight of the thorax and brings the thoracic spine into the neutral position. The patient relaxes the hyperactive lumbar and ventral muscles and feels normal respiration begin

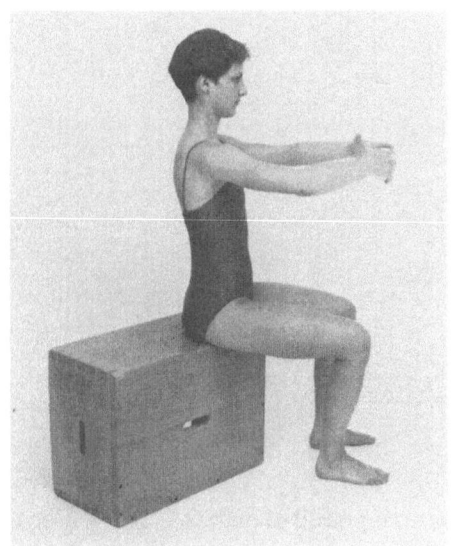

Fig. 81. Adaptation for thoracic spine problems with thoracic stability and flat back.
The weight of the arms, held horizontally
and in front of the midfrontal plane, stimulates extensional stabilization of the thoracic
spine

Cushioned Semisidelying Position, Preferably to the Right (Fig. 35)
See the Sleeper (p. 140).

Relief Posture for the Thoracic Spine in Supine (Fig. 82)
In the relief posture shown in Fig. 82a, elevation of the elbows is particularly important for the thoracic spine. Care should be taken that the elbows are barely
lower than the shoulder joint. The shorter the arm and the more ventral the
shoulder joint lies, the higher the elbow will have to be raised. The hands are best
folded over the abdomen.
In Fig. 82b, the arms are elevated. This position has acquired the name "the Little
Shepherd Boy". Basically, the head is level with the thorax, a few cushions are
placed only under the neck. The arms are flexed and externally rotated in the
shoulder joints, but *not* to end-stop; accordingly, they must be elevated. In this position, too, it is a good idea to either fold the hands or cross the forearms, in order
to avoid braking activity in the muscles of the shoulder joint. In both examples, BS

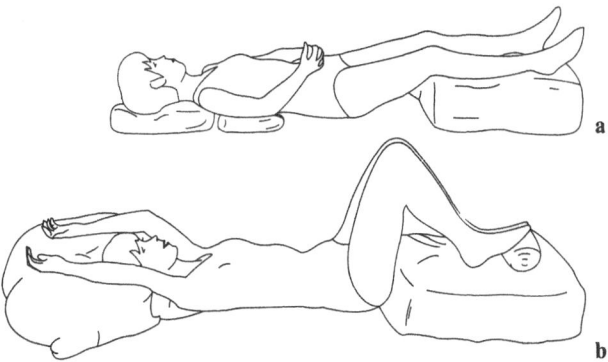

Fig. 82 a, b. Relief postures
for the thoracic spine (also
lumbar and cervical spine)
in supine

257

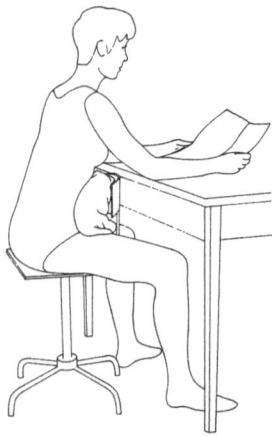

Fig. 83. Relief posture for the thoracic spine in sitting: work posture

arms is placed so that its weight has no effect on the thoracic spine and the muscle activity bridging between the two body segments can switch off.

In cases of pronounced thoracic flat back it is sometimes helpful slightly to elevate BSs thorax, head and arms, especially if the legs are not being elevated and there is restricted flexion in the lumbar spine and/or restricted extension in the hip joints.

Relief Postures for the Thoracic Spine in Sitting (Figs. 83, 84; see also Fig. 72)

Figure 83 shows a posture for sitting at work. The forwards-leaning long axis of the body is propped against an abdominal support. The thoracic spine is relieved by leaning the forearms on a desk of the proper height. Figure 84 illustrates how, with the long axis of the body vertical, the thorax can be suspended from the shoulder girdle by pressure activity of the hands against the seat (see also Fig. 72), making it

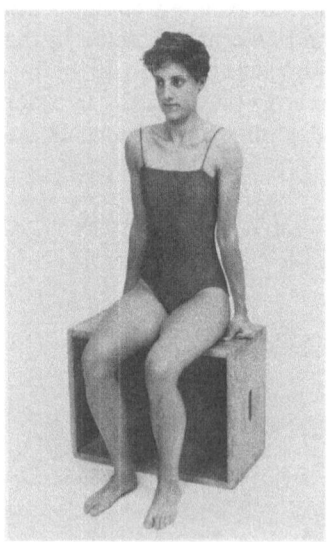

Fig. 84. Relief posture for the thoracic spine in sitting, using the arms for support

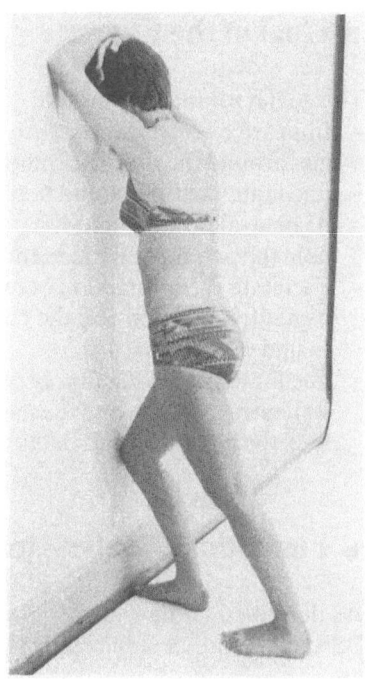

Fig. 85. Relief posture for the thoracic spine in standing

unnecessary to stabilize the thoracic spine against gravity. Unfortunately one cannot work in this position. With lateral arm supports at the right height, however, one could suspend the thorax from the shoulder girdle by pushing down with the elbows on the armrests, and the hands would be free.

Relief Posture for the Thoracic Spine in Standing (Fig. 85)
This relief posture in standing is easy to assume any time it is needed during the day. Notice the stride position with the front knee supported against the wall. The long axis of the back leg and of the body incline forwards enough for the forehead to be comfortably supported against the wall. The arms, with forearms crossed, are supported against the wall and on the patient's head. If constitutional factors (+ + upper body, short thighs) reduce the effectiveness of this posture, it can be attempted in the corner of a room. The hands are then crossed over the chest, the same stride position is taken up, and the shoulders and the forehead seek support against the two walls that form the corner.

5.4.2 Movement Levels for Mobilizing Massage Around the Thoracic Spine (Figs. 86–89)

The name "Movement Levels for Mobilizing Massage Around the Thoracic Spine" refers to the area in which the technique of mobilizing massage (see *Functional Kinetics,* pp. 301–311) is to be applied.

■ Goal of the Exercise

The goal is for the therapist to:
– Improve circulation, elasticity and contractility and normalize tone in the muscles around the thoracic spine through mobilizing massage
– Facilitate the interaction between the thoracic spine dynamically stabilized in its neutral position and the potentially mobile cervical and lumbar spines and help the patient to understand how it works
– Facilitate the interaction between the thoracic spine dynamically stabilized in its neutral position and the costal respiratory movements and help the patient to understand how it works
– Facilitate the interaction between the thoracic spine dynamically stabilized in its neutral position and the movements of the shoulder girdle on the thorax and help the patient to understand how it works

▶ Functional Analysis in Therapist Language

As described in the goal, Mobilizing Massage Around the Thoracic Spine treats BS thorax and the adjacent BSs pelvis, head and arms. The levels of movement are:
– Thoracic spine/lumbar spine, thoracic spine/cervical spine
– Thoracic spine/ribs
– Thorax/shoulder girdle

Movement Levels Thoracic Spine/Lumbar Spine, Thoracic Spine/Cervical Spine (Fig. 86)

Because the greatest demands around the thoracic spine are made on the extensor muscles, we want to treat these by mobilizing massage. To do this, we set the thoracic spine moving in small, rhythmic, lift-free movement excursions (about 60/minute) in flexion/extension and massage the muscles during the extension phase.

Procedure
The patient is positioned on his right or left side. The spinal column rests horizontally, roughly in the neutral position. The muscle tone in BSs pelvis, thorax and head must not be raised by the weights of the extremities.
The therapist exerts axial pressure perpendicular to the flexion/extension axis of a motion segment in the thoracic spine. The patient responds with counterpressure, deforming the thoracic spine into flexion. He must maintain this flexion even when following the therapist's instruction to break of the activity of the abdominal muscles. The autochthonous muscles are activated: they are the ones performing the flexional stabilization. The spontaneous movements of costal respiration are a sign to the therapist that this has occurred.

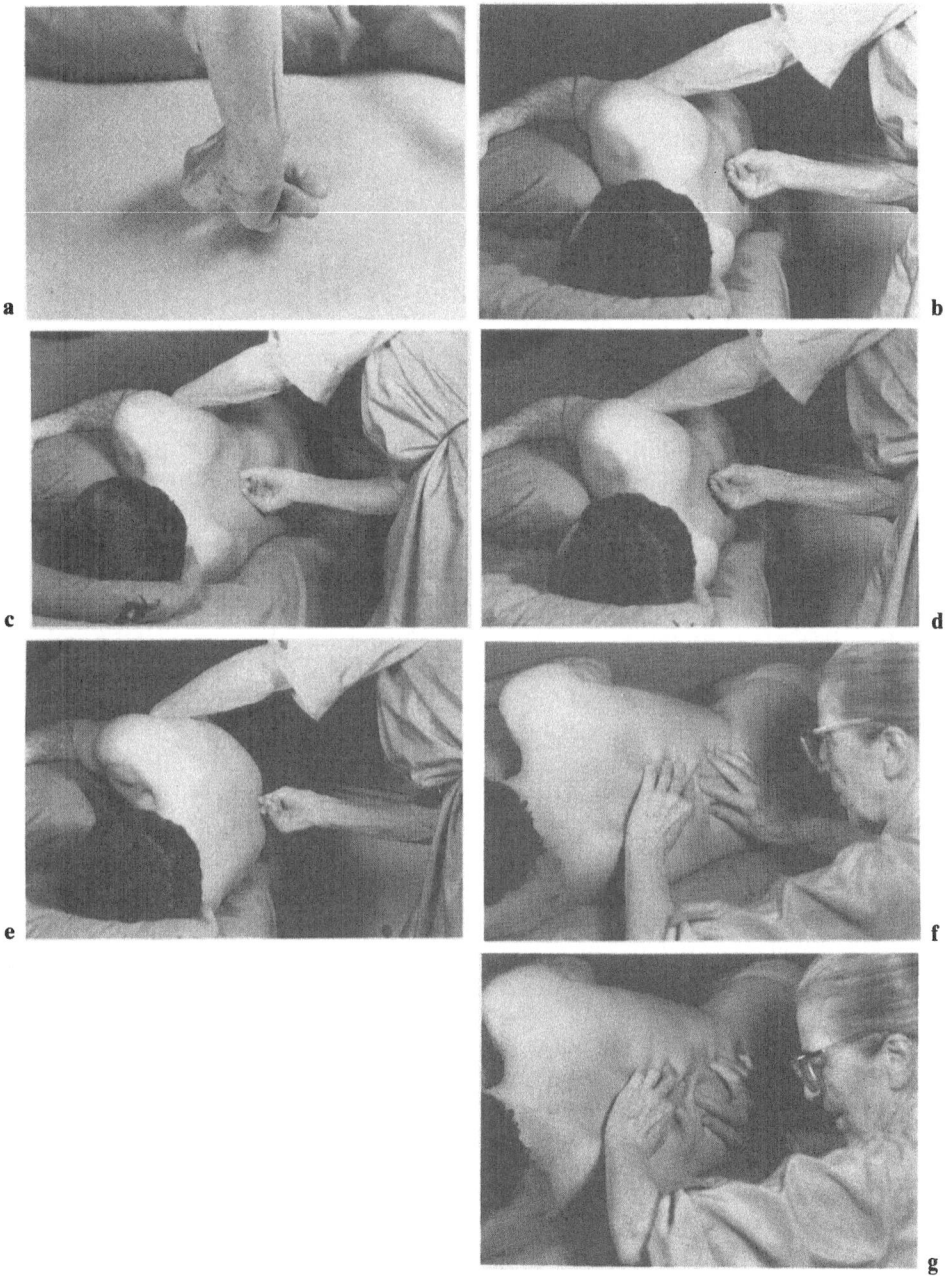

Fig. 86 a–g. Mobilizing Massage at Movement Level Thoracic Spine. **a** Position of the therapist's hand for applying axial pressure to bring about extension of the thoracic spine, **b, c** The patient yields to the pressure exerted by the therapist's hand. **d, e** The patient presses back, flexing his thoracic spine, **f, g** Mobilizing massage of the extensors of the thoracic spine

While the therapist instructs the patient to slowly relax the flexional activity, she continues gently to exert the axial pressure. The thoracic spine is passively extended to its neutral position, the therapist holding the patient's thorax in the side-lying position.

In the next phase, the patient is to activate the thoracic spine extensionally, beyond the neutral position if possible. He is instructed to move away from where he feels the therapist's hand pressing on his skin. The only way he can do this is to actively extend the thoracic spine. He must not hold his breath in doing this.

Finally the patient is instructed to stop all activity. During this relaxation phase, which can last up to 30 seconds, the therapist puts both hands around the patient's thorax, supporting the pelvis too if necessary, so that the patient feels secure. This makes it much easier to relax. The relaxation phase ends when breathing has spontaneously returned to normal.

This four-phase procedure is repeated about three times. Then the spinal column is moved through small flexion/extension movement excursions which are in part manipulated by the therapist, in part performed by the patient. The patient is instructed never to lose touch with the therapist's hand at the critical contact point. He must therefore yield to pressure by extension and, when the pressure is withdrawn, follow the therapist's hand by flexion. These movements are lift-free and should be carried out in an effortless way by the patient. Only thus can the mobilizing massage of the extensor muscles be applied in rhythm with the movement. In the extension phase, the therapist kneads the muscles together, the extension increases and the extensor muscles are relaxed, to be stretched again in the flexion phase. Either one side or the other or both sides at a time can be treated, depending on the patient's needs.

Naturally, before mobilizing massage is performed, a complete assessment of the patient's mobility must be made. The therapist must be aware of any partial stiffness and/or hypermobility in the spinal column and hip joints. In particular, she must know exactly where the one or more motion segments are in which flexion/extension is restricted. The axial pressure is exerted at the centre of the stiff area which is to be mobilized.

Depending on where the axial pressure is exerted, the following reactions will be seen:

- If the axial pressure is exerted on the lower thoracic spine in a ventral and, if necessary, somewhat cranial direction, there will be a continuing movement producing more or less pronounced total flexion in the lumbar/thoracic spine and extension in the cervical spine and in the pelvis in the hip joints.
- If the axial pressure is exerted on the midthoracic spine in a ventral and, if necessary, somewhat caudal direction, the continuing flexional effect, particularly on the lumbosacral transition, can be suppressed by active buttressing (flexional in the hip joints).
- If the flexional resistance is to affect the upper thoracic spine, the axial pressure should be applied to the sternum, somewhat below the jugular notch, in a dorsal/cranial direction. For the active phase of extension it is advisable to apply pressure in a ventral/caudal direction at the level of C7.

Movement Level Thoracic Spine/Ribs (Figs. 87, 88)

To mobilize the costovertebral joints, we employ the movements of inspiratory and expiratory costal respiration, reinforce them by manipulation, and also manipulate the buttressing movement in the thoracic spine.

The manipulations we will perform for buttressing are:

– For inspiration, flexion in the thoracic spine from cranial to caudal, ipsilateral concave lateroflexion in the thoracic spine and ipsilateral backward rotation of the pelvis in the lower thoracic spine
– For expiration, extension of the thoracic spine from cranial to caudal, ipsilateral convex lateroflexion of the thoracic spine and ipsilateral forward rotation of the pelvis in the lower thoracic spine.

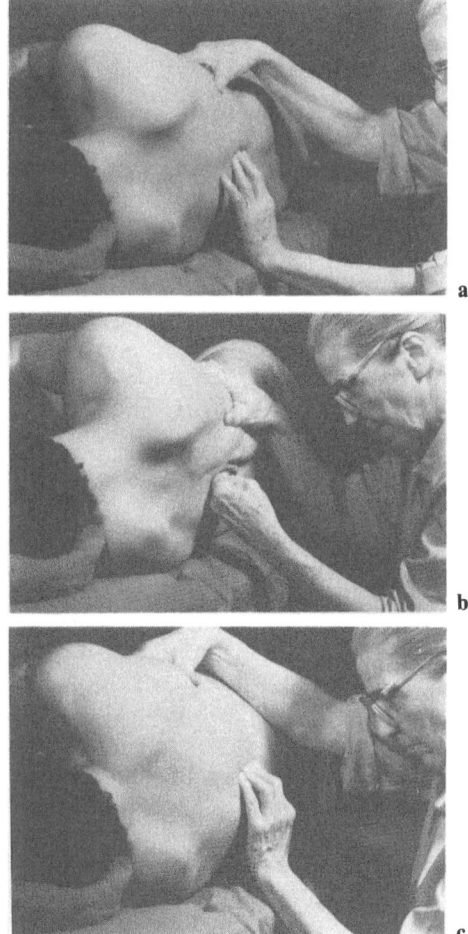

Fig. 87 a–c. Mobilizing Massage at Movement Level Thoracic Spine/Ribs. **a** Starting position. The therapist's left hand inhibits a continuing movement of lateroflexion of the thoracic spine. **b** Lowering the ribs (expiration). **c** Raising the ribs (inspiration)

263

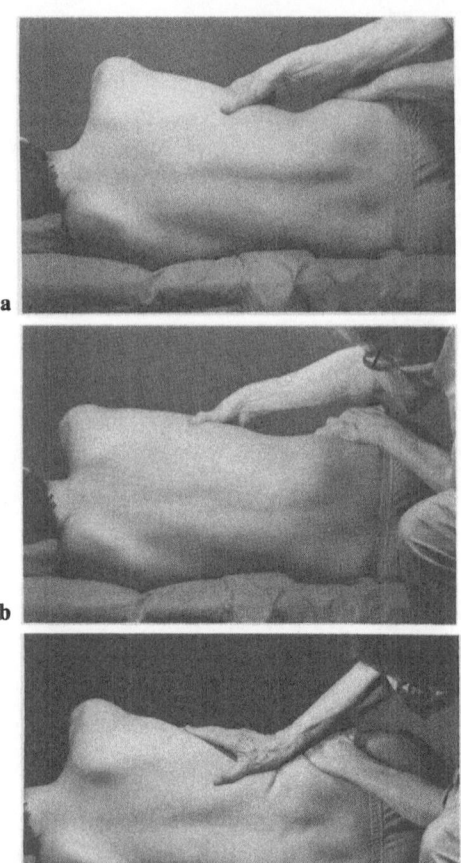

Fig. 88 a–c. Movement Level Thoracic Spine/Ribs. **a** Starting position. The therapist's left hand is ready to pull the pelvis dorsally/medially. This causes pelvis-positive rotation in the thoracic spine. The therapist's right hand can manipulate the ribs upward at the thoracic spine. When the ribs fall, the pelvis rotates ventrally. Raising the ribs (inspiration). **c** Lowering the ribs (expiration)

Procedure

The patient lies on his side. The weights BS head, upper leg and upper arm are positioned so that they do not activate the muscles of BS thorax against gravity.

During mobilizing massage of movement level thoracic spine/ribs, we must be very careful that the patient does not hyperventilate. To be on the safe side, plenty of pauses for normal breathing should be taken. The therapist places one hand on the upper side of the thorax, palpates the course of the intercostal spaces and identifies the direction in which the ribs move during inspiration and expiration. She remembers that this direction is not constant. Normally it goes in the lower region from caudal/dorsal to cranial/ventral and back again; in the mid and particularly in the upper region it runs primarily from caudal to cranial and back again. After the therapist has found the intercostal spaces that are to be mobilized, she palpates with her other hand the vertebrae that articulate with these ribs. This is where the undesired continuing movements will start most strongly, so this is where lateroflexional and/or rotational buttressing manipulation must be applied. The hand manipulating the rib movement is the one primarily responsible for the flexional/extensional buttressing.

Now the conversation with the patient can begin. "You feel quite peaceful and still. Don't breathe until you need air." During the initial inhalation, the hands of the therapist rest on the ribs and the spinal column. Then comes the first instruction, "Breathe in further," and she reinforces the increased inspiratory movement of the ribs by manipulation.

Now comes a twist that flexes the upper thoracic spine. At the same time, the other hand prevents the continuing movement of ipsilateral convex lateroflexion in the thoracic spine by pulling the spinal processes most clearly affected downwards into ipsilateral concave lateroflexion. If necessary, the hand can shift to the pelvis, pulling it dorsally/slighty cranially by rotation in the lower thoracic spine. This is always helpful if the increased inhalation has caused flexion in the lower thoracic spine.

The conversation with the patient continues: "Slowly let the air out through your nose." The therapist's hands do nothing except feel this movement. Then she says, "Breathe on out further, still through your nose," and reinforces the increased expiratory movement of the ribs by manipulation. Now comes a twist that extends the midthoracic spine. At the same time, the other hand prevents the continuing movement of ipsilateral concave lateroflexion in the thoracic spine by pressing on the spinal processes most clearly affected by the movement upwards into ipsilateral convex lateroflexion. If necessary, the hand shifts to the pelvis and pushes it ventrally/a little caudally by rotation in the lower thoracic spine.

At the end of the active exhalation, the patient is encouraged with, "Hold this position, but keep your throat relaxed." This pause in breathing is good training for the oblique abdominal muscles and reduces the risk of hyperventilation. Now the patient is ready to follow his next instruction. "Very slowly let go of your stomach and let the air flow in through your nose." Once again, the therapist's hands are concerned only with feeling inspiration commencing as the expiratory muslces relax.

This mobilization technique can basically be used on every costovertebral joint. However, the therapist must always bear in mind the changing direction of the costal movements from motion segment to motion segment and the many variations in thorax shape. If the problem is one of restricted movement in individual ribs, the mobilization and its buttressing are performed within the rib cage. Let us assume that the costovertebral movements of the sixth rib are blocked: the therapist reinforces the inspiratory movement of the six upper ribs, simultaneously holding back the lower ribs by expiratory manipulation. Then she reinforces the expiratory movement of the six upper ribs, simultaneously manipulating the lower ribs as for inspiration. This "wringing" of the thorax can, for example, bring instant relief of persistent pain between the shoulder blades. This technique works the intercostal muscles thoroughly. Vibration can be used as an adjunct to increase the effect.

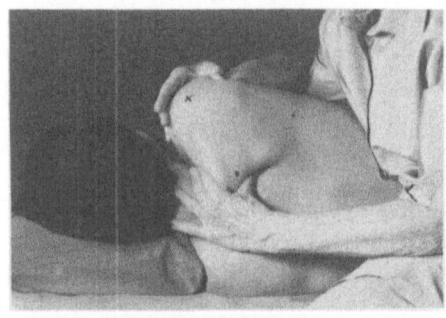

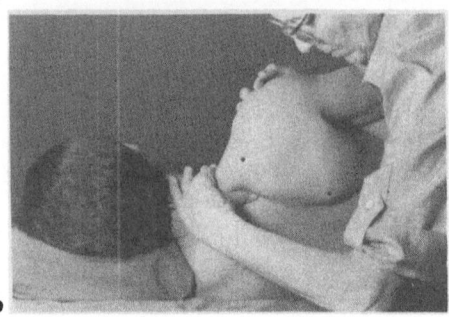

a

b

Fig. 89 a–i. Mobilizing Massage at Movement Level Shoulder Girdle/Thorax.
a, b Upper trapezius and levator scapulae

Movement Level Thorax/Shoulder Girdle (Fig. 89)

In order to mobilize by massage the muscles connecting the shoulder girdle to BS thorax and in part to BSs head and pelvis, we must call to mind the direction in which these muscles contract. We are going to slide the shoulder girdle along the thorax so that the muscles concerned relax through approximation of their insertions, and then stretch as they are moved away again. Obviously, stretching one muscle means relaxing its antagonist.

Unit 1
Acromion slides ventrally/caudally/laterally, lower scapular angle slides dorsally/cranially/medially.

Muscles Relaxed: Levator scapulae, rhomboids major and minor, pectoralis minor, superior anterior serratus lateralis.

Muscles Stretched: Descending and ascending trapezius, converging anterior serratus lateralis.

The patient rests on his side. With one hand the therapist slides the shoulder girdle by its acromion and with the other she grasps the levator scapulae and the rhomboids between fingers and thumb cranial to the upper scapular angle and massages them emphatically in the relaxed phase, perpendicularly to the lie of the fibres. Then the patient lies on his back. With one hand the therapist slides the shoulder girdle back by its acromion and with the other she grasps the pectoralis minor and

266

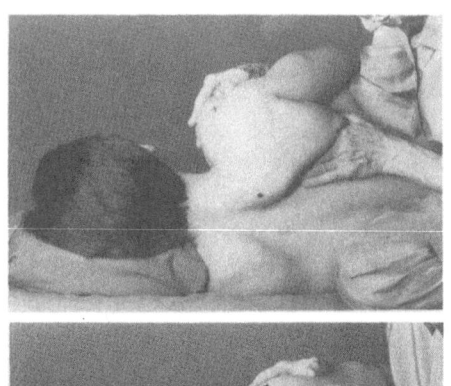

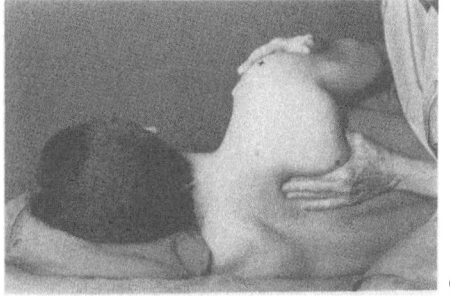

Fig. 89 a–i. Mobilizing Massage at Movement Level Shoulder Girdle/Thorax.
c, d Lower trapezius and latissimus dorsi

the superior anterior serratus lateralis between her fingers and thumb ventromedial to the axilla and massages them emphatically in the relaxed phase, perpendicularly to the lie of the fibres.

Unit 2
Acromion slides dorsally/cranially/medially, lower scapular angle slides ventrally/laterally/caudally. As these move, the scapula rotates around a point approximately in the middle of the infraspinatus.

Muscles relaxed: Descending and ascending trapezius, converging serratus lateralis.

Muscles stretched: Levator scapulae, rhomboids major and minor, pectoralis minor, superior serratus lateralis.

The patient lies on his side. With one hand the therapist slides the shoulder girdle by its upper scapular angle while with the other she reaches caudal to the lower scapular angle, underneath it if possible, to grasp the converging serratus lateralis and ascending trapezius between her fingers and thumb and massage them strongly in the relaxed phase, perpendicularly to the lie of the muscle fibres.
Then with one hand the therapist slides the shoulder girdle back by its lower scapular angle while with the other she grasps the descending trapezius cranial and medial to the acromion between her fingers and thumb and massages it strongly in the relaxed phase, perpendicularly to the lie of the muscle fibres.

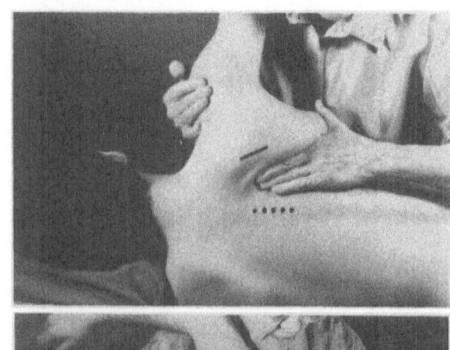

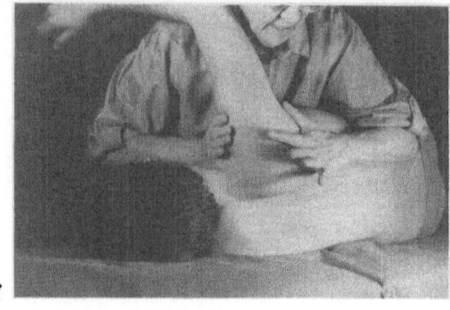

Fig. 89 a–i. Mobilizing Massage at Movement Level Shoulder Girdle/Thorax.
e, f Middle trapezius, rhomboids, pectorals

Unit 3

Acromion slides cranially/medially, the medial scapular margin makes a roughly parallel sliding movement.

Muscles relaxed: Sternocleidomastoid, descending trapezius, levator scapulae, rhomboids major and minor, serratus lateralis (diverging), pectoralis major (inserting at the humerus).

Muscles stretched: Subclavian, pectoralis minor, caudal tract of the converging serratus lateralis, ascending trapezius, caudal tract of the latissimus dorsi (inserting at the humerus).

The patient lies on his side. With one hand the therapist slides the shoulder girdle by grasping the dorsal and ventral muscles of the axillary margin between her thumb and fingers, coming from caudally. The weight of the patient's arm rests on the therapist's arm. With her other hand she grasps the descending trapezius cranial to the acromion and upper scapular angle, the rhomboids and the levator scapulae, or, cranial/dorsal to the manubrium sterni, the sternocleidomastoid, and massages these strongly in the relaxed phase, perpendicularly to the lie of the fibres.

Unit 4

Acromion slides caudally/laterally; the medial scapular margin makes a roughly parallel sliding movement.

Muscles relaxed: Subclavian, pectoralis minor, caudal tract of the converging serratus lateralis, ascending trapezius, caudal tract of the latissimus dorsi (inserting at the humerus).

268

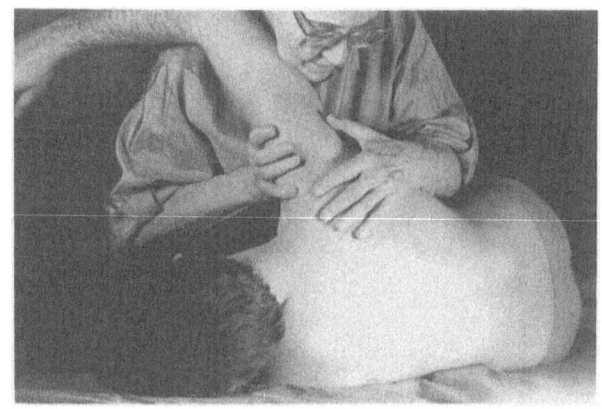

Fig. 89 a–i. Mobilizing Massage at Movement Level Shoulder Girdle/Thorax.
g Middle trapezius, rhomboids, pectorals

g

Muscles stretched: Sternocleidomastoid, descending trapezius, levator scapulae, rhomboids major and minor, diverging serratus lateralis, pectoralis major (inserting at the humerus).

The patient lies on his side. With one hand the therapist slides the shoulder girdle by approaching the pincer jaws from cranially and pulling them caudally. The weight of the patient's arm rests on the therapist's arm. With her other hand the therapist either grasps the ascending trapezius caudal and ventral to the lower scapular angle, the caudal tract of the latissimus dorsi and the caudal tract of the serratus lateralis, or she grasps the pectoralis minor and the subclavian caudal to the coracoid process and the clavicle between her fingers and thumbs, and massages them strongly in the relaxed phase perpendicularly to the lie of the fibres.

Unit 5
Acromion slides dorsally/medially, the medial scapular margin makes a parallel sliding movement.

Muscles relaxed: Descending and transverse trapezius, rhomboids minor and major, ascending trapezius, latissimus dorsi (inserting at the humerus).

Muscles stretched: Diverging serratus lateralis, levator scapulae, pectoralis major (inserting at the humerus), pectoralis minor, converging serratus lateralis.

The patient lies on his side. Using both hands, the therapist is able to press the acromion dorsally/downwards so that the pincer jaws open and the medial scapular margin is pressed against the spinal processes of the thoracic spine. This relaxes the entire trapezius, especially the transverse tract, and the rhomboids. Before the pincer jaws pull ventrally/upwards and close, the therapist can hook her fingertips under the medial scapular margin.
The therapist can also slide the shoulder girdle with one hand by laterally pressing the acromion dorsally/medially/downwards. The radial aspect of the index

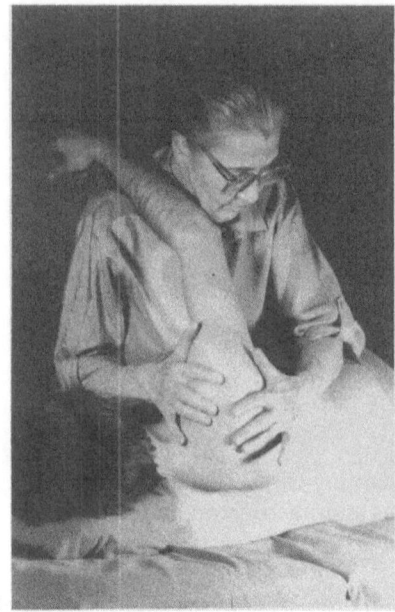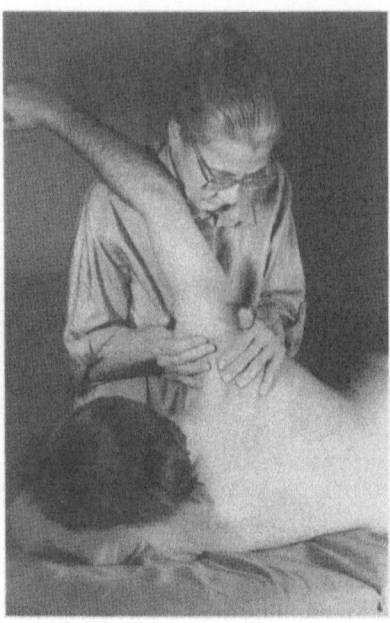

Fig. 89 a–i. Mobilizing Massage at Movement Level Shoulder Girdle/Thorax. **h, i** Middle trapezius, rhomboids, pectorals

finger and the middle portion of her other hand rest on the medial scapular margin and the thumb grasps the lower scapular angle. This way the therapist can turn the medial scapular margin over in her hand. The rhomboids and the transverse trapezius are massaged with little cranial and caudal gliding movements.

Unit 6
Acromion slides ventrally/laterally, the medial scapular margin makes a parallel sliding movement.

Muscles relaxed: Diverging and converging serratus lateralis, pectoralis minor.

Muscles stretched: Descending, transverse and ascending trapezius, rhomboids minor and major, latissimus dorsi (inserting at the humerus).

The patient lies on his side. The therapist uses one hand to displace the shoulder girdle by sliding the scapula ventrally/laterally from behind. With the other hand she pushes the radial aspect of her index finger, pointing cranially, and the middle portion of her hand under the lateral scapular margin from the front, grasps the diverging and converging serratus lateralis and massages them strongly in the relaxed phase, perpendicularly to the lie of the fibres. The radial aspect of her index finger, now pointing caudally, and the middle of her hand can also reach under the coracoid process and the shoulder joint from ventrally to grasp the pectoralis minor and the superior serratus lateralis and massage them in the relaxed phase perpendicularly to the lie of the fibres.

270

5.4.3 Balancing Up (Figs. 90, 91)

"Balancing Up" is an invented name. The image is of a beam balance or scales, with trays on either side in which one can play with weights and counterweights and try to balance them.

■ Goal of the Exercise

The goal is for the patient to learn to:
- Use the weights of his own body to extensionally stimulate the thoracic spine in its neutral position with variable intensity of economical activity
- Lower the intensity of economical activity to resting tone, particularly in the abdominal muscles, so that normal breathing with free costal respiratory movements returns spontaneously.

▶ Functional Analysis in Therapist Language

● Conception of the Exercise

In order to extensionally stimulate the thoracic spine in its neutral position with variable intensity of muscular activity, as specified in the goal, and at the same time keep tone in the abdominal muscles low, we start from the following considerations. The best form of the neutral position for the thoracic spine is when the long axis of the body has been functionally created by straight alignment of BSs pelvis, thorax and head. When this has been done, the only body weight that can extensionally stress the thoracic spine is that of the legs. Therefore, the arms join hands and create a sling in which the weight of the legs is suspended. For this the patient must be sitting on a stool of the right height. Only *one* leg is suspended in the arm sling; this way, the weights of BSs head, thorax, arms, pelvis and the one leg become a single movement system that can be balanced around the flexion/extension axis of the opposite hip joint with the spinal column in neutral position, while the free leg automatically acts as a counterweight to the movement system as it leans further backwards, or goes into supporting function as it leans forwards, thus regulating the movement of the "scales" (Fig. 90).

● Position and Activation in the Starting Position

Position in Space of the Critical Axes
Points of Contact Between the Body and the Environment
Components of Movement in Relation to the Neutral Position of the Joints
The starting position is upright sitting on a stool that is at least the height of the patient's lower legs. BSs pelvis, thorax and head are aligned in the long axis of the body, which is vertical. Sitting across the corner of the stool makes it possible to

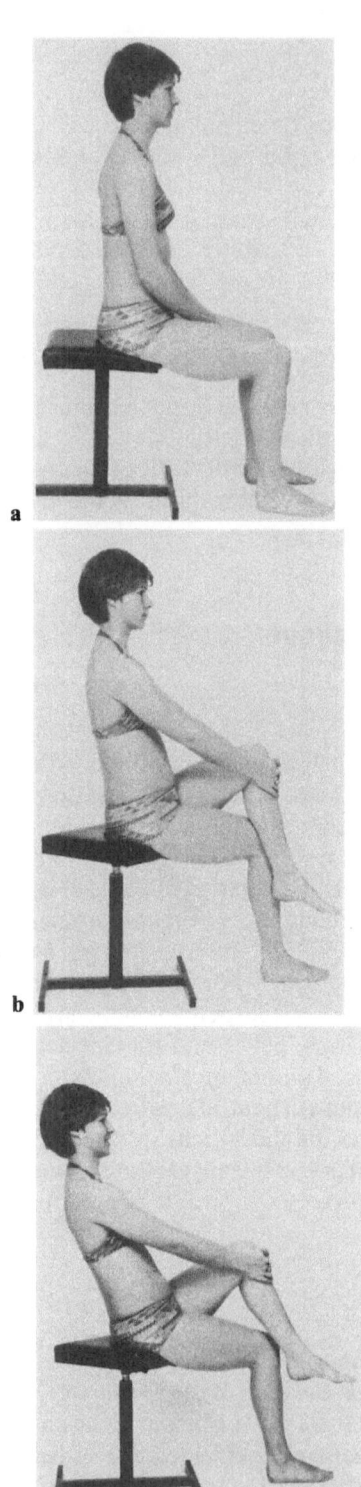

Fig. 90 a–c. Balanced Up. **a** Starting position, **b** phase 1, **c** phase 2 and end position

272

limit the points of contact between the body and the seat to the left and right ischial tuberosities.

The legs are in about 90° flexion in the hip joints/comfortable transverse abduction/zero rotation. The heels are under the knees and the soles of the feet are the body's points of contact with the floor. The functional long axes of the feet diverge in accordance with the straddle of the legs.

In BS arms, the shoulder girdle is in neutral position, the upper arms are parallel to the long axis of the body, the hands are folded and rest on the thighs close to the abdomen.

Movement Tolerances at the Critical Joints in Relation to the Intended Primary Movement

In the hip joints there is sufficient tolerance for flexion by the distal lever and sufficient tolerance for flexion and extension by the proximal lever.

Distribution of Body Weight on a Base Support or Suspension Device, Against a Supportive Device, or Over a Support Area, and the Resulting Activity States of the Musculature

When the patient sits on a stool, the weight of BSs pelvis, thorax, head and arms presses on the seat. BS legs is parked. The potential support area is therefore the smallest area encompassing the points of contact soles/floor and pelvis/seat. The pelvis is potentially mobile, in BS thorax the thoracic spine is extensionally dynamically stabilized, BS head balances in free play over the thorax, the shoulder girdle is parked on the thorax, the upper arms are suspended in free play from the shoulder girdle and the forearms are parked on the thighs with hands folded.

Intensity of Muscle Activity Required with Economical Activity
Respiration

In the starting position, the intensity of economical activity is low; the patient breathes normally.

● Actio – Reactio of the Movement Sequence

The movement sequence of Balancing Up has two phases: a set-up phase that prepares the body to allow the two "scale trays" to swing and reach balance, and a tipping phase. During this second phase, the horizontal direction components dominate, moving alternately backwards/slightly downwards and forwards/downwards. Owing to the predominance of unambiguous horizontal direction components, we can expect a clear reactio. The scales are balanced when the ventral and dorsal weights roughly balance each other out.

Set-Up Phase

The left leg is crossed over the right and the right leg is shifted under the left. The hands are clasped around the upper knee, and BSs pelvis, thorax and head, stabilized in the long axis of the body, lean so far backwards that the weight of the leg pulls the shoulder girdle ventrally/caudally in relation to the thorax. Neither the shoulder girdle nor the elbow joints exhibit any increased activity; the only activation is that of flexion in the wrists and flexion and adduction in the finger joints, keeping the hands clasped (Fig. 90 b). If crossing the legs causes the patient even the slightest effort, the legs are simply positioned close to each other (Fig. 91 a).

Tipping Backwards

The left leg is suspended in the arm sling (Figs. 90 c and 91 b).

Actio: The Primary Movement
The critical distance points of the primary movement, DPs right and left eyes, move backwards/a little downwards by flexion in the atlanto-occipital and atlanto-axial joints and extension in the right hip joint effected by the proximal lever. They move until the pressure under the sole of the right foot markedly diminishes. The leg hanging suspended in the arm sling is taken along in the movement.

Reactio: Activated Passive Buttressing
Activated passive buttressing occurs through the right sole's being nearly lifted off the floor. When this happens, the right leg becomes hung onto the pelvis by flexional activity in the hip joint. The position of the right heel relative to the right knee in the starting position will determine whether the lower leg is now suspended flexionally or extensionally from the knee.

Reactio: Change to the Support Area
When the "scales" tip backwards in Balancing Up, the support area shifts backwards a little and becomes smaller because the right sole is now nearly off the floor.

Tipping Forwards

The left leg is suspended in the arm sling (Fig. 91 c).

Actio: The Primary Movement
The critical distance point of the primary movement, DP hands clasped around the left knee, moves forwards/downwards with flexion in the right hip effected by the proximal lever, until the pressure under the right sole markedly increases. BSs pelvis, thorax and head, suspended as a stabilized unit from the hands via the shoulder girdle and arms, are carried along with the movement. The activity in the right hip joint that has triggered the movement starts as concentric isotonic flexion then changes into eccentric isotonic extension.

Reactio: Activated Passive Buttressing
Because the entire movement system suspended from the arm sling, BSs pelvis, thorax and head and the left leg, is transported en bloc forwards/downwards by

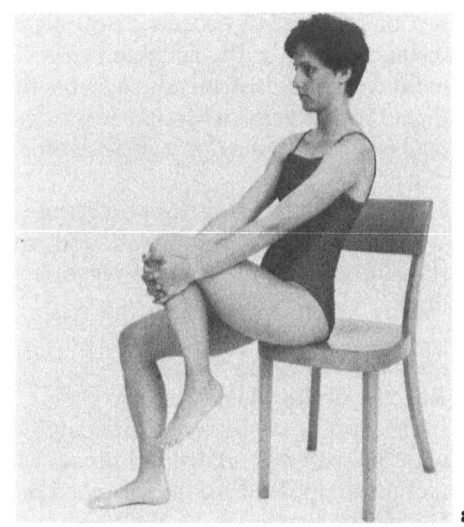

a

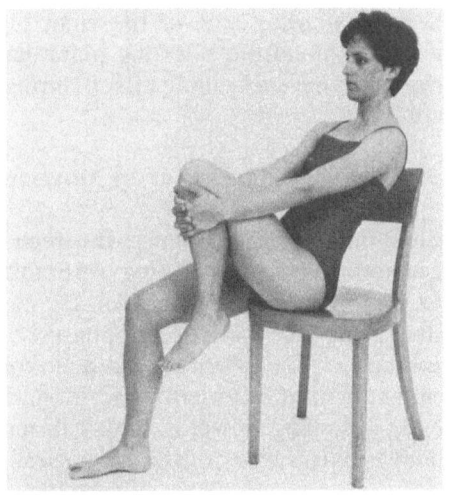

b

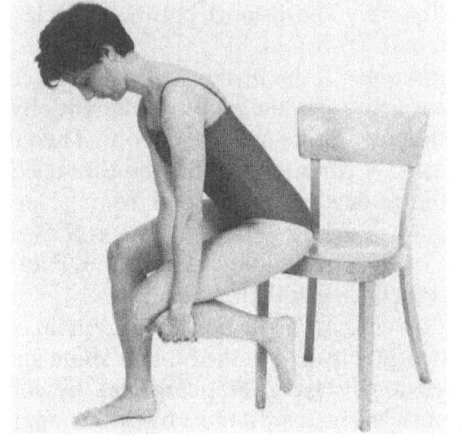

Fig. 91 a–c. Balanced Up, adaptation to improve performance. **a** Starting position. **b** Tipping backwards. **c** Tipping forwards, extended

c

flexion followed by eccentric isotonic extension in the right hip joint, none of the distance points of the activated passive buttressing move contrary to the movement direction. Instead, any weights that have an effect in a direction other than that of the movement become less as the long axis of the body approaches the vertical on its way from tipping backwards to tipping forwards.

Reactio: Change in the Support Area
When the "scales" tip forwards/downwards in Balancing Up, the support area shifts forwards and becomes bigger as the right leg moves into supporting function.

Actio: Accelerating Weights
Reactio: Braking Weights
In the starting position of Balancing Up the potential bisecting plane is identical with the patient's midfrontal plane, which is vertical, because the horizontal direction components of the intended primary movement go backwards/forwards. During the tipping phase, the bisecting plane goes roughly through the horizontal flexion/extension axis of the right hip joint. During tipping backwards, the weights behind the bisecting plane have an accelerating effect while those in front of it have a braking effect; during tipping forwards they are the other way around.

● **Conditio – Limitatio of the Movement Sequence**

Conditio: Constant Distances Between Body Distance Points
Limitatio: Active Buttressing and Stabilization
Conditio: The distance between DP navel and DP xiphoid process remains constant throughout both tipping phases.
Limitatio: If this distance is to remain constant, the thoracic spine must be dynamically stabilized in its neutral position, flexionally in tipping backwards, extensionally in tipping forwards, and with increasing intensity as the long axis of the body inclines further out of the vertical.

Conditio: The distance between DP clasped hands and DP right/left shoulder joint remains constant.
Limitatio: If this distance is to remain constant during both tipping phases, flexional activity in the elbow joints and, by continuing movement, retraction in the shoulder girdle must be cut out. Then the weight of the left leg hangs suspended directly from the thorax, the thoracic spine is extensionally stimulated and the thorax becomes suspended from the leg via the hands.

Conditio: The distance between DP left knee and DP jugular notch remains constant during both tipping phases.
Limitatio: If this distance is to remain constant, BS pelvis must be stabilized in its neutral position in the lumbar spine and the left leg must not become suspended flexionally from the pelvis and, by continuing movement, from the abdominal muscles. Instead, it must be extensionally stabilized in the left hip joint during the

backward tip. Only then can the movement system pelvis, thorax, head and left leg tip backwards and forwards en bloc with extension and flexion in the right hip joint. The activity of the abdominal muscles remains low, promoting normal breathing.

Conditio of Absolute and/or Relative Fixed Spatial Points
Limitatio by Limiting the Primary Movement, Activated Passive Buttressing
and/or Change in the Support Area
In Balancing Up there are only relative fixed spatial points.

Conditio: The contact maintained between the right sole and the floor is a relative fixed point throughout both tipping phases.
Limitatio: This checks the tip backwards by keeping the right leg from moving completely into free play, for then the contact between the right sole and the floor would be lost.

Conditio: While tipping backwards, the patient continues to look forwards.
Limitatio: This relative fixed spatial point is maintained by flexion in the atlanto-occipital and atlanto-axial joints adjusting to the backward tip.

Conditio: While tipping forwards, the patient continues to look forwards until the long axis of the body is vertical. As he tips on further forwards, he looks ventrally/downwards.
Limitatio: This relative fixed spatial point means that the atlanto-occipital and atlanto-axial joints move back into neutral position when the long axis of the body tips forwards into the vertical, and they keep this neutral position as the axis tips on further forwards because the patient is looking ventrally/downwards instead of straight ahead.

Conditio: The patient's plane of symmetry must not rotate in space as he tips forwards and backwards.
Limitatio: This relative fixed spatial point ensures that the tipping movement of the movement system pelvis, thorax, head, arms and left leg remains one of flexion and extension in the right hip joint and that no avoidance mechanisms of transverse abduction or adduction occur.

Conditio: The left knee joint does not leave the plane of symmetry as it moves backwards/upwards and forwards/downwards with the tipping of the scales.
Limitatio: This relative fixed spatial point ensures that the spinal column is stabilized against the possible avoidance mechanisms of rotation or lateroflexion. This stabilization is necessary because the weight of the left leg hanging from the clasped hands during forward tipping and the weight of BSs pelvis, thorax and head hanging from the left knee during backward tipping are unequal weights that have a tendency to deflect the tipping movement in the right hip into transverse abduction and adduction.

Conditio of Movement Speed
Limitatio of Economical Activity by Finding the Optimal Speed
Conditio: A good guide to speed is about 15 tips/minute.
Limitatio: This speed roughly matches a normal breathing phase of 4 seconds. The intensity of economical activity is the lowest at this speed. One is balanced up when the tipping movement stops without any braking muscle activity.

▶ Instruction in Patient Language

● Instruction Appealing to the Patient's Perception

In Balancing Up, the direction of the patient's gaze plays an important part because both what the patient sees in front of him and the attempt to keep a certain distance from it are extremely helpful to stabilization of the thoracic spine in neutral position.

● Verbal Instruction   ● Instruction by Manipulation

Position and Activation in the Starting Position
See Building Blocks (p. 204)

Actio and Conditio of the Movement Sequence (Tipping Backwards)

"Look straight ahead. As if in a dream, cross your left knee over your right and clasp your hands around it. Steer yourself backwards with your head until your arms are very long and you can feel the weight of your leg in your hands. Your back is long. The weight of your leg pulls your shoulders forwards. You can feel it pulling quite hard, but not unpleasantly so. Only your clasped fingers need to be strong.

Now your head moves farther backwards, until your left leg lifts up from the right one. Lift it only so far that the right sole remains comfortably on the floor. Your back stays straight; it doesn't hump anywhere. But now your body is leaning backwards quite markedly. You can't fall because your left leg keeps you balanced as long as you keep your hands clasped. Other than

Here the lengths of the arms, thighs and the "turret" are an important factor, and so is the relationship between the weight of the leg and that of the "turret". A patient with long arms and a heavy upper body can "shorten" his arms by gripping the wrist of one hand with the other. The arms can also be "lengthened" with a towel. The movement impulse begins with a minimal dorsal translation of the head. Instantly, continuing movement begins, with BSs head, thorax and pelvis en bloc effecting extension in the hip joint of the parked leg until a wavering equilibrium is established. The weight of the left leg is literally hung onto the thoracic spine, whose activation can be palpated. The therapist makes sure that there is no activity in the arms and shoulder girdle that might inhibit free breathing. The

that, your arms don't have to work at all. Your stomach is entirely relaxed and your breathing comes automatically. Now you're a set of scales that can tip gently to and fro. You can sit like this anywhere to relax."

gentle tipping to and fro of the scale beam made by BSs head, thorax, arms, pelvis and left leg about the flexion/extension axis of the right hip joint can be continued ad libitum.

► Adapting the Exercise to the Patient's Constitution and Condition

● Adaptation to Constitution: Role of Lengths, Widths, Depths and Distribution of Weights

In patients with a longer upper length, especially those with overweight around the thorax and shoulder girdle and when the legs are relatively light, the backward tipping movement will be relatively short. Patients with a longer lower length, heavy legs and a relatively light thorax and shoulder girdle, on the other hand, may tip backwards until the long axis of their body inclines at an angle of more than 45°.

The lengths of the arms and of the thighs are also of significance. The longer the arms, the greater the angle between the long axis of the body and the long axis of the left thigh. In patients with long thighs and heavy legs, the long axis of the arms becomes almost horizontal on tipping backwards.

● Adaptation to Condition

Increasing Performance (Fig. 91)
To dynamically increase the stabilization of the thoracic spine in its neutral position, the patient finds the position of equilibrium, pulls his left knee towards his sternum by flexional activity in the elbows, and then immediately releases the elbow flexors. The weight of the left leg extends the elbows with a jerk. This jerk must be absorbed by the thoracic spine by correctly coordinated extensional active buttressing.

In this variation, the legs should not be crossed.

If the forward/downward tipping is continued until the long axes of the arms are almost vertical and the long axis of the lower left leg is almost horizontal, the right leg goes into supporting function and the extensional stress on the spinal column increases considerably.

To add a good method of training the abdominal muscles for skill, we stop the patient in the equilibrium position between forwards and backwards tipping and have him unclasp his hands, with the conditio that no further movement take place. The abdominal muscles carry out the limitatio, spontaneously going into fall-preventing activity.

Instability/Hypermobility of the Spinal Column

There is a variation of Balancing Up that is especially beneficial for patients with unstable thoracic flat back. First the patient finds the position in which tipping stops. Then, he carefully retracts the shoulder girdle and just as carefully lets it go again, so that it is protracted by the weight of the leg hanging from the hands. This stimulates the thoracic spine to extensional active buttressing. This exercise helps the patient to become aware of the antagonism between keeping the spinal column stabilized in its neutral position and moving the shoulder girdle on the thorax, and can practice it.

5.4.4 The Corkscrew (Fig. 92)

"The Corkscrew" is an invented name, an association given rise to by the way the body is pulled out long and at the same time the pelvis twists against the thorax.

■ Goal of the Exercise

The goal is stabilization of the thoracic spine in its neutral position, even in patients with pronounced thoracic flat back, unstable spinal column and thoracic round back, by self-manipulated twisting of the thorax against the pelvis.

▶ Functional Analysis in Therapist Language

● Conception of the Exercise

Experience has shown that the functional problem in patients with back pain is very often that the thoracic spine has become destabilized, i. e. lost its dynamic stabilization in neutral position.

In patients with thoracic flat back, the stimulus to extend when the long axis of the body is vertical is not strong enough, especially in patients who lead a very sedentary life. This applies to generally unstable spinal columns as well. In the case of thoracic round back tending towards stiffening, there is too much resistance against reaching the neutral position.

In both cases, attempting to attain or hold the neutral position leads to avoidance mechanisms. In the case of the flat back, we see total extension of the thoracic and lumbar spine and retraction of the shoulder girdle, while in the case of thoracic round back there is hyperextension of the lumbar spine with flexion of the pelvis in the hips and retraction of the shoulder girdle.

Like in the Classic All-Fours Exercise, we want to exhaust the tolerance for rotation in the lower thoracic spine using buttressing movements, so that a strong extensional stimulus coming from BS head in the form of traction and dorsal transla-

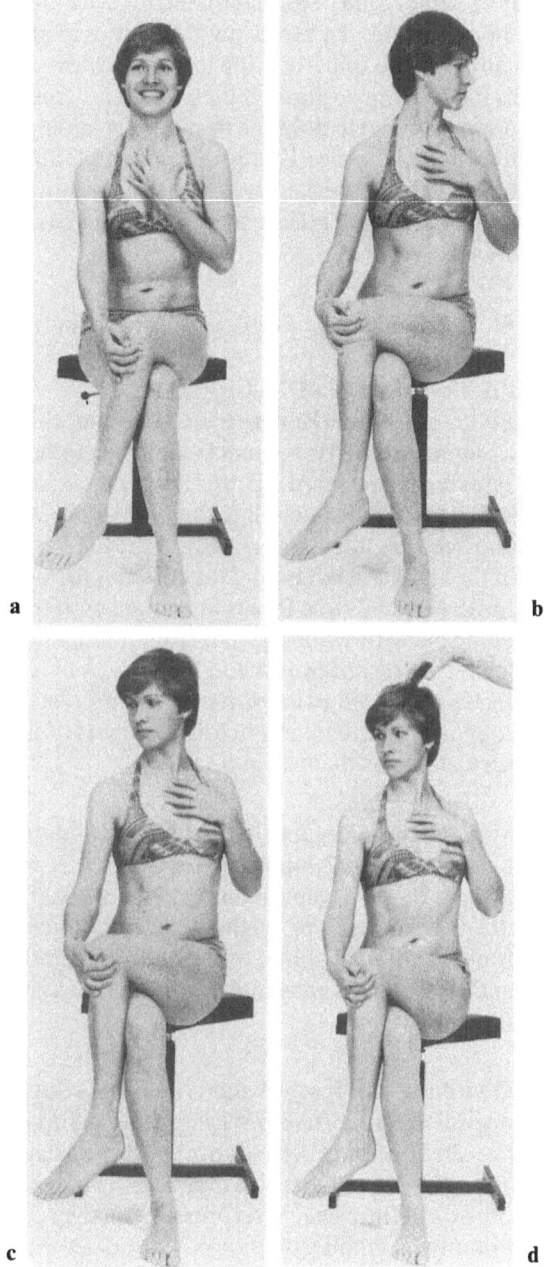

a

b

Fig. 92 a–d. The Corkscrew. a Starting
position, b phase 1, c phase 2, d phase 3 c

d

281

tion, rather than being dissipated in continuing movements, is concentrated on the thoracic spine. To avoid any difficulties in aligning the long axis of the body vertically with the spinal column in neutral position, we choose upright sitting on a stool as the starting position. If the patient crosses one leg over the other, he can use the opposite hand to hold the upper knee and pull his thorax forward with rotation in the thoracic spine. This rotation can be augmented by co-rotation of the head. Once in this "straitjacket", the patient is reminded to breathe freely again. The extensional stimuli arising from the head are unable to trigger any avoidance mechanisms.

● Position and Activation in the Starting Position

Position in Space of the Critical Axes
Points of Contact Between the Body and the Environment
Components of Movement in Relation to the Neutral Position of the Joints
The starting position is sitting across the corner of a stool that is as high as the knee is from the floor (including the heel of the shoe if one is worn). BSs pelvis, thorax and head are aligned vertically in the long axis of the body. In BS pelvis, the region of the right and left ischial tuberosities forms the contact with the seat.
In BS legs, the right foot is in contact with the floor with the sole a little to the left of the plane of symmetry. The functional long axis of the foot points forwards. The left leg is crossed over the right.
In BS arms, the palm of the left hand rests on the sternum. The index finger is roughly in the jugular notch. The fingers of the right hand clasp the left tibial tuberosity from medially (Fig. 92 a).

Movement Tolerances at the Critical Joints in Relation
to the Intended Primary Movement
Since the spinal column is roughly in neutral, we have full tolerance for rotation at the rotation levels of the thoracic and cervical spines. However, movement restrictions in the hip joints, especially restricted transverse adduction, and/or short and/or fat thighs, may make it difficult to assume the starting position (for adaptations, see p. 287).

Distribution of Body Weights on a Base Support or Suspension Device,
Against a Supportive Device or Over a Support Area,
and the Resulting Activity States of the Musculature
The weight of BSs pelvis, thorax and head, the shoulder girdle, the left arm and a portion of the right exerts pressure on the seat of the stool. BSs pelvis and head are potentially mobile, BS thorax is stabilized, the shoulder girdle is parked on the thorax, the left arm hangs suspended in free play from the shoulder girdle and from the manubrium sterni, the right arm hangs suspended from the shoulder girdle and from the suspension device of the left knee. The left leg is parked on the right and the right leg is in slight supporting function.
The support area is the smallest area encompassing the points of contact pelvis/seat and the right sole/floor.

Intensity of Muscle Activity Required with Economical Activity
Respiration
The intensity of economical activity is low. Breathing should be normal. DP vertex strives upwards and the eyes keep their distance from what they see.

● Actio – Reactio of the Movement Sequence

In the movement sequence of the Corkscrew, the emphasis is on lift-free rotation of the thorax in the thoracic spine. Since the horizontal components of direction in this rotation cancel each other out and there is a pronounced striving vertically upwards, no dominant reactio will appear.

The actio occurs in three phases. In this example, negative rotation of the thorax at the rotation level thoracic spine is analysed.

Actio: The Primary Movement
Phase 1
Negative rotation of the thorax in the lower thoracic spine with two primary movements. The critical distance point of the first primary movement, DP right hand, clasps the left tibial head from medially/ventrally and pulls it to the right/backwards. This movement involves flexion in the finger joints and wrist and, by proximally continuing movement, supination in the forearm, flexion in the elbow, and extension/external rotation in the shoulder. By further continuation, the right side of the thorax is pulled into the pincer jaws, opening them and adducting the thoracic spinal processes against the medial scapular margin. The thorax has rotated negatively in relation to the lower thoracic spine and the right pincer jaws.

In addition, the right hand pulling on the left tibial head causes the continuing movement of internal rotation of the lower leg in the left knee, transverse adduction in the left hip effected by the distal lever, distally arising transverse traction in the left iliosacral joint, and proximally arising transverse traction in the right iliosacral joint. The tendency of the pelvis to transversely adduct in the right hip (critical fulcrum) as a continuing movement is actively buttressed transverse adductionally by the distal lever, because DP right knee must push to the left/backwards. Simultaneously, the second primary movement is under way with a lower intensity of economical activity. DP right eye moves left/forwards, DP left eye left/backwards. As they go, the head rotates negatively in the atlanto-occipital and atlanto-axial joints and cervical spine. By continuing movement, DP right nipple moves left/forwards and DP left nipple moves right/backwards and the thorax rotates negatively in the lower thoracic spine. The active buttressing checking the movement occurs in both hips and keeps the caudal pointer of rotation of the thoracic spine, the pelvis, in place (Fig. 92 b).

Phase 2
In the second phase BS head moves back into or even beyond neutral position by positive rotation in the atlanto-occipital and atlanto-axial joints and the cervical spine, exhausting the tolerance for positive rotation until actively buttressed by the negative rotation of the thorax in the thoracic spine. During its positive rotation the head must be kept in the long axis of the body by dorsal translation: DP

vertex strives upwards and the head translates dorsally due to the efforts of the eyes to keep their distance from all they see. Both of these activities stimulate extensional stabilization of the thoracic spine. At the same time, the tone in the ventral and dorsal paravertebral waist muscles should be decreasing. When economical activity is reached, breathing returns spontaneously to normal (Figs. 92 c, d).

Phase 3
The gaze is directed forwards and the pull of the patient's right hand on his left knee is first reduced, then increased, like pulling a bowstring. A sudden release of the knee sets the thorax and arms off on an alternating rotating movement; the right hand has come to rest on the left. The thorax rotates at rotation levels thoracic and cervical spines, above the stationary pelvis and below the stationary head.

● Conditio – Limitatio of the Movement Sequence

Conditio: Constant Distances Between Body Distance Points
Limitatio: Active Buttressing and Stabilization
Conditio: The distance between DP right iliac spine and DP long axis of the right thigh remains constant.
Limitatio: If this distance remains constant, the avoidance mechanism of pelvic flexion in the right hip will be prevented and the pull of the right hand on the left tibial head will result according to plan in a continuing negative rotation of the thorax in the thoracic spine.

Conditio: The distance between the horizontal transverse plane through the right and left iliac spines and the horizontal transverse plane through the horizontal frontotransverse diameter of the thorax remains constant.
Limitatio: If these two planes remain equidistant, horizontal and parallel, avoidance mechanisms in the form of translation of the thorax to the right/to the left/forwards/backwards, flexion/extension, lateroflexion in the thoracic spine and flexion/extension/internal/external rotation of the pelvis in the hips will be prevented by active buttressing.

Conditio of Absolute and/or Relative Fixed Spatial Points
Limitatio by Limiting the Primary Movement, Activated Passive Buttressing and/or Change in the Support Area
Conditio: The point of contact right sole/floor is an absolute fixed spatial point.
Limitatio: This point is fixed by appropriate active buttressing in the tarsometatarsal and metatarsal joints of the right foot: pronation/supination/eversion/inversion.

Conditio: The point of contact right and left ischial tuberosity/seat, on which the pressure always remains the same, is an absolute fixed spatial point.
Limitatio: This fixed point guarantees the alignment of BSs pelvis and thorax in the long axis of the body and prevents all the avoidance mechanisms that would be

triggered by shifting weights horizontally or shifting the distribution of pressure within the support area.

Conditio: The right acromion is an absolute fixed spatial point.
Limitatio: This fixed point ensures that the distal-to-proximal continuing movement in the right arm causes the proximal pointer, the frontotransverse diameter of the thorax, to move in relation to the stationary distal pointer, the medial scapular margin, at movement level shoulder girdle/thorax.

Conditio: The point of contact left palm/sternum is a relative fixed spatial point.
Limitatio: This fixed point makes the left arm remain on the thorax throughout the exercise. Its weight takes the rotational swing of the thorax in the lower thoracic spine and cervical spine further at the end of the movement sequence, and reinforces extensional stimulation of the thoracic spine.

Conditio: DP vertex is an absolute fixed spatial point.
Limitatio: This keeps the head from horizontal ventral translation in the cervical spine as it rotates around the long axis of the body. To keep this point fixed in space, the head must constantly strive towards dorsal translation as it rotates. This, together with the pulling forwards of the xiphoid process, results in the upward striving of DP vertex (Fig. 92 d).

Conditio of Movement Speed
Limitatio of Economical Activity by Finding the Optimal Speed
Conditio: The movement is performed at a leisurely speed.
Limitatio: "Leisurely speed" will mean different things to different people and will naturally also depend on the amount of experience the patient has had with this exercise. Once it has been absorbed into the patient's movement repertoire, the whole sequence wants about 30 seconds. While learning the exercise, the patient must take time to consciously think about and fulfil each of the required conditios.

▶ Instruction in Patient Language

● Instruction Appealing to the Patient's Perception

In the Corkscrew exercise, the patient should be able to reproducibly create the dynamic stabilization of his thoracic spine specified in the goal by on the one hand maintaining a watchful but distanced perception of his surroundings, and at the same time feeling the weight of his hand on his chest and the normal process of his breathing.

Position and Activation in the Starting Position

"Sit over the corner of a stool, nice and upright. Your thighs don't touch the seat at all. Casually cross your left leg over your right. It's a good thing that you moved your right foot a little to the left. But the tips of your toes still point forwards. Now put your left hand on your chest. With the fingers of your right hand, clasp your left knee from the side. But don't let your right shoulder move forwards."

The therapist checks the sitting position carefully. If the patient cannot easily cross his legs, the exercise must be adapted, as it must also if the arm is too short to clasp the knee from medially without bringing the right shoulder forwards. Here, too, the exercise will need to be adapted if lowering the seat slightly doesn't compensate the problem.

Actio and Conditio of the Movement Sequence

"Look attentively over your left shoulder and take the shoulder backwards with you. With your right hand, pull the right side of your chest forwards, so you can look backwards better. You've seen what you wanted to. Now look over your right shoulder; your eyes are looking forwards and to the right. With your right hand, pull your rib cage still a little farther forwards. Your left hand stays on your chest while you grow a couple of inches. Stay tall, but let your stomach relax, and the small of your back too – neither of them has anything to do. When you can feel that relaxing has allowed your breathing to come very lightly, let go of your left knee suddenly and place your right hand over your left. Now look straight ahead and let your rib cage turn weightlessly to and fro, like a perpetual motion machine."

The therapist can facilitate rotation by manually turning BS head counterclockwise. She also makes sure the activity of the right biceps doesn't pull the left knee towards the body, but instead reinforces the negative rotation of BS thorax. During the subsequent positive rotation of BS head the therapist watches out for two things: (1) that the negative rotation of BS thorax remains in its extreme position and (2) that, as the head positively rotates, no avoidance mechanism in the form of right-concave lateroflexion in the cervical spine arises. If she is manipulating the movement, she can give a suggestion of left-concave lateroflexion, thus achieving maximum rotation in the cervical area. During the "self-extension", compressive resistance applied in the direction of the long axis of the body can be very helpful. This resistance continues to be applied while the abdominal and lumbar muscles are relaxed. If the hyperactivity in the lumbar muscles was high, the relaxation of these muscles will cause the long axis of the body to shift somewhat dorsally. When the patient lets go of his left knee, he must not let his spinal column collapse into flexion.

▶ Adapting the Exercise to the Patient's Constitution and Condition

● Adaptation to Constitution: Role of Lengths, Widths, Depths and Distribution of Weights

It may be impossible for the patient to cross his legs if his thighs are short and/or fat. The rule is that the lower half of the crossed leg should hang and swing freely. One good adaptation is to support the leg on a footrest such that the patient can comfortably grasp the knee from medially. The only way short arms can grasp the crossed knee is if the shoulder comes forwards or the lumbar and thoracic spine flexes. Neither of these is allowed in this exercise. However, by folding a towel four times we can make a sling for the knee that can be held together by the hand doing the pulling.

● Adaptation to Condition

The Corkscrew can be easily adapted to accommodate discomfort in the iliosacral region. In the same starting position, the patient leans his left arm on the seat close to and somewhat behind the left greater trochanter. The right arm crosses over the left thigh, pressing it to the right/backwards, with the forearm in supination and the palm facing laterally/forwards. The thorax has rotated negatively to end-stop in the lower thoracic spine.

5.5 Adapting Lift-Free/Reduced-Lift Mobilization of the Spinal Column to Special Problems of the Cervical Spine

In functional terms, the cervical spine is part of BS head. In upright economical posture, the cervical spine and the atlanto-occipital and atlanto-axial joints should be potentially mobile. They should also be so, particularly the atlanto-occipital and atlanto-axial joints – the mid and lower cervical spine to a lesser extent – when the virtual long axis of the body is inclined forward. Only in this way can this segment of the spine be prepared to meet the constant demands made on it for fine flexional, extensional, lateroflexional, translational and rotational movement. Moreover, this state of readiness means that the fall-preventing muscles are subjected to constant fluctuations in tone even when the multiplicity of tolerances for movement in the vertebral and intervertebral joints are not being used. This motor behaviour protects the cervical spine against premature wear and tear. However, it can only function if the adjacent thoracic spine is dynamically stabilized; otherwise, the muscles in the cervical and shoulder girdle region are called in to help with maintaining posture and become overstressed.
People with sedentary occupations using their hands and eyes a great deal subject

their cervical spine to very considerable stress even if their sitting posture is good. Stress caused by fleeting changes in position is easily tolerated, as long as there is no acute radicular symptomatology that makes any stress unbearable. However, driving for long stretches at a time, especially at high speed, without frequently checking the positioning of the head has the effect of constant slow-motion whiplash trauma.

Comparing the two lordotic segments of the spine, the lumbar and the cervical, we notice one important difference: the lumbar spine is the lowermost segment of the virtual long axis of the body. The postural statics of its superstructure, the thorax, depends considerably on its substructure, the pelvis and the legs. The legs are functionally constructed for a supporting function.

The cervical spine is the uppermost segment of the virtual long axis of the body. Its superstructure is the rigid head, which it must keep economically balanced above itself. Its substructure is the thoracic spine, which is inherently flexible and only functions properly when dynamically stabilized in its neutral position. This sensitive structure is subjected to the asymmetrical activities of the free-play arms as the hands go about their business at the end of their long levers.

Functionally belonging together with the cervical spine and cranially contiguous with it is the head, a bony receptacle whose connection to the cervical spine via the atlanto-occipital and atlanto-axial joints is extremely mobile in the service of the visual, auditory and olfactory senses, and which is functionally an extremity. It is obvious that even under normal circumstances the cervical spine is subjected to many different kinds of stress.

When, due to pathological changes or merely to the statics of posture, the position of the cervical spine relative to the other body segments and to gravity has become uneconomical, the process of wear and tear speeds up rapidly. We therefore try to identify the functional relationships underlying such problems and aggravating any pathological conditions already existing in this area.

Common Causes of Faulty Postural Stress

– Structural cervical kyphosis above a thoracic flat back, causing permanently raised tone in the muscles of the shoulder girdle, especially the levator scapulae and the upper rhomboids, with ischaemic pain and shearing stress to the passive structures in the motion segment immediately cranial to the kyphosis.
– Hollow back with cranial extension of the thoracic kyphosis and ventral/forward slippage of the cervical spine together with the head in the motion segment where the cervical lordosis starts. In addition to this shearing stress on the passive structures, there is always reactive hypertonia in the paravertebral cervical muscles and cranial muscles of the shoulder girdle.
– Thoracic flat back and flattened out cervical lordosis or even cervical kyphosis as far up as the atlanto-occipital and atlanto-axial joints and ventral translation in several motion segments of the cervical spine with a destabilized thoracic spine and hyperactivity of the scalene muscles and retractors of the shoulder girdle.

– Constitutionally extra-long upper length in patients whose desk, when they sit at work, is too low, and/or chair too high, or arms are too short, to keep the spinal column in its neutral position when vertical or leaning forwards. To shorten this overlength, they increase the extension of the pelvis in the hips, totally flexing the lumbar and thoracic spine and hyperextending the cervical spine or allowing it and the head to slip ventrally, which leads to overstressing of the passive and active structures of the lumbothoracic and cervical regions.
– Any visual impairment causing the eyes be brought nearer to the work. This causes the upper body to collapse at the hip and vertebral joints.
– Existing pathological changes caused by osteochondrosis, spondylosis, arthritis in the uncus, discopathies, herniated discs, scoliosis, spasticity, inflammation, partial stiffnesses, cervical rib syndrome, muscular disorders, contusions (whiplash), osteoporosis and many others. The disorders collectively referred to as cervical syndromes must be differentially diagnosed for functional determination of the correct therapy. Those particularly to be mentioned include scalenus syndrome, symptomatology of the costoclavicular and infraclavicular passage (Mumenthaler's or outlet syndrome), compression of the vertebral arteries with vertigo, scapulocostal syndrome; tennis elbow and carpal tunnel syndrome should be distinguished.
– Effects that functional respiratory disorders have on postural stress on the cervical spine. Every functional respiratory disorder is accompanied by destabilization of the thoracic spine. As a consequence, the weight of the thorax is no longer carried by the thoracic spine but hangs more from the scalene muscles, overstressing the first and second ribs and the levator scapulae.

5.5.1 Relief Postures for the Cervical Spine

The name "Relief Postures for the Cervical Spine" refers to the functional problem to be solved.

■ Goal of the Exercise

The goal is for the patient to find resting positions and work postures:
– That neutralize the weight of the head so that the cervical spine in its neutral position and the atlanto-occipital and atlanto-axial jonts do not have to be held together by muscle activity
– In which the cervical spine and the adjacent BS thorax are roughly in neutral position and the weight of the shoulder girdle and of the arms is so arranged that it causes no stress on either the active or the passive structures of the cervical spine and the atlanto-occipital and atlanto-axial joints.

▶ Functional Analysis in Therapist Language

● Conception of the Exercise

For sleep and rest we aim to find completely comfortable, "switched-off" positions. However, positions for sitting, standing and working are also needed. Work postures in which the long axis of the body inclines out of the vertical present the greatest problems because the hands must be free to engage in manual activities.

● Position and Activation in the Starting Position

These relief postures also apply in part to the lumbar and thoracic spines; here we will limit ourselves to aspects specific to the cervical spine.

Little Shepherd Boy Position, Preferably with the Hips in Neutral Position, Knees Flexed to 90°, Soles Touching the Base Support (Figs. 59, 93)

If the hips are freely mobile, the patient lies on his back on a bed or a treatment bench. There must be enough room beyond the head for the arms. The flexion creases of the knees are on the caudal edge of the bed or bench. The knees are flexed to 90°, the soles are on the floor or on a footrest at the right height. If the patient has good hip extension he can lie with his gluteal folds along the caudal edge of the bench, which is a good position for simultaneous stretching of the hip flexors, but the lumbar spine must be able to stay in its neutral position. The thoracic spine is slightly extended (Fig. 59).

The head rests on the base support. If, however, cervical kyphosis or thoracic round back cause shearing stress on the passive structures of the spinal column, or if there is any reactive muscle tension that would make parking function for all body segments impossible, the head will need to be elevated. If the head can stay on the base support, many patients find it comfortable to have a little padding under the cervical spine, especially if there is even the slightest cervical hyperlordosis.

The legs can also rest on the bench; if they don't require any special positioning, it's good to cross them. In acute syndromes of the lumbar spine, a pillow can be placed under the pelvis, bringing the lumbar spine into slight flexion. The legs can also be positioned on a square pillow such that the long axes of the thighs are vertical (Fig. 93).

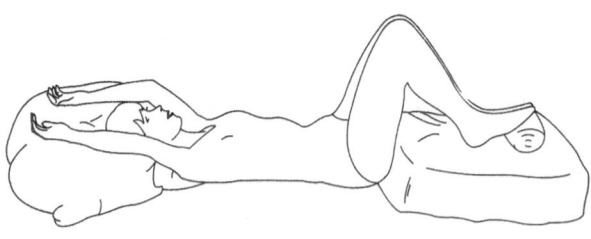

Fig. 93. Little Shepherd Boy: relief posture for the cervical spine

Positioning the arms on a pillow is important, bringing the forearms up to a horizontal level higher than the head. For this, elbows and hands must be well supported. The humeroscapular joints are flexed almost to end-stop, well rotated internally (but not to end-stop) and somewhat abducted. The elbows are flexed, the forearms pronated. In the shoulder girdle, the acromion is cranial/medial/dorsal to its neutral position. The muscle slings at the cervical spine are completely relaxed; the cervical spine and atlanto-occipital and atlanto-axial joints have been completely relieved of stress.

This relief posture is also the position of choice for patients with epicondylitis, carpal tunnel syndrome and arthrosis of the metacarpophalangeal joint of the thumb.

Relief Posture for the Cervical Spine in Sidelying (see Fig. 66)

The sidelying position described on p. 221 is also a relief posture for the cervical spine. Here the upper arm must be placed on a relatively high pillow so that the pillow bears its entire weight. This position is not as good for the lower arm. In addition, the head has a tendency in this position to slide ventrally/downwards, and if this happens the position is no longer suitable as a relief posture for the cervical spine.

Relief Postures for the Cervical Spine in Sitting (Figs. 94, 95)

Figure 94a shows a very good relief posture for the shoulder girdle, arms and cervical spine. It is also good for respiration. Moreover, in this position, the therapist can carry out mobilizing massage in the region of the neck and shoulder girdle.

This relief posture can also be taken up when knitting or sewing. For this, the table must be moved very close to the body, so that what the patient is knitting or sewing can be placed on the table. Another possible relief posture is to use a chair with armrests of a height for the elbows to be supported without flexing the thoracic spine or pulling the shoulder girdle up. A cushion of suitable shape can also be put on the patient's lap, and a footstool used to support short lower legs. A bed table elevated to the proper height and slightly angled can also be pulled up close. In either case, the weight of the arms and of the work they are doing is transferred to another base support.

If the patient's thighs are long and easily crossed, the table will not be needed, provided the projects being worked on are not too large or heavy.

Figure 94b shows the same sitting posture with the arms parked on the thighs and BSs pelvis and thorax inclined slightly backwards at the hips. The extent to which the patient leans back can vary, but as long as BSs pelvis and thorax are well supported against a backrest and the tendency to slide forwards on the seat of the chair is low, and as long as the long axis of BS head is vertical, relief of the cervical spine is ensured. As soon as the backrest is removed, however, faulty stress on the cervical spine will only be avoided by keeping the long axis of the body vertical. For this, BSs pelvis, thorax and head must be aligned as in Fig. 95.

291

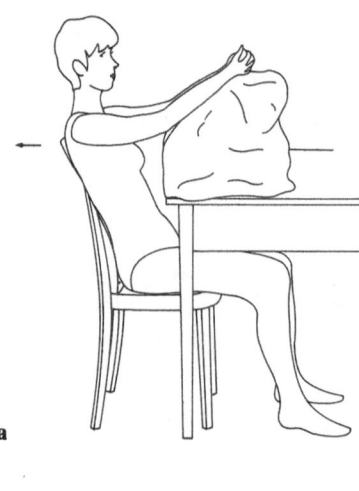

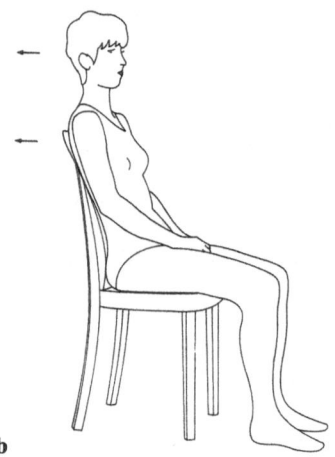

Fig. 94 a, b. Relief postures for the cervical spine in sitting with a backrest. **a** With arm support, **b** without arm support

Relief Postures for the Cervical Spine During Typing or Desk Work
(Fig. 96; see also Fig. 83)

We have already seen (Fig. 83) how an abdominal support can shorten by half the long lever at the end of which the hands are moving if BSs pelvis and thorax are well aligned in the long axis of the body and this axis is moderately inclined forwards at the hips. This dramatically reduces the intensity of activity in the muscles providing extensional anchoring in the lumbosacral area and the strain on the the extensor muscles of the back of the neck. It also makes coordination of movements of the shoulder girdle on a stabilized thorax much easier. Now both hands can function freely.

Figure 96 shows two variants of a posture for reading and writing. Leaning the head on the forehead is good for patients with a relatively stiff cervical spine if spontaneous improvement of the postural statics is not possible.

By supporting the head on the chin (Fig. 96 b) patients with mobile spinal columns can also learn better posture. Each time the wrist supporting the head leans against

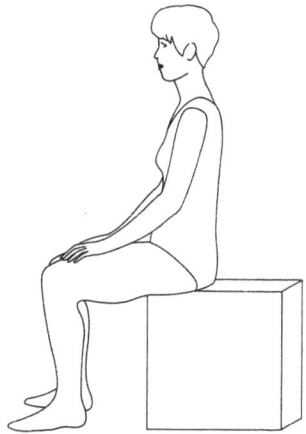

Fig. 95. Relief postures for the cervical spine (also for thoracic and lumbar spine), sitting upright without backrest

the sternum the patient has a learning experience, for this effectively manipulates the head into dorsal translation in the cervical spine and the atlanto-occipital and atlanto-axial joints into flexion. The weight of the head is supported ventrally to prevent its falling and the extensors of the atlanto-occipital and atlanto-axial joints automatically relax. The chin should never be supported from caudally, as this would manipulate ventral translation of the head and hyperextension of the atlanto-occipital and atlanto-axial joints.

Towel Trick (Fig. 97)
The towel trick can be explained as follows. First the patient learns to transfer the weight of his arms to a suspension device which he grips with his hands. For this we use a sturdy towel that the therapist holds at a suitable height. The only activity in BS arms is that of the hands holding on to the towel. The therapist can

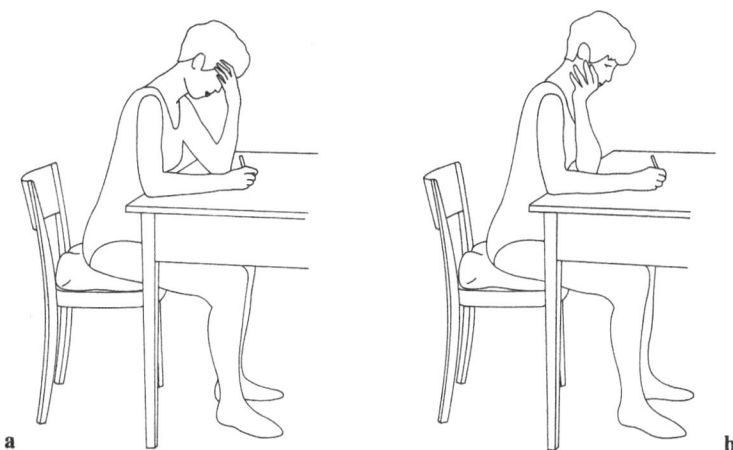

a b

Fig. 96 a, b. Relief postures for the cervical spine in sitting: postures for writing and working

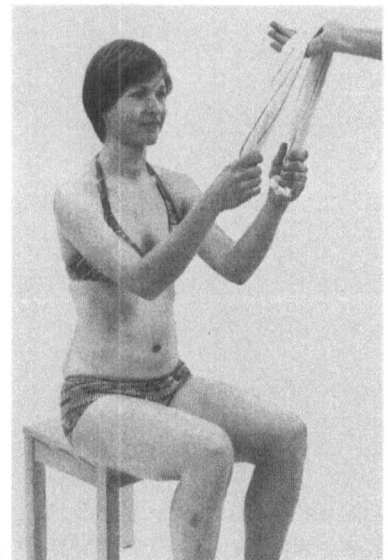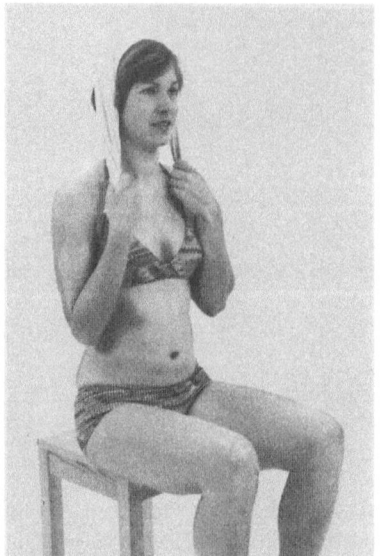

a   b

Fig. 97 a, b. The Towel Trick. **a** Preliminary exercise. **b** Using a towel, the weight of the arms is suspended from the head

check whether the arms and the shoulder girdle are relaxed by shaking the towel. Next, with the patient sitting upright, she uses the weight of the relaxed arms to compress the vertical long axis of the body and stimulate the carrier function of the thoracic spine, by hanging the towel, with the arms still dangling from it, over the top of the head, near the vertex. If the posture is correct, there is no fall-preventing activity in either the region of the shoulder girdle or the back of the neck. The patient can get up, walk about the house and, if he wants to, even dance.

5.5.2 Movement Levels for Mobilizing Massage Around the Cervical Spine

The name "Movement Levels for Mobilizing Massage Around the Cervical Spine" describes the sites for the mobilizing massage.

■ Goal of the Exercise

The goal is for the therapist to:
- Improve circulation, elasticity and contractility of the muscles in the region of the cervical spine and normalize their tone by mobilizing massage

294

- Facilitate the interaction between the head, potentially mobile in the atlanto-occipital and atlanto-axial joints and the joints of the cervical spine, and the thoracic spine, dynamically stabilized in its neutral position, and help the patient to understand how these work together
- Facilitate the interaction between the head, potentially mobile in the atlanto-occipital and atlanto-axial joints and the joints of the cervical spine, and the shoulder girdle, anchored by muscles to the stabilized thorax and to the potentially mobile atlanto-occipital and atlanto-axial joints and joints of the cervical spine, and help the patient to understand how these work together

▶ Functional Analysis in Therapist Language

As described above, mobilizing massage of the region of the cervical spine treats BS head, the adjacent BS thorax and, to a certain extent, BS arms. The movement levels concerned are:
- Cervical spine/upper thoracic spine, cervical spine/atlanto-occipital and atlanto-axial joints
- Cervical spine/shoulder girdle

Mobilizing massage in the cervical spine region presents special functional problems.

The transition between the lower cervical spine and the upper thoracic spine is a border between very mobile and much less mobile motion segments. It is practical to have less mobility in the upper thoracic spine because it has to carry the upper three pairs of ribs. However, cervical kyphosis, which is very common, extends this less mobile part cranially, and the low mobility soon becomes partial stiffness. The lordotic curvature begins usually at motion segment C5. Here we frequently see ventral slippage of the head from C5 onto C6.

The transition midcervical spine/atlanto-occipital and atlanto-axial joints (axis, atlas, occiput being part of the rigid skull) has the functional peculiarity that the atlanto-occipital and atlanto-axial joints often act as active buttresses to the rest of the cervical spine. This happens, for instance, when the gaze has to be kept horizontal.

Comparing the transition between the lower lumbar spine and the pelvis to that between the atlanto-occipital and atlanto-axial joints and the skull, we can say that the sacrum is like a rigid wedge pushed by the spinal column into the pelvic ring, which possesses in the symphysis and the two iliosacral joints, with their minimal cushioning effect, three shock absorbers. During walking, a key role is played by the transmission of the leg movements from the very mobile hips via the not quite rigid pelvis to the spinal column with its virtual long axis aligned in the plane of symmetry (see Klein-Vogelbach 1991). Thus, the rigid unit pelvis–sacrum functions between the very mobile hip joints and the joints of the lumbar spine, and the intrinsically sprung pelvic ring is part of the substructure of the spinal column.

The case is different in the cervical region. Here, the rigid head balances freely over the substructure of the cervical spine, which is particularly mobile in its most cranial portions. Where the pelvis moderates the leg movements and transmits them to the spinal column, the task of the cervical spine is to moderate the movements of the head as it turns eyes, ears, mouth and nose in every possible direction. The following presentation of mobilizing massage treats together the movement levels cervical spine/upper thoracic spine and cervical spine/atlanto-occipital and atlanto-axial joints/head, respectively, as they are treated in practice during massage.

Movement Levels Cervical Spine/Upper Thoracic Spine, Cervical Spine/Atlanto-occipital and Atlanto-axial Joints
Head in Ventral/Dorsal Translation (Fig. 98 a–c)

We start with ventral/dorsal translation because these two movements have more often than any others to be functionally reestablished in order to facilitate lateroflexion in the vertebral joints. Even when lateroflexion causes pain, the therapist or the patient himself can usually manipulate ventral and dorsal translation painlessly. We will focus here on dorsal translation of cranial gliding body head in relation to caudal gliding body thorax, and ventral translation of caudal gliding body thorax in relation to cranial gliding body head. In other words, the head is translated dorsally in relation to the cervical spine which in turn is translated dorsally in relation to the thoracic spine. The thoracic spine is translated ventrally in relation to the cervical spine which in turn is translated ventrally in relation to the head.

Procedure
The therapist sits at the head end of a treatment bench on a stool the height of her lower legs. The treatment bench is high enough above the stool that the patient's head can rest on the therapist's thighs. The patient lies on his back with his knees bent. The edge of the treatment bench is about at the level of T5, T4 or T3, depending on the patient's physical condition and on the length of the therapist's thighs.

The therapist's thighs are in comfortable transverse abduction, so that her knees can support the part of the patient's thorax that protrudes over the edge. The therapist can adjust the height of her knees from the floor as needed by having her soles on the floor, or just her forefoot, or just her toes. Her hands support the patient's neck and back of the head from underneath while her thumbs act as a kind of lateral splint for the neck. If possible, the therapist takes the stress off her own neck by resting her elbows on her thighs.

Now the patient's head is raised, with extension in the atlanto-occipital and atlanto-axial joints and ventral translation in the rest of the cervical spine. This relaxes the extensors of the atlanto-occipital and atlanto-axial joints and the sternocleidomastoid, and they can be given mobilizing massage. Next, the head is brought downwards, the atlanto-occipital and atlanto-axial joints move in flexion, the cervical spine – and, by continuing movement, the upper thoracic spine – in dorsal translation. The therapist intensifies this dorsal translation by pulling the scalene muscles and the levator scapulae dorsally with her thumbs.

Attention can be concentrated on a single motion segment. This should always be done if two or more motion segments are translating dorsally en bloc. The

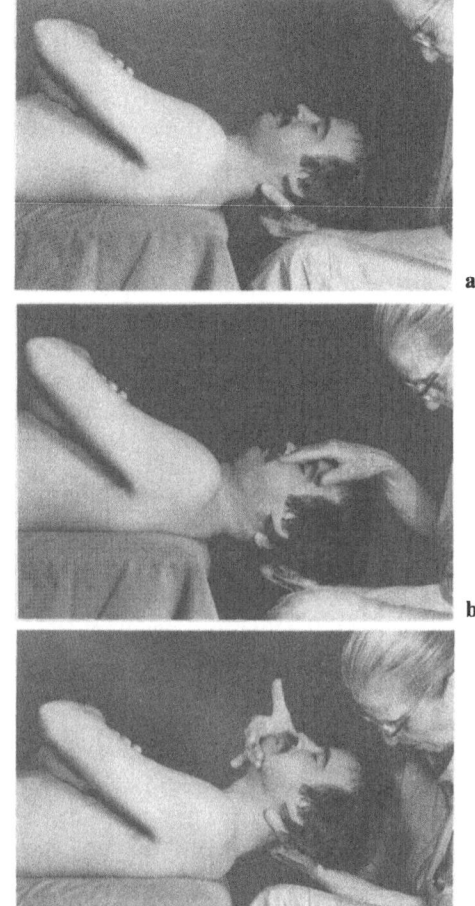

Fig. 98 a–c. Movement Level Upper Thoracic Spine/Cervical Spine/Atlanto-occipital and Atlanto-axial Joints. **a** Starting position, **b** Dorsal translation with flexion in the atlanto-occipital and atlanto-axial joints. **c** Ventral translation with extension in the atlanto-occipital and atlanto-axial joints

blocked segment is carefully mobilized during dorsal translation of the head by being fixed with ventral translational pressure. To do this, the therapist brings her legs together and places the patient's head on them, thus freeing both hands for massage. She must be careful that it is always the cranial hand that emphasizes the dorsal translation and the caudal hand that blocks it in the affected segment.

Movement Levels Cervical Spine/Upper Thoracic Spine, Cervical Spine/ Atlanto-occipital and Atlanto-axial Joints
Head in Translation to the Right/to the Left (Fig. 98 d–g)

Translation to the right/to the left, which takes place primarily in the vertebral–intervertebral disc articulations, is always to be recommended as a preliminary procedure in patients who have pain on flexion or extension of the vertebral joints.

297

Like dorsal/ventral translation, lateral translation helps in better alignment of the individual motion segments within the spinal segment concerned.

Procedure
The starting position is the same as that described above for dorsal/ventral translation. Starting with translation of the head to the right, the therapist begins by supporting the patient's head with one hand and pulling or pushing it to the right. As she does this, the atlanto-occipital and atlanto-axial joints move in left-concave lateroflexion and the head moves by right translation in the rest of the cervical spine. With her other hand the therapist keeps the patient's thorax in place by placing her hand in his axilla from above/right, as if she were pushing it to the left. To exhaust the tolerance for the same translation from the caudal end, by left translation of the thorax, the therapist shifts her knee with the patient's thorax on it to the left, holding the patient's head in place as if pushing it to the right. After practicing the movements, the version that provides the most extensive translation is chosen. If it is the head that is kept stationary during the massage, the therapist can exert light compression on the vertex by pressing against it with her stomach. When the thorax is now translated to the left, the muscles on the right side of the neck can be massaged. If it is the thorax that is kept in place, the therapist carefully wedges the patient's head between her thighs with a pillow. When the head is now translated to the right, the therapist again massages the muscles on the right side of the neck. For left translation of the head or right translation of the thorax, the sides are reversed accordingly.

Variation: The therapist sits with her right side against the head end of the treatment bench with the patient's head resting on her left thigh and his thorax on her right. By sliding her thighs parallel in opposite directions, with transverse abduction of one and adduction of the other in the hip joints, the therapist is able to translate both gliding bodies, thorax and head, to the right/left. This manipulation can also move just one of the gliding bodies while the other remains stationary.

Movement Levels Cervical Spine/Upper Thoracic Spine, Cervical Spine/ Atlanto-occipital and Atlanto-axial Joints Head in Distraction, Approximation, Rotation

Distraction or, less frequently, approximation is the preliminary to mobilizing massage for rotation. Compression to the cervical spine applied at the vertex should only be used if it reduces tone in all of the cervical muscles; i.e. BS head must be aligned in the long axis of the body, at least in relation to BS thorax.

Procedure
The starting position is the same as that described above for dorsal/ventral translation. To start with manual *distraction,* first the head is translated slightly dorsally. The patient can wrap his arms around the therapist's neck if that seems comfortable; it has the advantage of relaxing some of the muscles of the shoulder girdle in-

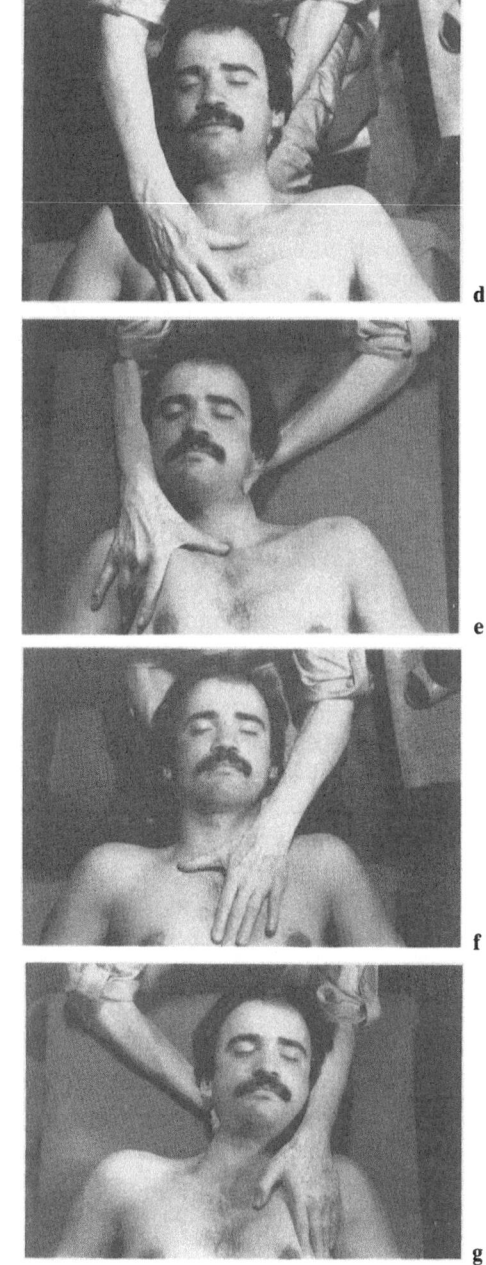

Fig. 98 d–g. Movement Level Upper Thoracic Spine/Cervical Spine/Atlanto-occipital and Atlanto-axial Joints. **d** Starting position for translation to the right. **e** Translation to the right by pushing. **f** Starting position for translation to the left. **g** Translation to the left by pushing

serting at the cervical spine (descending trapezius) or at least of loosening them up (levator scapulae). For distraction, both of the therapist's hands are under the back of the patient's head and neck. In pulling on the patient's head, the therapist seeks a hold on the patient's right/left mastoid process. If distraction is combined with prolonged expiration, it also arises caudally. Inspiration is effected by slowly relaxing the muscles of expiration (see Slow Motion Breathing, p. 146) and by compression applied at the vertex.

If the therapist wishes to keep dorsal translation and flexion in the atlanto-occipital and atlanto-axial joints well under control during distraction, she grasps the left and right zygomatic arches from above with one hand. No hold caudal to the lower jaw can be recommended for applying traction, since, first, this presses the teeth too hard against each other and, secondly, the lower jaw can be pushed out of position. If traction is to be applied only to the cervical spine, it is advisable to first slide C7 ventrally and then exert countertraction with the other hand at C7, pulling caudally. Distraction and approximation are performed alternately.

If *rotation* causes pain, we simply do not perform it at all at the start, or only very small movement excursions. Starting cranially with rotation body head, this must rest on the therapist's thighs or the treatment bench properly aligned in the long axis of the cervical and the upper thoracic spine. To make sure that there is no unwanted ventral translation when the head rotates, the therapist places one hand under the back of the patient's head and pulls it left when the head moves in head-positive rotation and right when the head moves in head-negative rotation. During the manipulated rotation, her other hand is free to massage the muscles of the front and back of the neck and the upper thoracic spine. If one wishes to manipulate rotation in the atlanto-occipital and atlanto-axial joints alone, the rest of the cervical spine is flexed out of the virtual long axis of the body. Now the head can be rotated positively and negatively in the atlanto-occipital and atlanto-axial joints without the rotation continuing caudally. If, on the other hand, one wishes to cut out the atlanto-occipital and atlanto-axial joints as far as possible, the hand that is rotating the head positively and negatively grasps the cervical spine caudally, blocks the atlanto-occipital and atlanto-axial joints, and permits rotation to start only at C3 or lower. In this way practically every motion segment can be attended to individually, and the mobilizing massage will accordingly have different effects.

To manipulate rotation in the cervical spine from caudally, there are two possibilities. The first requires an assistant. The patient lies on the table such that the thorax is no longer supported. His arms are laid out of the way on his thorax. His weight is borne by the assistant and his head lies on the therapist's thighs. To rotate the thorax positively in the cervical spine, the assistant turns the right side of the patient's thorax dorsally/medially and the left side ventrally/medially. The head stays where it is. This rotation of the thorax can again be limited to a particular level, while the mobilizing massage is performed.

In the second variant the patient must help. Thorax and head are lying on the treatment bench. By pressure activity of his elbows and head, the patient takes the weight off his thorax, which the therapist can then rotate around the long axis of the body. For this variant the headrest can be elevated to about 35°.

Movement Levels Cervical Spine/Upper Thoracic Spine, Cervical Spine/ Atlanto-occipital and Atlanto-axial Joints
Flexion/Extension (Fig. 98 h–j)

In almost all patients with a cervical syndrome, the flexion-/extensionally neutral position of the cervical spine has deviated from the normal neutral position of this potentially mobile lordotic segment of the spine. This may be due to an overall increase or decrease in the lordotic curvature or, which is more frequently the case in cervical syndromes, individual segments may be malaligned or one or more segments blocked. By first using lateral translational mobilizing massage we have already attempted to reduce blockages, and by using distraction and approximation, slight rotation, and dorsal/ventral translation we have tried to normalize as far as possible the position and movement of the cervical spine in the plane of symmetry, so that we can perform mobilizing massage during flexional and extensional movements of the vertebral joints.

Procedure

The patient is well positioned on his back on a treatment bench. His elbows should be somewhat higher than his shoulders. His hands are folded over his upper abdomen. The therapist sits at the head end of the treatment bench such that she can support her elbows on it or against her own body when pushing her hands, palms up, under the back of the patient's neck until the left side of the fingertips of her right hand and the right side of the fingertips of her left hand touch his neck in the region of T3–C7. With her wrists dorsiflexed, she pushes upwards with her fingertips and tells the patient not to resist the pressure. The cervicothoracic transition is deformed into extension. As she releases the pressure, the manipulated spinal

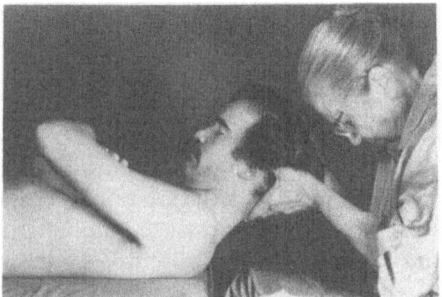

Fig. 98 h, i. Movement Level Upper Thoracic Spine/Cervical Spine/Atlanto-occipital and Atlanto-axial Joints. **h** Flexion, **i** extension

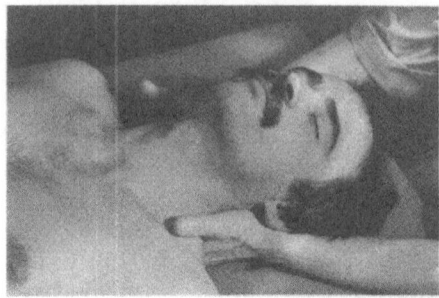

Fig. 98 j. Movement Level Upper Thoracic Spine/Lower Cervical Spine. Position of the Therapist's hands for treating cervical kyphosis

region flexes. This pressing and releasing is repeated in rhythm, the patient taking a slightly active part in the movement. During extension, the relaxed levator scapulae and the deep extensor muscles of the back of the neck are massaged (Fig. 98 j). Mobilization in the middle of the cervical spine is performed in a similar fashion. To mobilize the atlanto-occipital and atlanto-axial joints, the therapist places one hand on the patient's forehead and pushes the other under his cervico-occipital transition. With the hand on the forehead she manipulates little nodding movements, in which the patient also takes part, and performs mobilizing massage when the atlanto-occipital and atlanto-axial joints are extended. It is also possible to put both hands under the patient's neck and massage with the balls of the thumbs.

Movement Levels Cervical Spine/Upper Thoracic Spine, Cervical Spine/Atlanto-occipital and Atlanto-axial Joints
Lateroflexion

The neutral position in relation to lateroflexion means that there is no malalignment in the frontal plane. However, scoliotic postures and structural scoliosis are frequent in the cervicothoracic transition. By first using ventral and dorsal translational mobilizing massage, we have already attempted to reduce blockages, and by distraction, slight rotation and lateral translation of the cervical spine we have tried to realign the cervical spine symmetrically so that we can perform mobilizing massage on it, particularly on the concave side, during lateroflexional movements.

Procedure
The patient lies on his back with his elbows somewhat higher than his shoulders, hands crossed over his chest. The therapist sits at the head end of the treatment bench, supporting her elbows on it and keeping her own spinal column in roughly neutral position. Approaching from cranially, she grasps the back of the patient's neck in both hands, with her thumbs at about the level of the levator scapulae and the fingers lying ventrally on top of the upper thorax. By alternating pressure to the right and to the left, she causes the cervicothoracic transition to deform into lateroflexion, C7 being displaced laterally the farthest. The relaxed muscles on the concave side are massaged.

If the therapist slides her hands somewhat cranially, so that it is about C4 that is laterally displaced the farthest, one hand lies under the back of the patient's head and includes it in the movement while the other shifts the lateroflexional deformation of the cervicothoracic transition more cranially or more caudally, as necessary.

The small lateral movements in the atlanto-occipital and atlanto-axial joints are manipulated by the therapist as very small movements, accompanying them with mobilizing massage.

If particular attention is to be paid to the upper trapezius, one or both of the patient's arms are placed in the Little Shepherd Boy position (see p. 257). To massage the right side of the neck, the right arm is positioned as in the Little Shepherd Boy. The therapist grasps the right pincer jaws from the side and simultaneously with her right elbow presses the patient's right arm against his head. Her left hand slides under from the left to the right side of the patient's neck, pulls the cervical spine at about the level of C4 in right-concave lateroflexion to the left, and carries out mobilizing massage on the right side of the neck.

Movement Level Cervical Spine/Shoulder Girdle

The important muscles of the shoulder girdle inserting at the cervical spine are:
- Descending trapezius, originating on the occipital protuberance, at the upper third of the nuchal line, the nuchal ligament and on the spinal process of C7 and inserting on the lateral third of the clavicle and the acromion.
- Levator scapulae, originating on the transverse processes of the four upper cervical vertebrae and inserting on the medial margin of the scapula between the upper scapular angle and the scapular spine. These two muscles are antagonists: when the one fully contracts, the other is stretched.
- Rhomboids minor, originating at the nuchal ligament and the spinal processes of C7 and T1 and inserting on the medial margin of the scapula at the scapular spine.
- Sternocleidomastoid, originating on the manubrium sterni and the medial third of the clavicle and inserting on the mastoid process at the upper nuchal line and on the occiput. Inappropriate stress on these muscles plays a substantial role in cervical syndromes in, for instance, secretaries; it is revealed on examination by tenderness to pressure at the sites of origin and insertion, and also by ischaemic pain.

Procedure

The patient lies on his back. In order particularly to give mobilizing massage to the origin of the right upper trapezius, we place the patient's right arm in the Little Shepherd Boy position (see p. 257). With her right hand on the lateral margin of the scapula, the therapist pushes the acromion as close as possible to the right occipital protuberance, exerting particular pressure on the humeroscapular joint with the ball of her thumb. Then she slides her left hand, palm up, under the patient's neck from the left, manipulates little lateroflexional movements in the atlanto-occipital and atlanto-axial joints, and simultaneously massages the area of the origin of the upper trapezius. As her left hand approaches C7, she lateroflexes the cervical spine by pushing C7 laterally. Throughout the entire procedure the therapist continues to grip the patient's shoulder girdle and neck in a constantly adjusting clamp hold.

To massage the right levator scapulae and the right rhomboids minor, the patient is positioned on his left side. The therapist sits behind him and slides her left hand under the left side of his head, lifting it in right-concave lateroflexion and head-positive rotation. Simultaneously, with the ball of her right thumb on the scapular spine, she pushes the upper scapular angle cranially/ventrally/slightly laterally and the right scapula rotates positively. The manipulation of the head and the displacement of the scapula must be well coordinated so that the therapist can massage the insertion of the muscles with the fingers of her right hand and the origin with the thumb of her left.

For mobilizing massage of the right sternocleidomastoid, the patient is positioned on his back. The therapist sits at the head end of the treatment bench. She slides her right hand, palm up, under the back of the patient's head and, pulling it to the right, rotates the head negatively and lifts it in right-concave lateroflexion. Now she can massage the entire course of the muscle as well as its origin and insertion with her left hand.

5.5.3 Dizzy (Figs. 99–101)

The name "Dizzy" refers to the problem to be solved. The exercise was given this name when it helped a patient find relief from troublesome vertigo.

■ Goal of the Exercise

The goal is for the patient to learn to
- Stimulate local circulation in the region of the inner ear to relieve vestibular vertigo (Ear Pulling),
- Stimulate local circulation in the cervical region to relieve vertigo of vertebral origin (Neck Fist).

► Functional Analysis in Therapist Language

● Conception of the Exercise

This method of improving local circulation in the inner ear by pulling the auricle in the line of the eustachian tube, away from the uvula, as it were, was happened upon purely by chance. An attempt to alleviate otitis by stimulating the circulation of the inner ear led via a number of experiments to the observation that this can in fact be achieved by pulling on the ears in a particular way, and that this is something the patient can perform himself. A series of practical experiments with otosclerotic patients nevertheless proved unsuccessful – but one patient noticed that, while his hearing did not improve, his constant vertigo had disappeared. Since that time I have continued to use this simple exercise for patients suffering from vertigo unrelated to blood pressure, with varied success.

While performing Dizzy we can also improve circulation in the back of the neck by Neck Fist. The patient starts by stretching the muscles of the back of his neck by himself manipulating his cervical spine into maximum flexion. The stretched extensors are then actively contracted in maximum extension of the cervical spine. The shoulder girdle is also pulled up and back, contracting the levator scapulae, the descending trapezius and the upper rhomboids. After a slow and careful release of the muscle contraction, powerful isometric resistance by the flexors of the cervical spine causes the extensors to further relax reflexively.

● **Position and Activation in the Starting Position**

There is no particular starting position for Dizzy. It can be performed any time, sitting, lying down, walking or standing. Only one condition ought to be fulfilled: BSs pelvis, thorax and head should be aligned in the long axis of the body.

● **Actio – Reactio of the Movement Sequence**

The movement sequences in Dizzy are small and restricted to BSs thorax, head and arms. There are no significant horizontal displacements of weight. For this reason, spontaneous equilibrium reactions in the form of activated passive buttressing and/or change to the support area are not anticipated. The therapeutic objective is therefore achieved by fulfilling the conditio.

Ear Pulling (Fig. 99)

In Ear Pulling to stimulate circulation in the inner ear in cases of vestibular vertigo, the actio consists of a preliminary and a main primary movement.

The critical distance points of the preliminary primary movement, DPs tips of the index fingers and thumbs of the right and left hands, move symmetrically upwards/slightly backwards such that the right index finger reaches into the right ear and the left into the left ear and the thumbs come up from behind, so that the auricle can be gripped between them as if by a pair of pliers, as close to the skull as possible. By continuing movement, the wrists have extended by fulcrum displacement, the forearms have supinated, the elbows flexed by fulcrum displacement and the arms abducted and externally rotated in the humeroscapular joints, while the clavicles have dorsally rotated in the sternoclavicular joints (critical fulcra).

The critical distance points of the main primary movement, DPs right and left olecranons, move symmetrically laterally/backwards/upwards by abduction and slight flexion in the shoulder joints. By proximally continuing movement, the distal distance points of the sternoclavicular joints, DP acromions, move backwards/upwards, causing the medial scapular margins to approach the spinal pro-

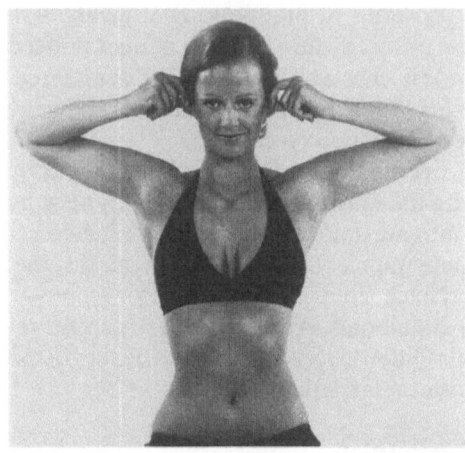

Fig. 99. Ear Pulling

cesses of the thoracic spine. By distally continuing movement, the auricles, held in a clamping grip, are flapped out from the head like jug-ears and firmly pulled backwards/outwards/upwards.

Neck Fist

The actio in Neck Fist has three phases.

Phase 1: Stretching the Extensor Muscles of the Back of the Neck (Fig. 100)
From the starting position of upright sitting on a stool, the critical distance point of the first primary movement, DP clasped hands, moves upwards/backwards with flexion in the wrists, supination of the forearms, and flexion and external rotation of the arms in the humeroscapular joints, and comes to rest with the palms on the occiput. Simultaneously, the critical distance point of the second primary movement, DP tip of the nose, has moved downwards with flexion in the atlanto-occipital and atlanto-axial joints, and the cervical and upper thoracic spines have flexed in a cranial-to-caudal continuing movement. DP occiput has thus moved forwards/upwards, so that the arms are brought into hanging activity, pulling the head downwards and stretching the extensor muscles of the back of the neck.
The critical distance point of the activated passive buttressing, DP C7, has moved backwards, with flexion in the cervical and upper thoracic spines by fulcrum displacement.
DPs right and left iliac spines are absolute fixed spatial points. They ensure that the stretching of the spinal extensors is limited to those of the cervical and upper thoracic regions.

Special Variant for the Atlanto-occipital and Atlanto-axial Joints: Of the two critical distance points of the primary movement, DPs right and left palm, one moves upwards with the thumb extended so that the thumb and index finger firmly touch the zygomatic arches while other moves backwards/laterally/upwards until the

306

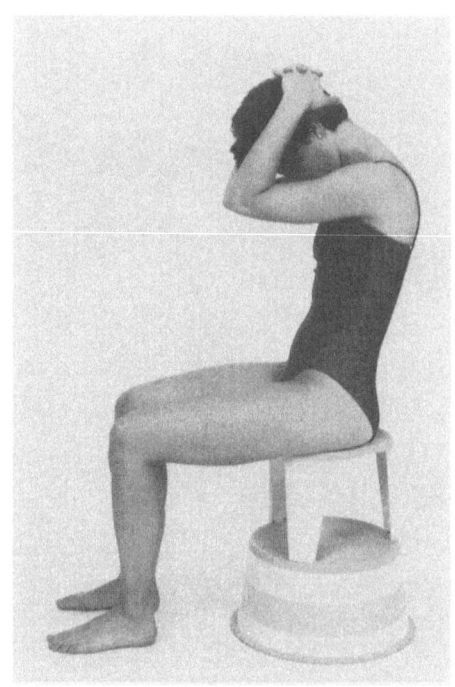

Fig. 100. Neck Fist: stretching the muscles at the back of the neck

palm is firmly on the occiput. In a nearly circular spiral with its centre roughly in the middle of the cervical spine, the one hand pulls the zygomatic arches downwards/first forwards, then backwards, while the other hand pushes the occiput upwards/slightly forwards. The resulting continuing movement flexes the atlanto-occipital and atlanto-axial joints and the cervical spine.

Phase 2: Maximum Contraction of the Muscles of the Back of the Neck
(Fig. 101 a, b)
From the end position of the stretch phase, the thumb or little finger of the right hand moves to the right acromion and that of the left hand to the left acromion.
The critical distance points of the primary movement of the contraction phase, DPs right and left olecranons, move upwards (cranially)/laterally/backwards (dorsally) by flexion, abduction and internal rotation in the humeroscapular joints. By continuing movement, DPs right and left acromions with the thumbs or little fingers touching them move upwards (cranially)/medially/slightly backwards (dorsally). Simultaneously, the critical distance point of the primary movement of the head, DP vertex, has moved in a nearly circular path backwards (dorsally)/first upwards, (cranially), then downwards (caudally), with extension in the atlanto-occipital and atlanto-axial joints and cervical and thoracic spine by continuing movement.

Phase 3: Reflexive Relaxation of the Extensor Muscles of the Back of the Neck
(Fig. 101 c)
By slow relaxation of the extensor muscles in the back of the neck and the muscles that elevate and retract the shoulder girdle, the head returns to its neutral position.

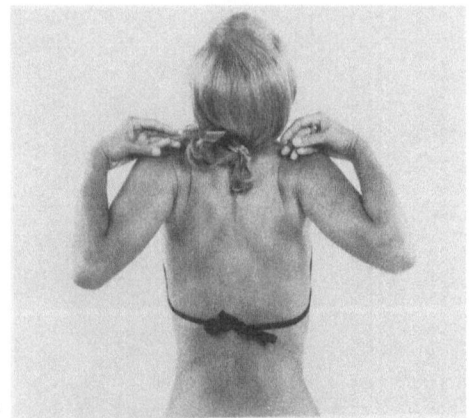

a

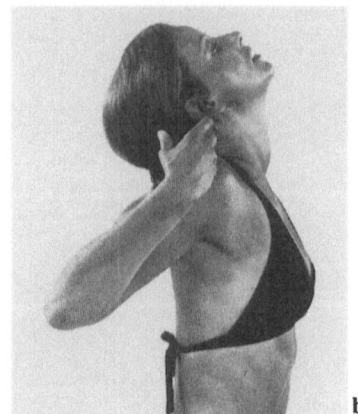

b

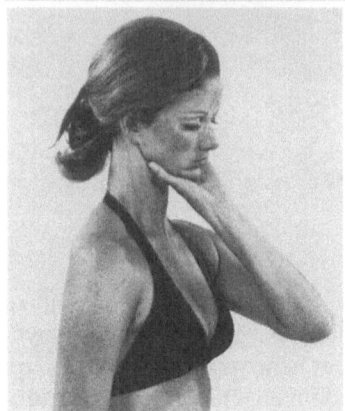

c

Fig. 101 a, b. Neck Fist: maximal contraction of the muscles at the back of the neck. **c** Reflexive relaxation of the extensor muscles at the back of the neck

At the same time, either or both palms, facing upwards by pronation and with the thumb extended, grasp the lower jaw.

The critical distance point of the primary movement, DP point of contact palm/caudal aspect of the lower jaw, is pulled forwards (ventrally) by the activity of the hands and simultaneously pressed upwards (cranially). The wrists go into extension by displacement of the fulcrum, the forearms into pronation effected by the distal pointer, the elbows into extension by continuing movement, the humeroscapular joints into flexion/adduction, the sternoclavicular joints into dorsal rotation, and the thoracic spine is flexionally activated from cranially (critical fulcrum without movement excursion, only cranially-arising activation of the rectus abdominis muscle).

● **Conditio – Limitatio of the Movement Sequence**

Conditio: Constant Distances Between Body Distance Points
Limitatio: Active Buttressing and Stabilization
In Dizzy the following distances are kept constant:

Ear Pulling

Conditio: The distance between DP tip of the chin and DP jugular notch remains constant.

Limitatio: This ensures that, during the primary movement of the preliminary phase of Ear Pulling, when the index-finger-thumb pliers grasp the auricle, the natural extensional movement of the head in the atlanto-occipital and atlanto-axial joints is actively buttressed flexionally. During the main primary movement in Ear Pulling, the tendency to react to the pull upwards/backwards with ventral translation of the head is turned into ventral-translational active buttressing. These two active buttressings keep the cervical spine in its neutral position and ensure that the direction of the pull on the ears is optimally directed to the inner ear.

Conditio: The distance between DP navel and DP xiphoid process remains constant during the main primary movement of Ear Pulling.

Limitatio: To keep this distance constant, the continuing movement of flexional deformation of the thoracic spine in reaction to the pull on the ears must be turned into active buttressing. The pull on the ears can have its best effect only if active resistance has set up in the straight abdominal muscles.

Variant of Phase 1

Conditio: The distance between DP navel and DP xiphoid process remains constant during the stretching of the muscles of the back of the neck.

Limitatio: To keep this distance constant, the thoracic spine must be further extensionally stabilized in its neutral position, so that when the cervical spine is manipulated into flexion to stretch its extensors, the intended effect of the stretch on the cervical spine muscles is not dissipated by an unwanted continuing movement flexing the thoracic spine cranial-to-caudally as well.

Phase 2

Conditio: The distance between DP symphysis and DP navel remains constant during the maximum contraction of the muscles of the back of the neck.

Limitatio: To keep this distance constant, the lumbar spine must be actively buttressed flexionally and the hip joints extensionally. If extension is restricted in the upper thoracic spine, the extension in the atlanto-occipital and atlanto-axial joints and cervical spine initiated by DP vertex will cause, by an unwanted continuing movement, flexion of the pelvis in the hip joints and extension of the lumbar and thoracic spine coming from caudally. The cranially arising extension of the upper thoracic spine and contraction of the muscles of the shoulder girdle inserting on the cervical spine by raising and retracting the shuolder girdle will not then take place in the maximally effective way that we are striving for.

Phase 3

Conditio: The distance between DP C7 and DP T12 remains constant during the reflexive relaxation of the muscles of the back of the neck.

Limitatio: To keep this distance constant, the extensional activity of the thoracic spine in its neutral position must be increased. This extensional stabilization of the thoracic spine should be seen as active buttressing of the tendency of the pelvis to extend in the hip joints, bringing total flexion of the lumbar and thoracic spine, an unwanted continuing movement which otherwise would be triggered by the hands on the lower jaw resisting the flexion in the atlanto-occipital and atlanto-axial joints and the cervical spine. Only if the continuing flexional movement is transformed into flexional activation without any movement excursion is perfect reflexive relaxation of the extensor muscles of the back of the neck and the shoulder girdle possible.

Conditio of Absolute and/or Relative Fixed Spatial Points
Limitatio by Limiting the Primary Movement, Activated Passive Buttressing and/or Change in the Support Area
In Dizzy there are absolute and relative fixed spatial points.

Conditio: In Ear Pulling, the head is an absolute fixed spatial point.
Limitatio: This absolute fixed point will be maintained if the pliers formed by the index fingers and thumbs are closed on the right and left auricle with a steadily increasing pull. Only then are the ears truly pulled away from the head rather than the head from the ears, and the feeling of intense warmth in the inner ear arises, signalling unmistakably that the circulation has been stimulated.

Variant of Phase 1
Conditio: The points of contact thumb, 2nd, 3rd and 4th fingers of one hand/skull caudal to the zygomatic arches and palm of the other hand/occiput are relative fixed spatial points during the stretching of the muscles of the back of the neck.
Limitatio: Not being allowed to shift these points of contact guarantees that the pulling of the one hand on the occiput and the pushing of the other on the zygomatic arches acts directly and precisely to cause flexion in the atlanto-occipital and atlanto-axial joints and cervical spine, rather than merely causing tissue to slip around on its bony underlay.

Phase 2
Conditio: The points of contact DP right thumb or little finger/DP right acromion and DP left thumb or little finger/DP left acromion are relative fixed spatial points during the contraction of the muscles of the back of the neck.
Limitatio: These relative fixed points facilitate the contraction of the muscles of the back of the neck and of the shoulder girdle by the continuing movement of DPs right and left acromions.

Phase 3
Conditio: The point of contact palm/caudal aspect of the lower jaw is an absolute fixed spatial point during the reflexive relaxation of the muscles of the back of the neck.
Limitatio: This absolute fixed spatial point ensures spontaneous reflexive relaxation of the extensor muscles of the neck and the muscles of the shoulder girdle inserting on the cervical spine, because it means that, with the hand or hands pulling and pressing on the lower jaw at the precise moment when BS head has returned to its neutral position after the contraction of the muscles of the back of the neck, there is

310

no extensional recoil in the atlanto-occipital and atlanto-axial joints, which would destroy the reflexive relaxation of the antagonistic muscles that we are aiming for.

Conditio of Movement Speed
Limitatio of Economical Activity by Finding the Optimal Speed
Conditio: The speed in Ears Pulling is slow. The preliminary movement takes about 8 seconds, the pulling of the ears about 5 seconds, and the holding of the ears in this position another 3 seconds.
Limitatio: The intensity of economical activity in the target area is high and increasing. The same is true of the cutting in of the active buttressings. The patient should nevertheless continue to breathe normally and slowly.

Conditio: The speed in Neck Fist during the stretching and maximum contraction of the extensor muscles of the neck is slow: 5 seconds for the movements and 5 seconds for holding each completed position. BS head takes 4 seconds to return to its neutral position for the reflexive relaxation of the extensor muscles of the neck. There is no movement when the hand starts to pull and press, but the position is held for about 5 seconds, until the patient can feel by the increase in the flow of saliva that the exercise has been successful.
Limitatio: The intensity of economical activity is also high in Neck Fist, but normal breathing should remain slow.

▶ Instruction in Patient Language

● Instruction Appealing to the Patient's Perception

When learning Dizzy, the patient can easily monitor whether what he is doing is having the proper effect. In Ear Pulling, what he has to wait for is the unmistakeable feeling of warmth in the region of the inner ear; in Neck Fist it is the increased salivary flow that signals success. In the maximum contraction of the muscles of the back of the neck and those of the shoulder girdle which insert on the neck, the feeling of warmth will not appear until the exercise has been repeated a few times. The patient should keep his mouth open during the exercise, touching his lower teeth with his tongue and breathing through his nose.

● Verbal Instruction ● Instruction by Manipulation

Actio and Conditio of the Movement Sequence (Phases 2 and 3)

"Put your right index finger in your right ear and your left index finger in your left ear. Your thumbs come up and grip the ears from outside. Really clamp that ear cartilage between your thumbs and index fingers. Now flap the

It is a good idea for the therapist to do the pulling on the patient's ears first until he can feel the inner ear get warm. It always does. The easiest way is to have the patient sitting on a chair in front of a mirror with the therapist

ears out so that they stick out at right angles to your head; make yourself jug ears. Now start to pull your ears outwards/backwards/upwards, slowly but steadily, away from your uvula, with your elbows moving backwards and upwards. It almost hurts. Then let go slowly and feel whether there isn't a fine but quite perceptible warmness in your inner ears. If there is, you did the exercise right and it worked. Do this twice every hour and every time you feel as if you are going to get dizzy again.

Now there's more. Bring your hands, lightly closed, up to your shoulders, and pull your shoulders up and backwards until your neck completely disappears. This will work fine if you look up, open your mouth, and pull your neck in until you almost get goose pimples on your back; you can give a big groan. Then release the tension very slowly, look straight ahead again and let your shoulders drop down onto your rib cage, but without letting your rib cage collapse – it has to absorb the weight of your shoulders.

Now push your hand, opened flat like a plate, under your chin with your thumb pointing out on one side and your fingers on the other. You try to pull your chin upwards and forwards, but it won't go, it doesn't budge from the spot."

standing behind him, so the patient can see how the ear pulling is being done. This manipulation of the ears is often helpful in cases of vestibular vertigo and should be done by the patient twice an hour and always at the slightest sign of vertigo.

To help the patient bring about really powerful contraction of his shoulder muscles and the muscles of the back of his neck, the therapist can at first apply massive manual resistance. Standing behind the sitting patient, with one hand she applies strong resistance to the extension of the head while with other she hangs onto the raised shoulders either side of C7 and pulls backwards and downwards.

The therapist instructs the patient and shows him how to apply resistance to the chin so that the ventral muscles of the neck have to work hard; the insertion of the sternocleidomastoid is visible and can be palpated as a check to see whether the muscles of the back of the neck have reflexively relaxed. These two types of resistance are repeated two to three times until the patient can feel the reactive warmth of the circulation in his neck and laryngeal region.

▶ Adapting the Exercise to the Patient's Constitution and Condition

It is unnecessary to adapt Dizzy for constitution.
As to condition, the only contraindication for the exercise is if the patient experiences pain while performing it.

5.5.4 Lockjaw (Figs. 102 and 103)

"Lockjaw" is a descriptive name. It indicates the problem to be remedied by this exercise.

■ Goal of the Exercise

The goal is for the patient to learn to move the temporomandibular joints freely and with precision in all directions.

▶ Functional Analysis in Therapist Language

● Conception of the Exercise

To be able to move the temporomandibular joints freely and precisely in all directions, we must first remember that we can distinguish between three types of jaw movements: movements of biting, grinding and gnawing (see *Functional Kinetics,* pp. 173–175). Normally these movements are initiated at the distal lever, the mandible. To functionally circumvent a mechanism which has become habitually faulty, however, we will play "upside-down world". We start by moving the proximal lever instead of the distal one; that is, we move the head but not the mandible and bite, grind and gnaw with head movements alone (although these are of course transmitted to the atlanto-occipital and atlanto-axial joints). Then we move the distal lever, but with the long axis of BS head turned through 180°, i.e. with the head down. When the distal lever of the temporomandibular joint, the mandible, bites, grinds and gnaws in this position, it does so against gravity.

● Position and Activation in the Starting Position

Our chosen starting position for Lockjaw is upright sitting. To get ready to mobilize the mandible from the proximal lever, BSs pelvis, thorax and head will first have to be aligned in the virtual long axis of the body, which is vertical. When the patient manipulates this himself, his fingers should grasp the right and left mandibular angles and fix them in position.

Turning the long axis of the head segment through 180° for the second form of the exercise is easy so long as the patient has good hip mobility and is sitting with legs straddled on a relatively high stool. The arms should hang down with the palms on the floor and BS head should hang down (Fig. 103). An alternative is for the patient to lie prone on a treatment bench with BSs pelvis, thorax and head hanging vertically with flexion of the pelvis in the hip joints (Fig. 58 a).

● Actio – Reactio of the Movement Sequence

In Lockjaw, the horizontal displacements of weight are so small that no reactio in the form of activated passive buttressing or change to the support area is anticipated.

Biting: Opening and closing the mouth (Fig. 102 a, b).
The critical distance point of the primary movement, DP tip of the nose, moves cranially/dorsally as the mouth opens; the atlanto-occipital and atlanto-axial joints and joints of the cervical spine extend, and the temporomandibular joints open, with the upper teeth moving cranially/dorsally away from the lower. As the mouth closes, DP tip of the nose moves ventrally/caudally, the atlanto-occipital and atlanto-axial joints and joints of the cervical spine flex, and the temporomandibular joints close, with the upper teeth moving ventrally/caudally towards the lower.

Grinding: The jaws slide right and left in relation to each other (Fig. 102 c, d). In grinding, the critical distance point of the primary movement, DP tip of the nose, moves laterally to the right/dorsally. The movement is one of head-positive rotation in the atlanto-occipital and atlanto-axial joints and joints of the cervical spine, and laterotranslation in the temporomandibular joints. The right upper teeth slide

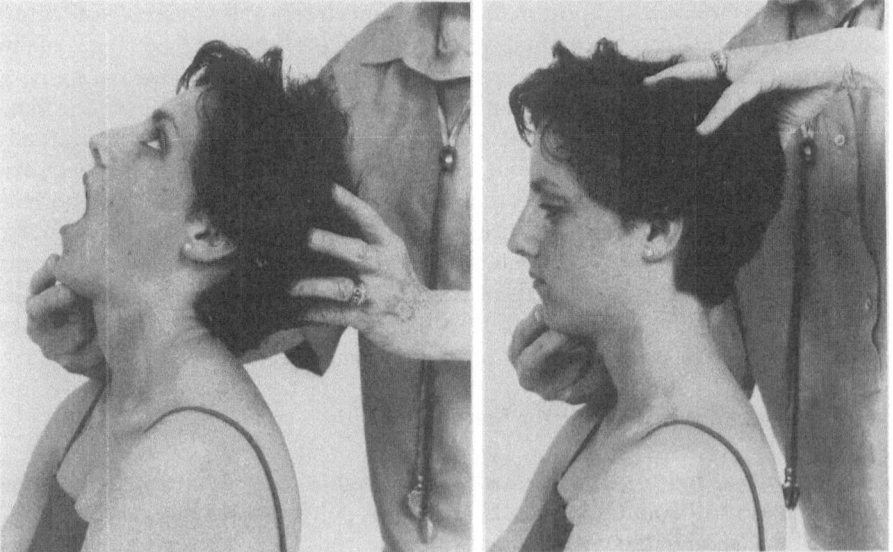

a   b

Fig. 102 a–f. Lockjaw. It is always the proximal lever that moves. **a, b** Opening and closing the mouth

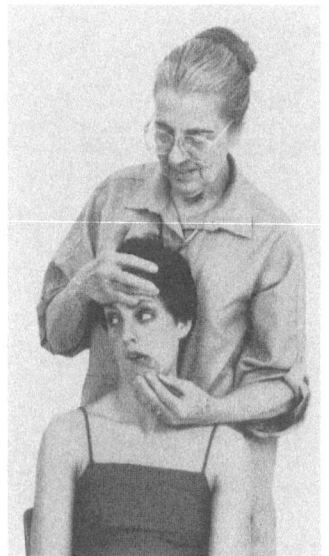
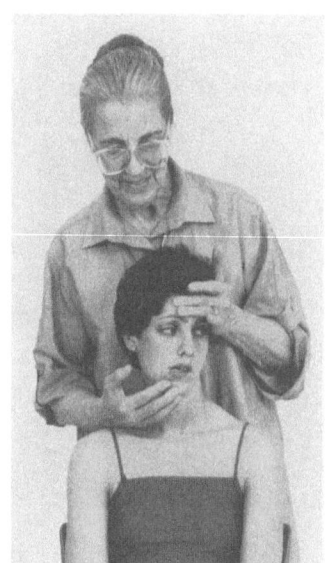

c   d

Fig. 102 a–f. Lockjaw. **c, d** Grinding movement to right and left

laterally/to the right of the lower and the left upper teeth medially/to the right of
the lower. (The opposite applies for a movement to the other side.)

Gnawing: The jaws slide ventrally and dorsally in relation to each other (Fig. 102 e,
f). In gnawing, the critical distance point of the primary movement, DP tip of the
nose, moves dorsally. The movement is one of dorsal translation in the cervical
spine and translation in the temporomandibular joints, with the upper teeth sliding
dorsally in relation to the lower. In the ventral gnawing movement, DP tip of the
nose moves ventrally by ventral translation of the cervical spine and translation in
the temporomandibular joints, with the upper teeth moving ventrally to the lower.

● **Conditio – Limitatio of the Movement Sequence**

Conditio: Constant Distances Between Body Distance Points
Limitatio: Active Buttressing and Stabilization
Conditio: In *biting* effected by the proximal lever, the distance between DP navel
and DP xiphoid process remains constant.
Limitatio: If this distance is kept constant, the thoracic spine is stabilized in its neutral position in active buttressing. This active buttressing is flexional when the
mouth opens and extensional when the mouth closes.

Conditio: In *grinding* effected by the proximal lever, the distance between the line
connecting the right and left zygomatic arches and the transverse plane through
the sternoclavicular joints stays the same.
Limitatio: If this distance is kept constant, flexion, extension and lateroflexion in
the atlanto-occipital and atlanto-axial joints and in the cervical spine are actively

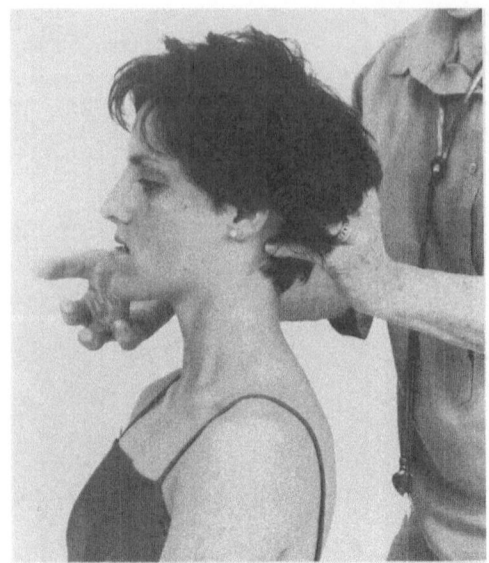

e

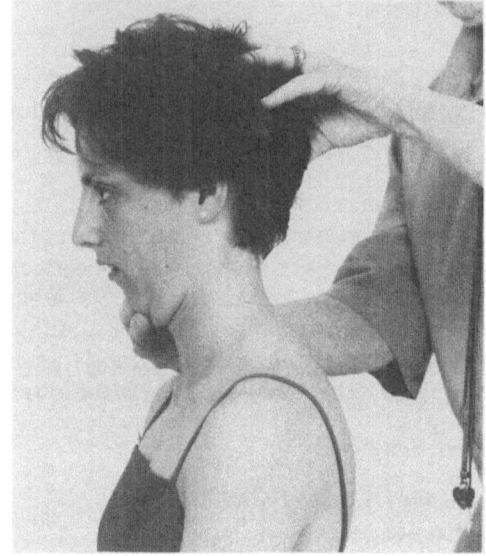

f

Fig. 102 e, f. Dorsal and ventral gnawing movement

buttressed and the laterotranslational grinding movements in the temporoman-dibular joints will not be circumvented by avoidance mechanisms.

Conditio: In *gnawing* effected by the proximal lever, the distance between DP navel and DP xiphoid process remains constant.
Limitatio: This causes the thorax to actively buttress the dorsal translation of the head ventral translationally and the ventral translation of the head dorsal transla-tionally.

316

Conditio of Absolute and/or Relative Fixed Spatial Points
Limitatio by Limiting the Primary Movement, Activated Passive Buttressing and/or Change in the Support Area
Conditio: DP mandibular angle and the fingertips holding it constitute an absolute fixed spatial point when the mouth opens and closes and in grinding and gnawing movements effected by the proximal lever of the temporomandibular joints.
Limitatio: To keep this point fixed, the mandible must, during opening of the mouth, be actively buttressed by activation as if for opening by the distal lever; during closing it must be actively buttressed by activation as if for closing by the distal lever. In grinding movements to the right, the mandible must be actively buttressed by activation as if for a grinding movement to the left by the distal gliding body, and vice versa when the sides are reversed. In dorsal translational gnawing it must be actively buttressed by activation as if for ventral translation of the distal lever, and vice versa if the sides are reversed.

Conditio of Movement Speed
Limitatio of Economical Activity by Finding the Optimal Speed
Conditio: The movement speed is slow and the intensity of economical activity very low. The patient breathes in and out through his nose and must not hold his breath.
Limitatio: These very precise and unfamiliar movements of the temporomandibular joints must be performed slowly and at low intensity because the body is having to learn to movement that it doesn't need in normal motor behaviour, but which for that very reason can loosen up a habitual blockage.

▶ Adapting the Exercise to the Patient's Constitution and Condition

This exercise does not need adaptation.

Mobilization of the Temporomandibular Joints Effected by the Distal Lever with the Long Axis of the Head Turned Through 180° (Figs. 58a, 103).
As long as the patient is able to assume the starting position, he will have no problem with the actio and conditio. The critical distance point of the primary movement is the tip of the chin. The patient is familiar with the movements of the mandible. No conditio need be fulfilled, as the movement is effected by the distal lever and no continuing movement takes place. If the patient finds it easy to assume the starting position, these movements of the mandible should be performed as often as possible to the prescribed extent, particularly the opening of the mouth, which in this position must be performed against gravity. This makes the eccentric isotonic work of the masseter muscle in opening and its concentric isotonic work in closing superfluous.

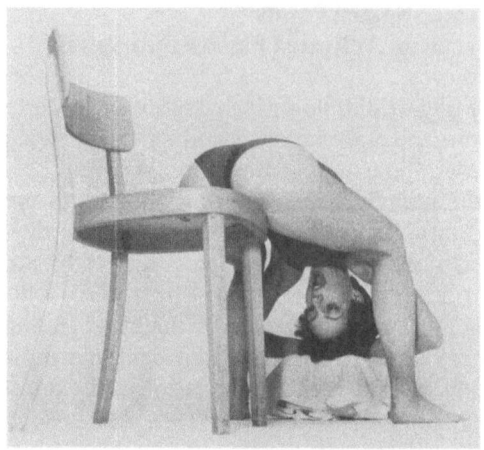

Fig. 103. Lockjaw. Opening the mouth with the long axis of the body inverted 180°

5.5.5 The Cork (Fig. 104)

The name "The Cork" refers to the aid used in this exercise.

■ Goal of the Exercise

The goal is for the patient to learn to alleviate symptoms of cervical syndromes in the region of the larynx, pharynx and the ear by moving the tongue.

▶ Functional Analysis in Therapist Language

● Conception of the Exercise

When training movements of the tongue, we first start with extreme exaggeration of normal tongue movement. For this we choose sticking out the tongue ventrally/caudally, then moving it laterally to the right and left, while saying "ah" and "eh" to tense the soft palate. After this warm-up exercise, we will train the tongue movements of articulation by wedging a cork between the patient's upper and lower teeth and having him speak.

● Position and Activation in the Starting Position

The starting position can be any position. It is best to start with the patient sitting upright; later on he can walk around.

- **Actio – Reactio of the Movement Sequence**

In the Cork, the horizontal displacements of weight are so small that no reactio in the form of activated passive buttressing and/or change to the support area is anticipated.

Warm-Up Training for the Tongue (Fig. 104a): Sitting properly upright, the patient vocalizes on any vowel at a comfortable speaking pitch. The critical distance point of the primary mvoement, DP tip of the tongue, moves ventrally (forwards)/caudally (downwards). As it does, DP tip of the chin moves caudally (downwards)/dorsally(backwards), opening the lower jaw. Continuing to vocalize, the patient changes initial vowel to "eh", and the soft palate responds by tensing. Then the tongue returns to where was during the initial vowel. This to-and-fro movement can be repeated ad libitum, with varying initial vowels. The actio always changes the vowel into the "eh", causing more or less pronounced lip movements by continuing movement. DP tip of the tongue can also be moved right and left as the patient vocalizes the "eh" and the voice pitch be altered up and down.

Talking with a Cork in the Mouth (Fig. 104b): With the patient sitting upright, a cork is wedged between his upper and lower teeth. The cork can be between 1.5–4 cm long, depending on how far the patient can open his mouth – he should only open it just over halfway – and on the specific movements of the tongue and lips to be practised. Practising "l" for instance, needs a longer cork than practising "d" or "p". The subsequent procedure is simple. The patient reads aloud, recites something memorized or simply improvises for about 2 minutes. Then he takes the cork out of his mouth, repeats what he just said, or just talks, and feels at once how easy

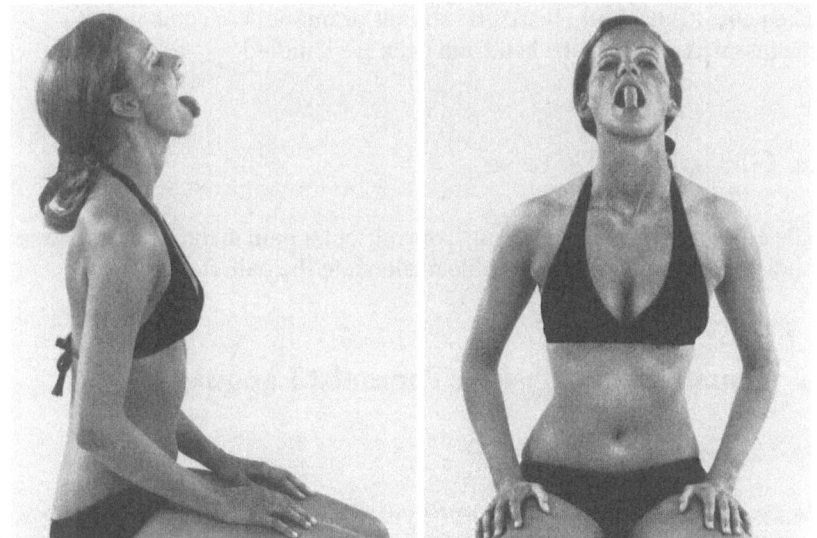

a   b

Fig. 104a, b. Lockjaw. **a** Tongue exercise. **b** Articulating with cork

it now is to articulate. Frequently when the patient is talking with the cork between his teeth, he will salivate so much that a napkin should be kept at hand. The feeling of warmth and relaxation at the base of the tongue and in the larynx brings instant relief to the patient with discomfort in the region of the larynx, pharynx and oesophagus.

- ● **Conditio – Limitatio of the Movement Sequence**

It is useful for the patient to sit up straight and proper while he is assimilating the exercise; particular care should be taken that the spinal column is in the neutral position. In this way, the necessary stabilization and active buttressing occur automatically. As soon as the patient is familiar with the exercise, it can be performed in any situation of daily life, so to speak, and should be several times a day. It doesn't have to take long.

Conditio of Movement Speed
Limitatio of Economical Activity by Finding the Optimal Speed
Conditio: Performed slowly, the "eh" exercise for training the tongue has a beat of about 1 second. It is important, however, that the tongue whips out and stops in the extreme position.
Limitatio: The whipping out of the tongue causes the intensity of economical activity in the muscles of the tongue, lips and pharynx to be very high. The same is true of talking with the cork in the mouth.

5.5.6 Pull Your Head Off (Fig. 105)

The name "Pull Your Head Off" sounds dramatic. We came up with it to refer to the intensity at which the head and neck are handled.

■ Goal of the Exercise

The goal is for patients suffering from muscular pain in the neck and occipital neuralgia of postural origin to be able to alleviate the pain themselves.

► Functional Analysis in Therapist Language

- ● **Conception of the Exercise**

Because a muscle which is tense (hypertonic) and therefore causing ischaemic pain cannot be relaxed voluntarily, the reflexive relaxation of antagonists must be made use of. We did this for hypertonia of the dorsal muscles of the neck, for instance, in Dizzy (see p. 304). Cervical syndromes of postural origin and occipital neuralgias result from chronic faulty posture, which causes abnormal tone in the fall-preventing muscles and functional respiratory disorders. The discomfort and pain, the body's alarm signals, are saying "Do something!" This is what Pull Your Head Off is all about.

In employing massive self-applied resistance, "cramped" muscles are called upon to fully contract against massive but primitive, i. e. simple, resistance. Only afterwards is the attempt made to relax these muscles. The muscles involved here have no fall-preventing work to do in the neutral position when the patient is upright, but should rather make it possible for BS head and the shoulder girdle parked on the thorax to be potentially mobile.

● Position and Activation in the Starting Position

The starting position is upright sitting on a stool. The exercise can also be performed while standing upright.

● Actio – Reactio of the Movement Sequence

Actio: The Primary Movement
Reactio: Activated Passive Buttressing
Reactio: Change in the Support Area

Actio: The patient starts by placing his hands, one on top of the other, folded, or simply touching, on the back of his neck so that the sides of the little fingers are immediately caudal to the mastoid processes. The long axes of the forearms are roughly parallel in the sagittal planes of the shoulders.

The critical distance point of the primary movement, DP vertex, moves backwards/downwards. As it goes, the atlanto-occipital and atlanto-axial joints extend and, by continuing movement, the cervical, thoracic and lumbar spine extends and the pelvis, as proximal lever, brings about flexion in the hips. The arms hanging from the neck go with the movement. In the second primary movement, the shoulder girdle is raised as far as possible by critical DPs right and left upper scapular angle moving cranially. A little later the third primary movement, or rather primary activity, begins, as critical DPs right and left olecranons pull strongly forwards, compelling the extensional movement of the spinal column to stop but, because of the resistance they are applying, raising the intensity of the extensional activity without any movement excursion. Thus, the dorsal cervical and cranial shoulder girdle muscles contract to their maximum. Next, resistance is applied against the ventral cervical muscles (Fig. 105 b), as described for Phase 3 of Dizzy (see p. 307).

Reactio: The critical distance points of the activated passive buttressing, DPs right and left iliac spines, move forwards (ventrally)/downwards (caudally) with flexion effected by the pelvis in the hips and extension in the lumbar spine.

The potential enlargement of the support area in the starting position of upright sitting, in which BS legs is parked on the floor with contact point soles of the feet/floor, becomes effective when the legs go into slight supporting function.

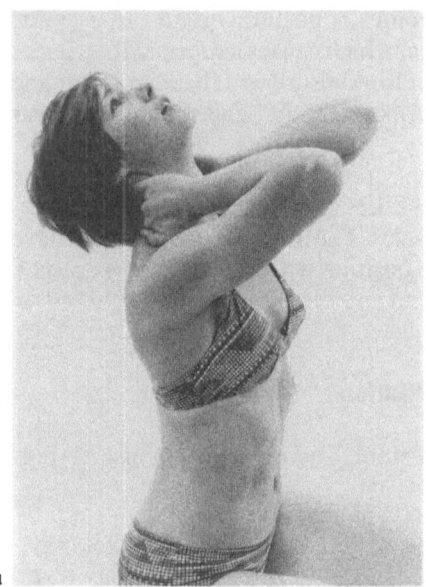

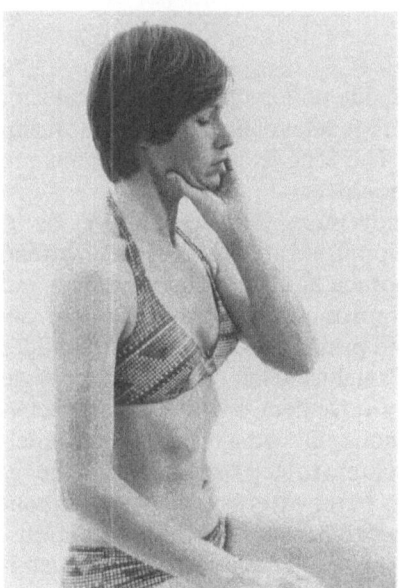

Fig. 105a, b. Pull Your Head Off. **a** Massive resistance to the contracted dorsal muscles. **b** Resistance to the ventral muscles of the front of the neck

Actio: Accelerating Weights
Reactio: Braking Weights

The actio with its horizontal direction component moves backwards, taking with it the weight of the head. Simultaneously it also brings weight forwards by bringing the long axes of the arms up roughly horizontal. The reactio causes weight to be brought forward by the flexion of the pelvis in the hips.

Since in the starting position the bisecting plane coincided with the midfrontal

322

plane of BSs pelvis, thorax and head, it shifts slightly forwards, against the direction of movement. This can also be seen by the change in the legs from parking to supporting function. All weights behind the bisecting plane have an accelerating effect on the movement sequence and all those in front of it have a braking effect. The high intensity of activity of the extensors of the atlanto-occipital and atlanto-axial joints and the cervical and thoracic spines, directed in the direction of movement, compensates cranially for the preponderance of braking weight.

● **Conditio – Limitatio of the Movement Sequence**

In Pull Your Head Off, the conditios of constant distances between distance points and fixed spatial points are not very important. The distance between the tips of the elbows can be regarded as a constant. This facilitates the forward direction of the activity of the arms which creates the resistance.

The points of contact between the body and the base support (seat and floor) are absolute fixed spatial points. The limitatio that arises from the conditio normally occurs spontaneously.

Conditio of Movement Speed
Limitatio of Economical Activity by Finding the Optimal Speed
Conditio: The speed of the movement is slow. When the tension is at its highest, the mouth should be open. Respiration may be accompanied by groaning.
Limitatio: Because the weights are evenly distributed and activity and counteractivity offset each other, the high intensity of economical activity can safely be increased individually for each patient, as long as breathing is not pressured.

5.5.7 Blockhead (Fig. 106)

"Blockhead" is an invented name. It refers to the way the head obstinately resists the forces attacking it.

■ Goal of the Exercise

The goal is for the patient to learn himself to alleviate pain in the neck and shoulders due to cervical syndromes, restrictions of movement, paraesthesia in the arms and hands, and discomfort in breathing and swallowing.

▶ Functional Analysis in Therapist Language

● Conception of the Exercise

In cases of cervical syndrome with many different symptoms and various pain on movement, we can attempt to release the muscles from the complicated function of fall-preventing by applying to the patient's head resistance to all possible movement components, to which resistance he must react without moving. In this simple manner it is possible to activate all muscles, hypertonic as well as hypotonic. Since it is often impossible to align BS head properly in the vertical long axis of the body, these resistances can be applied in the whatever is the best attainable position at the time. Such activation against resistance, with the position being simply held and no movement allowed, is successful after only a few trials and is almost always pain-free. If there is pain, the therapist should treat this appropriately, through distraction, etc. In this way, the patient learns to respond with normal protective reflexes, automatically and without delay, to the many "mini whiplash traumas" of daily life. The faster and more precisely the resistances can be applied, the quicker the reaction to prevent the possible unwanted movements.

● Position and Activation in the Starting Position

The starting position is sitting or standing upright.

● Actio – Reactio of the Movement Sequence

The actio lies in the patient's own hands providing the resistance. The horizontal displacements of weight are insignificant. There is no reactio in the form of activated passive buttressing or change in the support area.

Sagittotransverse Resistance: Extensional/Flexional in the Atlanto-occipital and Atlanto-axial Joints, Dorsal/Ventral Translational in the Cervical Spine
(Fig. 106 a, b)
The critical distance points of the primary movement, DPs right and left palms, move cranially/dorsally towards the middle of the occiput, with pronation in the forearms, flexion in the elbows, and flexion/abduction/external rotation in the shoulders. The acromions move cranially/medially/dorsally in the sternoclavicular joints. All of this occurs in the form of a co-rotational continuing movement flowing from distal to proximal. As soon as the palms approach the occiput, the hands fold and press the head directly forward, causing extensional activation of the atlanto-occipital and atlanto-axial joints and ventral translational activation of the cervical spine.
Of the critical distance points of the antagonistic primary movement, DPs right and left fists, DP right fist moves forwards/slightly downwards towards the tip of the chin. The wrist goes into dorsiflexion by displacement of its fulcrum, and the forearm into slight supination effected by the distal pointer. By continuing movement, the humeroscapular joint goes into slight extension/adduction/considerable

324

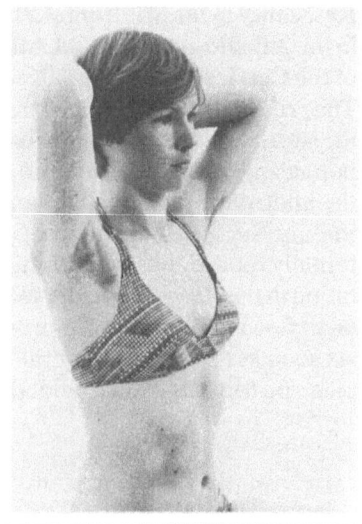

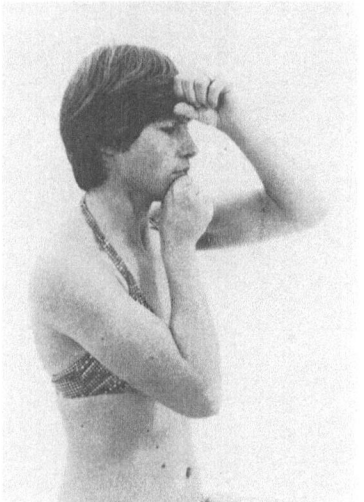

Fig. 106 a–h. Blockhead. **a** Resistance to dorsal translation. **b** Resistance to ventral translation

internal rotation and the acromion moves caudally/ventrally by ventral rotation in the sternoclavicular joint, until the thumb/index finger side of the fist reaches the tip of the chin from ventrally.

Meanwhile, DP left fist has been moving forwards/slightly upwards towards the middle of the forehead. The wrist goes into dorsiflexion by displacement of its fulcrum. By continuing movement, the humeroscapular joint goes into extension/transverse flexion/internal rotation and the acromion moves ventrally by ventral rotation in the sternoclavicular joint until the thumb/index finger side of the fist reaches the middle of the forehead from ventrally.

When it reaches the forehead, the left fist presses backwards on the chin, while the right fist pushes the chin backwards not quite as hard, without mobilizing the mandible in a gnawing movement.

Resistance in the Midfrontal Plane: Right-/Left-Concave Lateroflexional in the Atlanto-occipital and Atlanto-axial Joints and in the Joints of the Cervical Spine (Fig. 106 c, d)

The critical distance point of the primary movement, DP right palm, moves out of the starting position upwards/backwards towards the vertex such that the metacar-pophalangeal joint of the third finger rests on the vertex and its volar aspect is in the midfrontal plane on the head. By continuing movement, the wrist flexes, the forearm supinates, the elbow flexes, the humeroscapular joint flexes/abducts/ex-ternally rotates, and the acromion moves cranially/medially/dorsally by dorsal rotation in the sternoclavicular joint, in the form of a co-rotational continuing movement flowing from distal to proximal.

As soon as the long axes of the hand and of the third finger are in the midfrontal plane on top of the head, with the fingers cupping the left side of the head and the

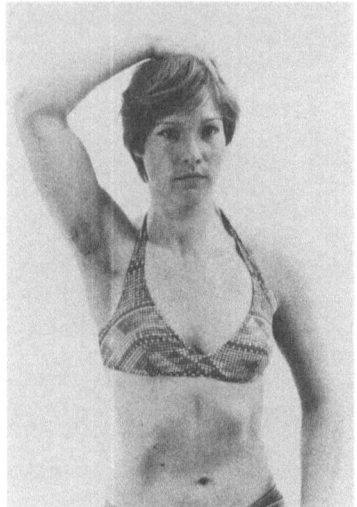

c

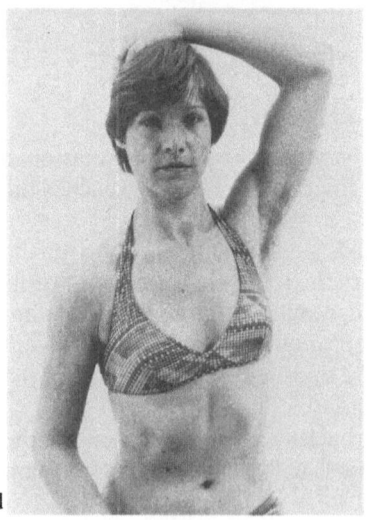

d

Fig. 106 a–h. Blockhead. **c** Resistance to left-concave lateroflexion, **d** Resistance to right-concave latero-flexion

wrist resting on the right, the fingertips pull precisely upwards/to the right and simultaneously the radial aspect of the wrist on the right side of the head presses downwards/to the right, causing right-concave lateroflexional activation of the atlanto-occipital and atlanto-axial joints and joints of the cervical spine. The opposite can be done with the left hand.

Resistance in the Transverse Planes: Head-Positive/-Negative Rotational in the Atlanto-occipital and Atlanto-axial Joints and in the Joints of the Cervical Spine (Fig. 106 e, f)

The critical distance point of the primary movement, DP right palm, moves out of the starting position upwards/forwards/medially towards the forehead such that the long axes of the hand and of the third finger lie more or less in a transverse

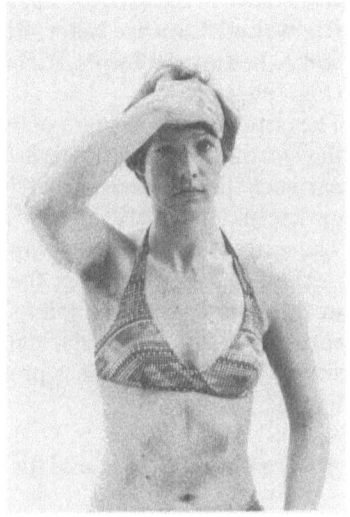

e

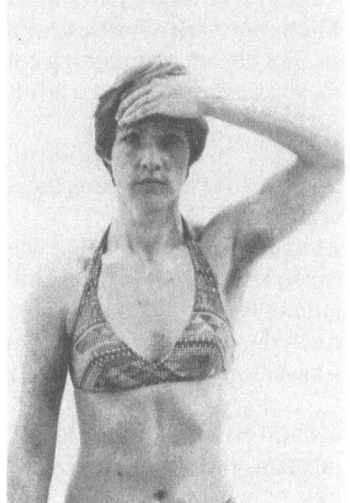

Fig. 106 a–h. Blockhead. **e** Resistance to negative head rotation. **f** Resistance to positive head rotation

f

327

plane of the forehead. By continuing movement the wrist flexes, the forearm supinates, the elbow flexes and there is flexion/abduction/external rotation in the humeroscapular joint. The acromion moves cranially/medially about a sagitto-transverse axis in the sternoclavicular joint in a co-rotational distal-to-proximal continuing movement.

As soon as the right hand is resting over the forehead with the fingertips cupping the left side of the forehead and the wrist resting on the right side of the forehead, the fingertips pull the forehead forwards/to the right, while simultaneously the radial aspect of the wrist presses the right side of the forehead backwards/to the right, which would effect head-positive rotation in the atlanto-occipital and atlanto-axial joints and the joints of the cervical spine. The opposite can be done with the left hand.

Resistance in the Frontotransverse Direction:
Right-/Left-Concave Lateroflexional in the Atlanto-occipital
and Atlanto-axial Joints, Right/Left Laterotranslational in the Cervical Spine
(Fig. 106 g, h)

The critical distance point of the primary movement, DP right palm, moves out of the starting position upwards/backwards/laterally to the right towards the right ear, such that the long axis of the hand points upwards, the thumb rests behind the auricle and the index finger rests just in front of the ear.

The movement continues with extension/ulnar abduction in the wrist, supination in the forearm, flexion in the elbow, flexion/slight abduction/external rotation in the humeroscapular joint. The acromion moves cranially/dorsally by dorsal rotation in the sternoclavicular joint. As soon as the palm reaches the right side of the face, it presses precisely to the left. The opposite is done by the left hand.

● Conditio – Limitatio of the Movement Sequence

Conditio: Constant Distances Between Body Distance Points
Limitatio: Active Buttressing and Stabilization

In Blockhead, maintaining constant distances is the key to achieving the goal of the exercise, for this goal is fulfilled by the reactively occurring limitatio.

Conditio: In the application of dorsal and ventral translational resistances in a sagittotransverse direction, the distance from DP jugular notch to DP tip of the chin remains constant.

Limitatio: This means that when the hands press forwards, they are actively buttressed flexionally in the atlanto-occipital and atlanto-axial joints and dorsal translationally in the cervical spine. When the hands press backwards, they are buttressed extensionally in the atlanto-occipital and atlanto-axial joints and ventral translationally in the cervical spine.

Conditio: In the application of right/left lateroflexional resistance in the midfrontal plane, the distance from DP right/left sternoclavicular joint to DP right/left earlobe remains constant.

328

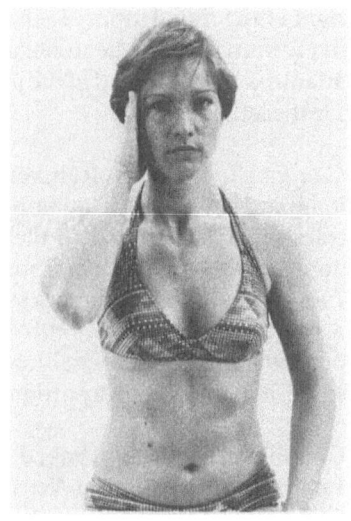

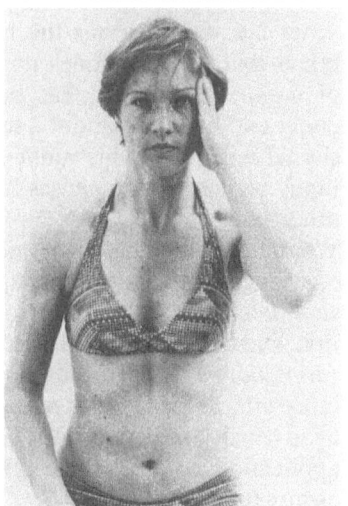

Fig. 106 a–h. Blockhead. **g** Resistance to lateral translation to the right. **h** Resistance to lateral translation to
the left

Limitatio: If these distances remain the same, the pull upwards/to the right of the
right fingertips on the left side of the head and the pressure downwards/to the right
of the radial aspect of the wrist on the right side of the head will be actively buttressed by left-concave lateroflexional activity in the atlanto-occipital and atlanto-
axial joints and joints of the cervical spine, and the other way around for the left
hand.

Conditio: In the application of head-positive and head-negative rotational resistance to the middle of the forehead in the transverse plane, the distance between
DP jugular notch and DP tip of the nose remains constant.
Limitatio: If this distance remains constant, the rotational pull forwards/to the
right of the right fingertips on the left temple and the pressure backwards/to the

right of the radial aspect of the wrist against the right side of the forehead are actively buttressed by head-negative rotational activity in the atlanto-occipital and atlanto-axial joints and in the joints of the cervical spine, and the other way around for the left hand.

Conditio: In the frontotransverse application of right- and left-concave lateroflexional resistances in the atlanto-occipital and atlanto-axial joints and right and left translational resistance in the cervical spine, the distances between DP jugular notch and DP right/left earlobe remain constant.

Limitatio: If these distances stay the same, the pressure from the right hand towards the left is actively buttressed right-concave lateroflexionally in the atlanto-occipital and atlanto-axial joints and right lateral translationally in the cervical spine, and the other way around for the left hand.

Conditio of Movement Speed
Limitatio of Economical Activity by Finding the Optimal Speed
Conditio: The movement of the hands towards the head is slow and tentative. After a few repetitions the hands can start to move faster, but care must be taken that the head does not move to meet the hands. As soon as the point of contact hand/head has been established, the hand presses quickly, precisely and hard, for about 2 seconds. When the resistance is removed, the head should not move. This sudden, precise, strong resistance is repeated about five times with 1-second pauses in between. Then the resistance is applied on the other side.

When the patient has mastered the exercise well, it is a good idea to apply all the resistances with one hand first, working to a 1-second beat through flexion/extension, left-concave lateroflexion, dorsal/ventral translation, right lateral translation, and then go through them all again with the other hand.

Limitatio: Suddenly increasing the economical activity makes the exercise much more effective and helps to develop the reactivity of the muscles of the neck and head which is so important. The patient should not hold his breath with the sudden application of the resistance. Inspiratory and expiratory whistling will if necessary ensure that he does not.

▶ Instruction in Patient Language

● Instruction Appealing to the Patient's Perception

To enable the patient to check whether he is performing the exercise properly and thus that it is having its intended effect, he should be guided to palpate the reflexively relaxing side at the moment the resistance is applied. For this the dorsal/ventral translational resistance is applied with only one hand; to apply lateroflexional resistance, the other hand presses on the same side upwards and towards the opposite side.

5.6 Adaptation of Lift-Free/Reduced-Lift Mobilization of the Spinal Column for Economical Strength and Skill Training

A spinal column which has been mobilized under lift-free or reduced-lift conditions is, so to speak, ready to bear a reasonable amount of stress. As soon as a high intensity of economical activity can be achieved, we should start to practice bearing increasing amounts of stress under conditions of reduced lift. If the spinal column has already been damaged as a result of faulty postural statics, training to bear more stress will have to be planned wisely and according to the patient's needs.

Bearing stress demands strength. Economy demands skill. Therefore, bearing stress economically means combining strength with skill. Skill in movement is the ability to choose the speed of movement well and to be in control of it. Starting out slowly and then getting faster is not always the way to learn the right speed. The synthesis of strength, skill and mastery of the movement speed depends on a capacity for fine differentiation.

Basic Principles of Stress Training for the Spinal Column

A person whose spinal column is about to be subjected to increased stress should be standing firmly on his or her legs. These constitute the substructure of the spinal column and provide the body's contact with the floor. The axes of the legs must be properly aligned above each other in a way that ensures that the ankles, knees and hips are physiologically stressed and held by the fall-preventing musculature. Only then is the spinal column able to stay in its neutral position when the long axis of the body inclines out of the vertical and thus the lifting stress involved in bending down and lifting weights can be kept as low as possible.

The weights of the pelvis, thorax, head, and the organs contained within them connect directly to the spinal column. In addition to the autochthonous muscles of the back, a powerful coat of muscles covers BSs pelvis, thorax and head. While in lift-free/reduced-lift mobilization of the spinal column we try to involve chiefly the autochthonous muscles, when stress is stepped up demands also have to be made of this muscular coat. Sometimes it is used like a corset, sometimes like a flexible tube. The patient is to learn how to use it economically.

The increases in the movement speed start at the periphery, in the extremities, the arms and legs. Whether they have a horizontal direction component and lead to locomotion, or have a vertical direction component and accelerate the body weight upwards against gravity, or whether the rise in speed demands a very high degree of skill, or whether all these possibilities are combined, the swift movements of the extremities all, by continuing movement, affect the central body segments pelvis and thorax. Because of the increased speed, the muscular coat referred to above is either used as a corset, to stabilize and actively buttress, or as a flexible tube along which continuing movement makes use of the available potential mobility.

5.6.1 Once Every Hour (Fig. 107)

The name "Once Every Hour" merely indicates that this exercise can and should be repeated hourly during the day.

■ Goal of the Exercise

The goal is for the patient to be able to interrupt inappropriate tone (hypertonia or hypotonia) due to chronic postural stress in muscles of the pelvis, thorax, neck and shoulder girdle, and to be able to do so in minimal time, even at work, by simple, strong, massive contractions of the abdominal and back muscles.

▶ Functional Analysis in Therapist Language

● Conception of the Exercise

We will let gravity be the decisive factor in choosing between the dorsal or the ventral muscles of the spinal column.

To stimulate fall-preventing activation of the spinal extensors in a sitting position, the centre of gravity must be shifted forwards by flexion of the pelvis in the hip joints and an additional voluntary mass contraction of all the extensors of the entire spinal column at the same time until all the available tolerance for extension is used up. This brings the legs into supporting function.

To stimulate fall-preventing activation of the spinal flexors in a sitting position, the centre of gravity must be displaced backwards by extension of the pelvis in the hip joints and an additional voluntary mass contraction of all the flexors of the entire spinal column until all the available tolerance for flexion has been used up. This brings the legs into free play.

Between these two extreme positions, we align the long axis of the body vertically and emphasize the relationship between the position of the vertical spinal column and gravity by traction of the spinal column upwards, initiated by the arms. Overactivation of the muscles around the lordotic spinal segments must be voluntarily reduced.

● Position and Activation in the Starting Position

Position in Space of the Critical Axes
Points of Contact Between the Body and the Environment
Components of Movement in Relation to the Neutral Position of the Joints
The starting position is upright sitting on a stool or chair. If the chair has a backrest, the patient turns through 90°.
The distance between the hip joints and the floor must not be less than the distance between the knee joints and the floor. If it is much more, i. e. if the hips are signifi-

cantly higher from the floor than the knees are, the patient should sit on the front edge of the chair or over the corner of the stool so that only his ischial tuberosities and not the dorsal aspects of his thighs touch the seat.

BSs pelvis, thorax, head are aligned in the vertical long axis of the body.

In BS legs, the hips joints are comfortably transversely abducted, flexed 90° or less, and neutral as to rotation. The knee joints are flexed to 90° or less, the lower legs are neutral as to rotation in the knee joints. The functional long axes of the feet are each parallel to the long axis of the ipsilateral thigh. The soles of the feet are in contact with the floor.

In BS arms, the palms rest on the thighs with the long axes of the metacarpals pointing forwards. The thumbs point medially/forwards.

Movement Tolerances in the Critical Joints in Relation
to the Intended Primary Movement

We are assured of tolerance for extension of the pelvis in the hip joints because in the starting position the hip joint is flexed to 90°. If there is not enough tolerance for flexion, it can be increased from the distal lever by raising the seat.

Since the spinal column is in neutral position, the existing tolerances for extension and flexion can be made use of.

In addition, we expect end-stop flexion and extensive extension/adduction in the shoulder joints and large extension and flexion in the elbow joints.

Distribution of Body Weight on a Base Support or Suspension Device,
Against a Supportive Device or Over a Support Area,
and the Resulting Activity States of the Musculature

The seat of the chair is the base support for BSs pelvis, thorax and head. The pelvis is potentially mobile in the hip joints and the joints of the lumbar spine and the head is potentially mobile in the atlanto-occipital and atlanto-axial joints and in the cervical spine. In BS thorax, the thoracic spine is dynamically stabilized in neutral position. The shoulder girdle is parked on the thorax. The arms, hanging from the shoulder girdle, are parked with the palms on the thighs. The floor is the base support for BS legs; they are parked on it ready to extend the support area forwards.

Intensity of Muscular Activity Required with Economical Activity
Respiration

In the starting position, the intensity of economical activity is low. Breathing should be normal.

Potentially Accelerating and Braking Weights in Relation to the Bisecting Plane
of the Intended Primary Movement

The horizontal direction components of the intended to-and-fro movement are forwards and backwards. For this reason, the bisecting plane in the starting position coincides with the midfrontal plane of BSs pelvis, thorax and head, which is vertical. The critical fulcrum of the primary movements is the flexion/extension axis of the hip joints. Roughly speaking, the upper body length supplies the accelerating weights and the lower body length the braking weights. When the long axis of the body moves forwards, the accelerating weights are in front of the bisecting plane and the braking weights are behind it, and the other way around when it moves backwards.

● Actio – Reactio of the Movement Sequence

Once Every Hour is a constant-location, three-phase movement. Phases 1 and 2 are to-and-fro movements with horizontal direction components forwards/backwards and corresponding extensions of the support area. In phase 3 the vertical direction component dominates and the reactio is minimal.

Actio: The Primary Movement
Reactio: Activated Passive Buttressing
Reactio: Change in the Support Area

Phase 1: Forwards
Actio: The critical distance points of the primary movement, DPs right and left iliac spines, move forwards/downwards with flexion by the proximal lever in the hip joints and extension by the caudal lever in the lumbar spine. Simultaneously, DPs right and left palms have gone into supported leaning on the ventral aspects of the thighs close to the hip joints, below the shoulder joints, with the long axes of the hands pointing medially/slightly forwards. DP tip of the nose has already begun a buttressing movement to the primary movement, moving forwards in space but dorsally/cranially in relation to the body, with extension in the atlanto-occipital and atlanto-axial joints and, by continuing movement, extension in the cervical and thoracic spine, exhausting extension in the spinal column to end-stop.

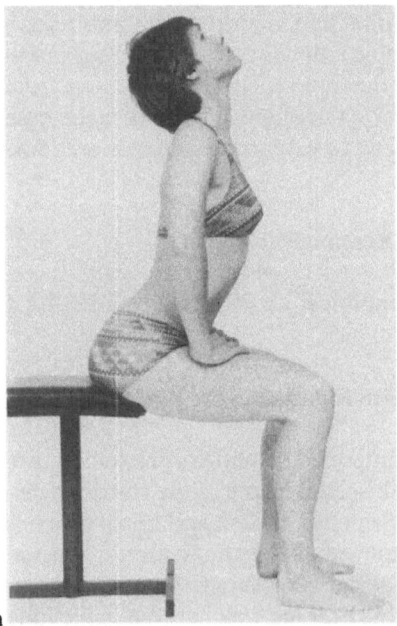

Fig. 107 a–c. Once Every Hour. **a** Massive extension of the spinal column

a

334

Reactio: The support area is moved forwards when BS legs begins to bear weight and DPs right and left ischial tuberosities lose contact with the seat. The support area is now the smallest area encompassing the points of contact dorsal aspects of the thighs around the trochanters/seat and soles/floor.

Phase 2: Backwards
Actio: The critical distance points of the second primary movement, DPs right and left iliac spines, move backwards/first upwards, then downwards, with extension by the proximal lever in the hip joints and flexion by the caudal lever in the lumbar spine. The palms leave the thighs when DPs right and left olecranons move medially/backwards. The elbows flex by displacement of their fulcra and there is extension/adduction/internal rotation by the distal lever in the humero-scapular joints. By proximally continuing movement, DPs right and left acromions move backwards in space but ventrally/medially/caudally in relation to the body by ventral rotation in the sternoclavicular joints. Meanwhile, the hands have formed a pattern fist (PNF), the wrists go into flexion/ulnar abduction and, by continuing movement, the forearms into pronation. These arm movements reinforce the buttressing movement that has already started in response to the primary movement, bringing DP tip of the chin backwards/downwards in space but caudally/first ventrally, then dorsally in relation to the body, with flexion in the atlanto-occipital and atlanto-axial joints and, by continuing movement, the cervical and thoracic spine, until the full tolerance for flexion in the spinal column is exhausted to end-stop.
Reactio: The critical distance points of the activated passive buttressing, DPs right and left toes, almost lose contact with the floor and the weight of the legs becomes

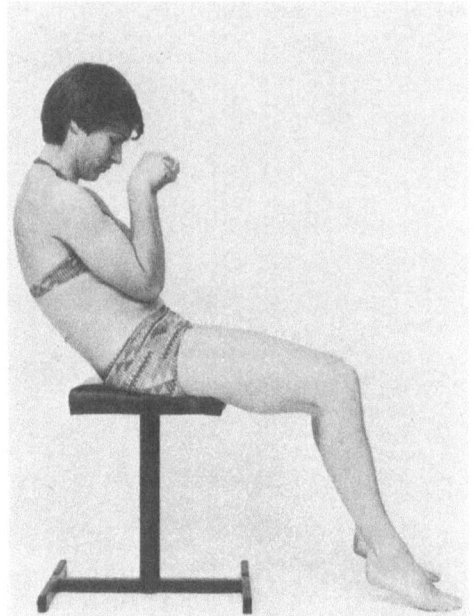

Fig. 107 a–c. Once Every Hour. **b** Massive flexion of the spinal column

b

335

suspended from the pelvis by flexional activity in the hip joints, thus turning into an activated passive buttress.

The support area moves backwards a little and becomes smaller because the soles have almost left the floor altogether. It is the smallest area encompassing the points of contact between the coccyx, ischial tuberosities, dorsal aspects of the thighs and the seat.

Phase 3: Traction

Actio: The critical distance point of the primary movement, DP right hand, grasps the left wrist dorsally and pulls it upwards. The movement continues with pronation in the forearms, extension in the elbows, and flexion/adduction/internal rotation of the upper arms in the humeroscapular joints. DPs right and left acromions move cranially/medially/dorsally in the sternoclavicular joints, the thoracic spine extends cranial-to-caudally, the ribs move as in inspiration and the pelvis flexes in the hip joints, causing the lumbar spine to extend.

Reactio: The support area extends forwards again and becomes bigger when the pressure of the soles on the floor increases and BS legs returns to slight supporting function.

Actio: In the concluding movement phase, critical DP coccyx approaches the seat by moving downwards, caudally/ventrally in relation to the body. The movement

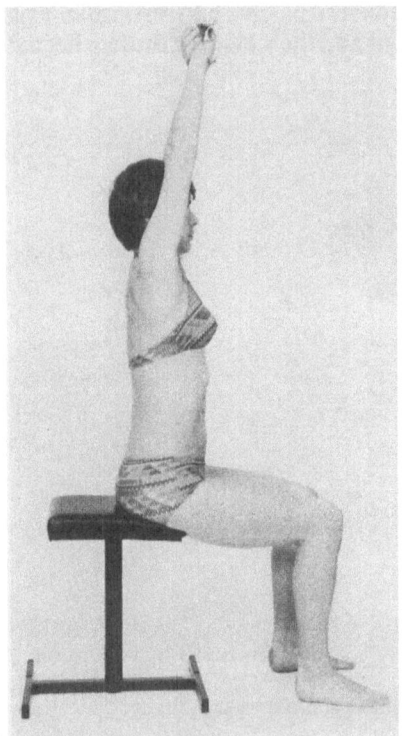

c

Fig. 107 a–c. Once Every Hour. **c** Traction of the vertical spinal column

336

continues with extension in the hip joints and flexion at the lumbosacral junction in the lumbar spine.

Reactio: The support area moves backwards a little and BS legs is back in parking function.

Actio: Accelerating Weights
Reactio: Braking Weights

During the movement forwards the bisecting plane shifts forwards; during the movement backwards it shifts backwards. During the traction movement the bisecting plane is again identical with the patient's midfrontal plane, which is vertical.

● **Conditio – Limitatio of the Movement Sequence**

Conditio: Constant Distances Between Body Distance Points
Limitatio: Active Buttressing and Stabilization

In Once Every Hour, there are absolute and relative fixed spatial points.

Conditio: The point of contact feet/floor is an absolute fixed spatial point during all three phases of the exercise.

Limitatio: During the forward movement, the absolute fixed point relates to contact between the soles of the feet and the floor. This fixed point prevents the support area from becoming either larger, by pushing the feet forwards, or smaller, by pulling them back, as the legs are activated in supporting function. Either of these would make full flexion of the pelvis in the hip joints difficult or even impossible, and the desired full extension of the pelvis at the lumbosacral articulation until the ischial tuberosities lift up off the seat would no longer be assured. The cranial/dorsal buttressing movement initiated by the nose with extension in the atlanto-occipital and atlanto-axial joints and joints of the cervical spine and in the thoracic spine cranial-to-caudally, completes the exhaustion to end-stop of tolerance for extension in the whole of the spinal column.

During the backward movement, the absolute fixed point relates to contact between the forefeet and the floor. The necessity of maintaining this contact checks the extent of the backward movement and stimulates the buttressing movement which, by cranial-to-caudal flexion in the atlanto-occipital and atlanto-axial joints and joints of the cervical and thoracic spine, reduces the accelerating primary weight.

During traction, the absolute fixed point again relates to contact between the soles and the floor. This facilitates a smooth transition from the activity state of supporting to that of parking in BS legs.

Conditio: During the forward movement, the contact point palms/ventral aspects of the thighs is a relative fixed point.

Limitatio: This relative fixed point should be so positioned at the beginning of the forward movement that, when the end position is reached, the long axes of the hands will point medially/slightly forwards and the shoulders will be above the palms. The hands will thus be in the best position to relieve stress on the lumbar region, if necessary, by pressure activity.

Conditio: During all three phases of the exercise the contact point body/seat is maintained and is restricted to the ischial tuberosities and the area slightly cranial and caudal to them.

Limitatio: This relative fixed point checks the forward primary movement, thus preventing too much weight from coming to rest over the legs, which would reduce the extension in the spinal column. Equally, it checks the backward primary movement, ensuring that the lumbosacral articulation does not touch the base support, which would displace too much weight backwards and thus reduce the flexion in the spinal column.

Conditio of Movement Speed
Limitatio of Economical Activity by Finding the Optimal Speed

Conditio: The optimal speed is found by starting out very slowly and gradually speeding up. It is advisable to start with the forward movement and move alternately backwards and forwards a few times before going from a backward movement into the traction phase to conclude the exercise. The traction phase requires at least three times as much time as a backward or forward movement.

During the forward and backward movements the primary movement is in the hip joints, followed by the coordinated arm movements and then, finally, by the cranial-to-caudal buttressing movements, which are essential to the achievement of massive flexion and massive extension to end-stop in the whole spinal column. Maximum increases in intensity are brought about by the movements of the pelvis in the hip joints; at the end of the forward movement this is when the ischial tuberosities are lifted up from the seat of the chair, accompanied by a "groaning sigh" from the patient, while at the end of the backward movement it is when the pelvic floor is tensed ("swallow your intestines"), the lower abdomen contracted to the maximum and the lumbosacral junction flexed, accompanied by Double Panting (see p. 151).

During the traction phase, reducing the intensity of economical activity in the ventral and dorsal muscles connecting the pelvis to the thorax takes a little time. Triggering the yawn reflex is the best way to find the position in which the pelvis regains its potential mobility in the hip joints and lumbar spine and the legs go back into parking function.

Limitatio: The optimal speed for this demanding, partly steered game playing with the intensity of economical activity is 1 second for the backward and forward movements and 3–5 seconds for the traction. The juxtaposing of high- and low-intensity economical activity with reduced lifting stress allows patients who work in a stereotypically sedentary posture to experience something radically different and stimulates the circulation around the spinal column.

▶ Instruction in Patient Language

● Instruction Appealing to the Patient's Perception

The patient will assimilate the exercise best if the therapist performs it with him, dramatically exaggerating the groaning in the extension phase, the Double Panting in the flexion phase, and the yawning in the traction phase.

▶ Adapting the Exercise to the Patient's Constitution and Condition

There are no difficulties in adapting this exercise to the patient's constitution and condition.

5.6.2 The Penguin (Fig. 108)

"Penguin" is an invented name: the teetering gait the patient learns in this exercise looks just like the way penguins walk.

■ Goal of the Exercise

The goal is for the patient to learn to:
- Maintain his balance around the long axis of the body even under difficult conditions
- Make use of the automatic twisting of the subtalar foot-plate under maximum stress
- Bring about maximum contraction of the extensors and external rotators of the hip joints
- Improve the lifting capacity of the triceps surae

▶ Functional Analysis in Therapist Language

● Conception of the Exercise

To train the patient's ability to keep his balance around the long axis of his body under difficult conditions, we position the axis vertically, reduce the support area by having the patient stand on tiptoe, and use the arms to lengthen the body and make the postural statics top-heavy. To make the subtalar foot-plate twist, and to contract the extensors and external rotators of the hip joints, we have the patient stand on tiptoe with the functional long axes of the feet markedly diverging and the heels pressing together. Because the flexion/extension axes of the body are horizontal, the activation directed upwards imposes pure positive lifting stress.

In this starting position, tolerance for upward movement is needed only in the talocrural joints and in the arms. The primary movement impulse is assigned to the arms; their pulling upwards pulls the patient onto tiptoe, and the destabilization of the long axis of the body is now complete.

Once the patient is in this position, he stands alternately on each leg by pulling up the toes of the opposite foot, thus calling into play not only the extensional and flexional but also the lateroflexional, abductional, adductional and rotational stabilizers in the hip joint.

● Position and Activation in the Starting Position

Position in Space of the Critical Axes
Points of Contact Between the Body and the Environment
Components of Movement in Relation to the Neutral Position of the Joints
The starting position is upright standing. All flexion/extension axes are horizontal. In BS legs, the soles of the feet form the contact with the floor.

The functional long axes of the feet diverge markedy. The heels are touching. The knee joints are in neutral position and the hip joints are neutral as to flexion/extension and in slight adduction and external rotation.

The virtual long axis of the body has been optimally constituted by perfect alignment of BSs pelvis, thorax and head, all in neutral position.

BS arms is in neutral position, the long axes of the arms roughly parallel to the long axis of the body.

Movement Tolerances at the Critical Joints
in Relation to the Intended Primary Movement
Because the starting position is upright standing with external rotation and adduction in the hip joints, the feet have the required tolerance for plantarflexion, inversion and pronation, and for extension in the metatarsophalangeal joints.

The arms are in neutral position and therefore have all the tolerance for flexion, abduction and internal rotation needed for raising the shoulder girdle and flexing the elbows in the intended primary movement.

Distribution of Body Weight on a Base Support or Suspension Device,
Against a Supportive Device, or Over a Support Area,
and the Resulting Activity States of the Musculature
The support area is the smallest area encompassing the points of contact between the soles of the feet and the floor. BS legs is in supporting function, BSs pelvis, thorax and head are aligned in the long axis of the body, the pelvis has reduced potential mobility, BS thorax is dynamically stabilized and BS head is potentially mobile and in free play. In BS arms the shoulder girdle is parked on the thorax and the arms hang from the shoulder girdle in free play.

Intensity of Muscle Activity Required with Economical Activity
Respiration
The intensity of economical activity in the starting position is on the whole low, somewhat higher in the hip joints. Because the thoracic spine is dynamically stabilized in its neutral position, breathing is normal.

● Actio – Reactio of the Movement Sequence

The Penguin is a two-phase constant-location movement sequence involving changes in the pressure distribution within the support area. The dominant direction component is vertical, directed upwards. The horizontal direction components are minor; in the first phase, they are directed forwards/outwards; in the second phase to the right/left.

Actio: The Primary Movement

Phase 1
The actio consists of symmetrical, simultaneous, accelerating arm movements directed upwards/outwards/slightly forwards.
The critical distance points of the primary movement, DPs right and left olecranon, move upwards/right/forwards and upwards/left/forwards as fast as possible

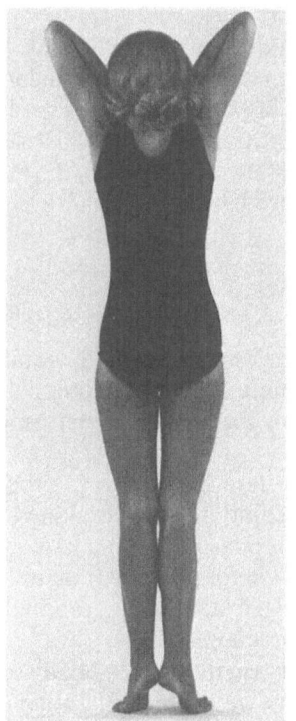
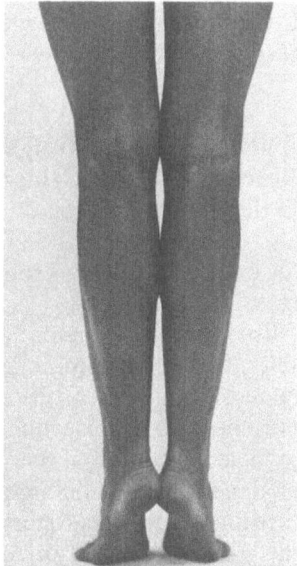

a   b

Fig. 108 a–e. The Penguin. **a, b** Phase 1

until they are well above the level of DP vertex. The elbows go into flexion by fulcrum displacement, while the upper arms flex/abduct/internally rotate in the humeroscapular joints. By continuing movement, DPs right and left acromion move cranially/medially in the sternoclavicular joints. In the acromioclavicular joint, the pincer jaws close. The continuation of the movement exerts traction on the spinal column and on the legs, coming from cranially and causing the thoracic spine to extend, the lumbar spine to flex, the hip joints to extend, the knee joints to extend, the talocrural joints to plantarflex by fulcrum displacement, the subtalar and calcaneonavicular joints to invert/pronate and the metatarsophalangeal joints – particularly that of the big toe – to be extended by their proximal levers. The long axis of the body shifts upwards/forwards, but without the heels' losing contact with each other (Fig. 108 a, b).

Phase 2
The actio consists of shifting weight right and left alternately within the support area, alternately relieving the stress on the left and right forefoot. As the stress is removed from each foot, that foot lifts up from the floor by dorsiflexion in the talocrural joint, but the heel does not lose touch with the supporting leg. With this movement the long axis of the body shifts towards the side of the supporting leg. To change supporting legs, the foot in free play is brought down to touch the floor again by plantarflexion in the talocrural joint (Fig. 108 c–e).

Reactio: Change in the Support Area
The horizontal forward direction component in phase 1 of the Penguin is brought into effect by the full extension in the metatarsophalangeal joint of the big toe effected by the proximal lever, because this causes the heels to leave the floor and the support area to move forwards and become 80% smaller.

In the alternating one-legged stance in phase 2 of the Penguin, the support area, already been dramatically reduced, becomes smaller to the right or left by another 75%.

Actio: Accelerating Weights
Reactio: Braking Weights
In the starting position of the Penguin, the midfrontal plane, which is vertical, is also the bisecting plane of phase 1. The bisecting plane then shifts forwards; in the end position it goes roughly through the metatarsophalangeal joints of the big toes.

All of the body segments or parts of them in front of the bisecting plane have an accelerating effect and those behind it have a braking effect on the movement sequence. In the end position of phase 1, the plane of symmetry, which is vertical, becomes also the bisecting plane for phase 2. It then shifts to the right or left and, in the end position of one-legged standing, goes roughly through the metatarsophalangeal joint of the right or left big toe.

Moving to one-legged standing on the right, all body segments or parts of them to the right of the bisecting plane have an accelerating effect and those to the left have a braking effect on the movement sequence. Moving to one-legged standing on the left, these are reversed.

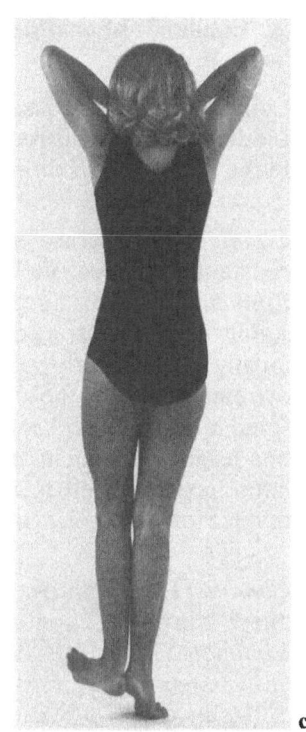

c

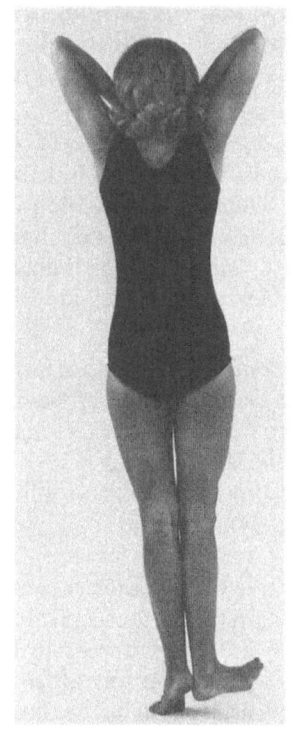

d

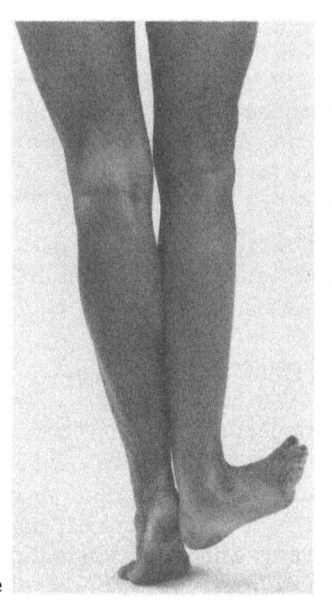

Fig. 108 c–e. Phase 2   e

343

● **Conditio – Limitatio of the Movement Sequence**

Conditio: Constant Distances Between Body Distance Points
Limitatio: Active Buttressing and Stabilization
In the Penguin, the following distances remain constant:

Conditio: The distance between DP tip of the chin and DP jugular notch remains constant during both movement phases.
Limitatio: If this distance is to remain constant, the cervical spine will have to be stabilized in its neutral position dorsal translationally in the cervical spine and flexionally in the atlanto-occipital and atlanto-axial joints, in order to withstand the extreme raising of the shoulder girdle and the traction exerted on the thoracic spine in phase 1 and keep the head aligned in the long axis of the body. In right one-legged standing in phase 2, the cervical spine must be stabilized left-concave lateroflexionally/left translationally to keep it in its neutral position, and the reverse for left one-legged standing.

Conditio: The distance between DP right heel and DP left heel remains constant in phase 1; in phase 2, contact must be maintained in the area of the heels.
Limitatio: This is achieved by external rotation/adduction in the hip joints.

Conditio of Absolute and/or Relative Fixed Spatial Points
Limitatio by Limiting the Primary Movement, Activated Passive Buttressing and/or Change in the Support Area
There are absolute and relative fixed spatial points in the Penguin.

Conditio: The points of contact right and left metatarsophalangeal joints of the big toes/floor are absolute fixed spatial points in phase 1.
Limitatio: During the primary movement of the elbows upwards/outwards/forwards, these fixed points keep the forwards horizontal direction component small, i.e. only as great as is needed to allow the heels to move upwards/forwards as far as they can without taking a step forward.

Conditio: The long axis of the body remains vertical.
Limitatio: This relative fixed spatial point requires in the end position of phase 1 a continuously connected series of active buttressings of the flexion/extension tolerances as follows:
- In the talocrural joints, plantarflexional fulcrum displacement forwards/upwards
- In the knee joints, extensional fulcrum displacement backwards
- In the hip joints, extensional fulcrum displacement forwards
- In the lumbosacral articulation, flexional fulcrum displacement backwards
- In the thoracocervical articulation with critical DP jugular notch, fulcrum displacement forwards/upwards with extension in the thoracic spine and ventral translation by the thorax in the cervical spine

- In the cervico-occipital articulation with critical DPs right and left eyes, fulcrum displacement backwards with dorsal translation by the head in the cervical spine and flexion in the atlanto-occipital and atlanto-axial joints

By this series of active buttressings all the fulcra which might otherwise jeopardize the vertical position of the long axis of the body in relation to in front/behind are stabilized.

In phase 2, the focus is on the active buttressing in the frontal and transverse planes. For standing on the right leg, this is: pronation/eversion in the subtalar and calcaneonavicular joints, external rotation in the hip joint by both pointers, abduction in the hip joint by medial fulcrum displacement, right translation effected by the thorax, right-concave lateroflexion in the lumbar and thoracic spines, thorax-positive rotation in the thoracic and cervical spines, head-negative rotation in the cervical spine and in the atlanto-occipital and atlanto-axial joints.

Conditio: The constant distance between the supporting heel and the floor is a relative fixed spatial point.
Limitatio: In the end position of phase 1, this applies to both heels, in the end position of phase 2, only to the heel of the supporting leg. It has the effect that the full plantarflexion in the talocrural joints and the associated maximum contraction of the triceps surae at the distal joint cannot be relinquished. The resulting vertical stress on the midfoot helps the pronational twisting of the foot.

Conditio: This functional long axis of the free-play foot always points outwards.
Limitatio: This relative fixed spatial point guarantees, by an increase in adductional/external rotational activity in the free-play hip, that the heels or the areas around the heels remain in contact even in the supporting-leg/free-play leg phase.

Conditio of Movement Speed
Limitatio of Economical Activity By Finding the Optimal Speed
Conditio: The speed in phase 1 is the fastest possible acceleration.
Limitatio: This speed in the primary movement forces the patient to keep the movement direction exact and reactively stimulates the stabilizing effect of the long axis of the body and the axes of the legs, united through the heel contact. This high intensity of economical activity is intentional and aimed at fulfilling the goal of muscular strength and contractility that in upright posture are directed against gravity. However, time must be taken to allow breathing to return to normal.

Conditio: For the teetering in phase 2, we take half the speed of normal gait, i.e. about 60 steps per minute.
Limitatio: At this rate, the patient has time to dorsiflex the free-play foot to the maximum and can still make a smooth transition between steps, so that there is not too much trouble about balancing on one foot. A series of 6–12 steps gives the best training effect.

▶ Adapting the Exercise to the Patient's Constitution and Condition

● Adaption to Constitution: Role of Lengths, Widths, Depths and Distribution of Weights

Because the exercise is performed standing upright, the distribution of weights is not significant, but lengths and widths are. Sometimes, if the legs are relatively short, the distance between the greater trochanters wide, and that between the hips narrow, the patient will not be able to keep his heels together, especially if his thighs are relatively fat. In this case, the exercise will have to be performed with the patient standing in a slight straddle, with thighs touching medially in phase 2.

A minor discrepancy in leg length can be compensated by reducing the plantar-flexion in the talocrural joint on one side. If there is a major discrepancy, one has to start thinking about adjusting the height of the base support on one side. Whether the goal of the exercise can be met at all in such a case is something which must be decided individually for each patient.

● Adaptation to Condition

Poor Physical Fitness
For patients who cannot correctly perform the Penguin because of poor physical fitness we make the following adaptation. In the starting position, the patient touches a wall about 40 cm away with his hands at about the level of his frontotransverse diameter of thorax. He touches the wall a little to the right and left of where his plane of symmetry intersects it. The impulse of the primary movement is provided by his swiftly raising his shoulder girdle. As soon as he is standing on his toes, the shoulder girdle is dropped down into neutral position again. To practice phase 2, the hands are moved to about the width of the pelvis apart.

Increasing Performance
For patients who wish to increase performance, the primary movement can be speeded up and the teetering slowed down. Ultimately the patient can abandon the constant location and move forward step by step, keeping the free-play heel in contact with the supporting leg, by each time laterally rotating the tip of the supporting foot until the long axis of the free-play foot points forwards.

Restricted Movement
Any movement restrictions preventing the patient from reaching the neutral position in the starting position can to a small extent be reduced by intensifying the continuous series of active buttressings. If restrictions exist at movement levels hip joints and lumbar spine, these levels will have to be left out of active buttressing, particularly if there is pain. In this case, the extensionally activated knee pushing backwards will be followed by the thorax pushing forwards.

5.6.3 Clip-Clop (Fig. 109)

The name "Clip-Clop" is simply onomatopoeic. Rhythmic repetition of the name generally sets a good speed for the movement sequence.

■ Goal of the Exercise

The goal is for the patient to learn to make his legs into a solid substructure for economical motor behaviour of the spinal column, i. e.:
– Activate the fall-preventing muscles by functional alignment of the axes of the feet and legs in standing
– Maintain this functional alignment when transferring load from right to left
– Adjust this functional alignment to track width

▶ Functional Analysis in Therapist Language

● Conception of the Exercise

Our basic assumption is that if the spinal column is to be able to coordinate dynamic stabilization economically with lift-free and reduced-lift behaviour, it has to have a good substructure.

The inherently mobile system of BS legs has 27 skeletal parts in the foot alone; to these are added the tibia, fibula, patella and femur. Of the axes of the feet and legs – the position of which in space in any posture determines which muscles are called upon to prevent falling and to maintain the posture – only the axes of the thighs and lower legs are unalterable, bony axes. All the other axes are only virtual axes. They are changeable because they are comprised of inherently mobile components and are only optimally functional when these individual components are aligned in a particular order. These are the axes of pronation/supination and inversion/eversion, and also the anatomical and functional long axes of the feet.

On the basis of these assumptions we can proceed to create the functional alignment of the axes of the feet and legs postulated in the goal that will automatically bring about muscular bracing in the arches of the feet and fall-preventing activity in the quadriceps. To simultaneously train economical motor behaviour in the spinal column, we have the long axis of the body vertical in the starting position. In this context, it is worth repeating that the long axis of the body is another which is not a true bony axis but a virtual one.

● **Position and Activation in the Starting Position**

Position in Space of the Critical Axes
Points of Contact Between the Body and the Environment
Components of Movement in Relation to the Neutral Position of the Joints
The starting position is upright standing on the floor. BSs pelvis, thorax and head are aligned in the vertical long axis of the body.
BS arms is in neutral position.
In BS legs, the soles of the feet are the points of contact between the body and the floor. The feet are somewhat more than the width of the pelvis apart. The functional long axes of the feet diverge moderately. They point in the same direction as the knees, whose flexion/extension axes are parallel to those of the metatarsophalangeal joints of the big toes. The lower legs as proximal levers have effected dorsiflexion in the talocrural joints, the knees are moderately flexed by forward fulcrum displacement, and the thighs are moderately flexed/abducted/neutral as to rotation in the hip joints (Fig. 109 a).
Figure 109 b illustrates the following changes. In BS arms the fingers are now supported on the ventral aspects of the thighs close to the hip joints. The wrists are extended/radially abducted, the forearms pronated, the elbows flexed, the shoulder joints abducted/internally rotated.
In BS legs, the toes, in extension effected by the proximal lever, touch the floor with their flexor aspects. The forefeet are pronated, the subtalar and calcaneonavicular joints inverted, the talocrural joints plantarflexed by fulcrum displacement, and the knee and hip joints in increased flexion.

Distribution of Body Weight on a Base Support or Suspension Device,
Against a Supportive Device, or Over a Support Area,
and the Resulting Activity States of the Musculature
The base support in the starting position of Clip-Clop is the floor. The support area is the smallest area encompassing the points of contact between the soles of the feet (or, later, the toes) and the floor.
BS legs is in supporting function. While the soles are in contact with the floor, there is tension in the muscles of the long arches of the feet.
BSs pelvis and head are potentially mobile; the thorax is in neutral position and dynamically stabilized in the thoracic spine.
In BS arms, the shoulder girdle is parked on the thorax; the arms hang from it in free play or are in slightly supported leaning on the ventral aspects of the thighs.

Intensity of Muscle Activity Required with Economical Activity
Respiration
Because the patient is standing with his knees flexed more than normal, the intensity of economical activity for the supporting function in BS legs is higher than usual. This affects particularly the vastus medialis muscle, because in the attempt to keep its flexion/extension axis parallel to that of the metatarsophalangeal joints of the big toe, the knee must turn laterally, causing the vastus medialis to face forwards. This causes greater demands on it for fall-preventing activity.

348

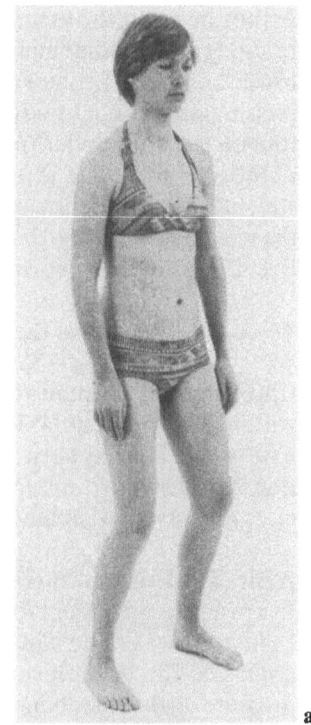

a

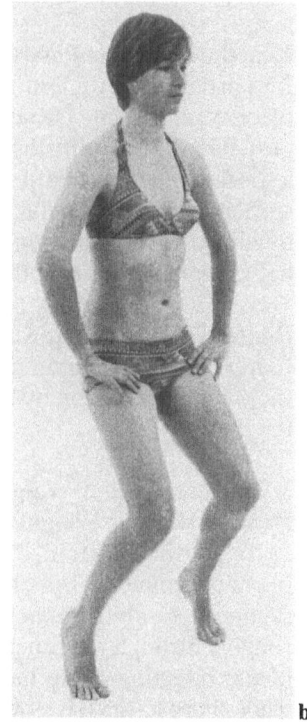

b

Fig. 109 a, b. Clip-Clop, starting position. **a** Standing on the soles of the feet, **b** standing on the toes

In the same way, the functional alignment of the axes of the feet and legs causes the bridging activity that guarantees the long arch of the foot to intensify in order to brace the arch. The lateral rotation in the knee joints is compensated by the buttressing pronational twist of the forefoot, which keeps the main pressure of the foot on the floor under the balls of the big toes, thereby taking stress off the balls of the little toes. The extensional activity in the toes allows room for a shifting of weight forwards; if this activity were flexional, it would prevent this or ensure that the weight were shifted backwards.

Breathing should be normal.

● **Actio – Reactio of the Movement Sequence**

Clip-Clop is a constant-location movement sequence with a shifting of pressure within the support area. The actio goes alternately right and left, in order to alternate weight bearing between the right and the left leg and set the "clip-clop" in motion. Because the direction component of the primary movement is horizontal, a clear reactio is anticipated.

Actio: The Primary Movement

In a primary movement to the right, the critical distance point DP right greater trochanter moves right. The right hip joint adducts through displacement of its fulcrum and the distal lever, the thigh, inclines laterally with the adduction. The pressure on the floor beneath the right sole or tip of the foot increases and the right leg supports more weight.

Reactio: Activated Passive Buttressing

In a primary movement to the right, the critical distance point of the activated passive buttressing, DP sole or toes of the left foot, is almost lifted off the base support, but without quite losing floor contact. By continuing movement the lower left leg is flexionally suspended from the thigh at the knee joint, the thigh is flexionally suspended from the pelvis in the hip joint, and the pelvis is in its turn suspended abductionally from the right thigh at the right hip joint and left-concave lateroflexionally from the thorax in the spinal region. The left leg has gone into free play.

Reactio: Change in the Support Area

In a primary movement to the right, the support area expands just a very little to the right, but is dramatically reduced by the near-lifting of the left sole or toes off the floor.

Actio: Accelerating Weights
Reactio: Braking Weights

In the starting position, the potential bisecting plane is identical with the patient's plane of symmetry, which is vertical. In a primary movement to the right, the bisecting plane shifts to the right and, when the left leg has gone into free play, goes roughly through the functional long axis of the right foot. All weights to the right of the bisecting plane have an accelerating effect on the movement sequence, while those to the left slow it down.

- **Conditio – Limitatio of the Movement Sequence**

Conditio: Constant Distances Between Body Distance Points
Limitatio: Active Buttressing and Stabilization
Conditio: The distance between DP xiphoid process and DP right/left iliac spine remains constant.
Limitatio: If this distance remains constant, in a primary movement to the right BSs thorax and arms will also move right, and unwanted activated passive buttressing by the thorax slipping to the left will be avoided.

Conditio: The distance between DP jugular notch and DP right/left earlobe remains constant.
Limitatio: If this distance remains constant, in a primary movement to the right the head will also move right, and unwanted activated passive buttressing by the head translating to the left will be avoided.

Conditio of Absolute and/or Relative Fixed Spatial Points
Limitatio by Limiting the Primary Movement, Activated Passive Buttressing and/or Change in the Support Area
Clip-Clop has both absolute and relative fixed spatial points.

Conditio: The points of contact soles or toes/floor are absolute fixed spatial points.
Limitatio: This means that the width of the track in the starting position is kept the same throughout the movement sequence. This checks the extent of the primary movement, and the foot in free play does not move along in the direction of the movement as if preparing to take a step.

Conditio: The point of contact ball of the big toe of the supporting leg/floor is an absolute fixed spatial point.
Limitatio: If the ball of the big toe of the supporting leg keeps its contact with the base support and allows no reduction of pressure, the pronational active buttressing of the primary movement is accentuated and the muscular bracing of the long arch of the supporting foot intensified.

Conditio: The supporting knee joint may not move backwards or against the direction of movement.
Limitatio: This relative fixed spatial point guarantees optimal fall-preventing activity by the vastus medialis muscle and economical stressing of the ligaments of the knee joint.

Conditio: The malleoli of the supporting foot may not move either laterally or medially.
Limitatio: This relative fixed spatial point stabilizes the malleolar arch over the talus by eliminating lateral movement, supports the concentration of pressure under the ball of the big toe in the supporting phase, and markedly activates the medial triceps surae. By eliminating medial movement it prevents the arch in the

351

supporting leg from flattening as a result of increased eversion in the subtalar and calcaneonavicular joints.

Conditio: The line connecting the right and left iliac spines remains horizontal. It may only perform a parallel shift to the right or left.
Limitatio: This relative fixed point will be maintained if, during the shift to the right or left, the adduction in the hip joint is effected only by the distal lever. This way, the vertical long axis of the body also undergoes parallel shifting to the right or left, without lateroflexion in the lumbar spine.

Conditio of Movement Speed
Limitatio of Economical Activity by Finding the Optimal Speed

Conditio: Clip-Clop requires a brisk speed. We start with the pace of normal gait, 120 load-shifts per minute, and speed up to twice that rate.
Limitatio: The pace of normal gait permits the lowest intensity of economical activity, because it is unhurried yet fast enough that one needn't balance too long on one leg nor lift the free-play leg entirely off the base support. Thus, the right–left displacements of the long axis of the body remain small (about 2–3 cm). The more the tempo is speeded up, the higher the intensity of economical activity. This is desirable as a training effect. The long axis of the body shifts laterally less and less with the alternating weight displacements, and in the end ceases to shift at all.

▶ Instruction in Patient Language

● Instruction Appealing to the Patient's Perception

The fact that the gaze is directed forwards and the ventral aspects of BSs pelvis and thorax face forwards is a useful aid to awareness of the vertical position of the long axis of the body and the potential mobility of the pelvis and head when the thoracic spine is dynamically stabilized in neutral position. By placing one hand on his abdomen and the other on his thorax, the patient can easily feel what is happening during the primary movements. A conscious awareness of his knees and feet pointing slightly outwards will emphasize the location-constancy of this exercise even when the movement is performed rapidly.

● Verbal Instruction   ● Instruction by Manipulation

Position and Activation in the Starting Position

"Stand upright with your legs fairly wide apart. Face straight ahead. Your stomach and chest are facing straight ahead too. Your knees face out to the

The patient will have to practice assuming the starting position a few times. Any hyperactivity in BSs pelvis, thorax and head will have to be reduced until

sides a little, but not more than your feet do. Now let the upright tower of your body sink down into its knees a bit, as if you were sitting down on a high barstool."

breathing returns to normal, but the dynamic stabilization in the thoracic spine must not thereby be lost. The patient must try out the potential mobility for flexion/extension of the pelvis in the hip joints and the joints of the lumbar spine. During hip and knee flexion, particular attention should be given to the alignment of the axes of the feet and legs.

Actio and Conditio of the Movement Sequence

"You feel you have very strong legs. You're standing there with your legs wide apart. Your toes and your knees point in exactly the same direction. You're more strongly aware of the floor under your forefeet than under your heels. Your toes are open fans. Your body is upright and long. You don't feel any tension in your abdomen. Your breathing comes all by itself. Lean your hands gently on your pelvis and feel your body swaying very gently in the hip joints. Now your legs get lively. Alternating rapidly, you push first one sole then the other against the floor. You don't need to lift either leg off the floor. Just keep pushing them down, faster and faster; 'clip clop' go your feet. It sounds like a drum roll. You start breathing faster; you'd better whistle. When your legs get tired, you simply stop, straighten your knees and wait until the tiredness has subsided. Afterwards you feel a pleasant tingling in your legs. That's good. Now start from the beginning again. Go up on tiptoe once or twice, without straightening your knees. You can even try doing Clip-Clop on your toes; that will make your calves work too."

If the patient has weak knee extensors or even pain in his knees, we will make do with just a slight knee and hip flexion – just enough to ensure that the quadriceps are activated. Patients with foot problems should perform the exercise with shoes on. The movements make great demands on the feet; the therapist should make sure beforehand that the arches of the feet are activated, and if necessary help the patient become aware of this activation by preliminary exercises. It is important that the knees always face outwards over the long axes of the feet and that the weight is not carried only on the lateral borders of the feet. The best way to do this is to tell the patient to take the pressure off the balls of his little toes when he points his knees out to the sides.

▶ Adapting the Exercise to the Patient's Constitution and Condition

● Adaptation to Constitution: Role of Lengths, Widths, Depths and Distribution of Weights

One relatively frequent constitutional problem is that the patient's greater trochanters and iliac spines are wide apart but the frontotransverse diameter of his thorax and his shoulders are narrow. Depending on the patient, the therapist may allow or even direct translation of BSs thorax, head and arms to the right in relation to the pelvis during a primary movement to the right.

● Adaptation to Condition

Poor Physical Fitness or Wish to Increase Performance

To train the axes of the feet and legs to bear stress, a maximum increase in speed and a pattern of 30 seconds exercise, 30 seconds rest is recommended.

If the exercise is performed on the toes, the distance from the heels to the floor can be varied, but it must stay the same during each movement sequence.

A good small-scale exercise is to rapidly alternate between standing on the soles to standing on the toes, by fulcrum displacement of the flexion/extension axes of the talocrural joints forwards/upwards and backwards/downwards, keeping the knees and hips flexed. The same exercise can also be performed alternately by the right and by the left foot, or by both together but moving in opposition to each other. This demands positive and negative lift of particularly the triceps. To increase the strain on the quadriceps, the flexion in the knee and hip joints should be increased. The long axis of the body, however, must always remain vertical.

Pain Arising During the Exercise a Contraindication

If patients with patellar chondropathy experience pain during or after this exercise for stress training of the quadriceps, they should stop the exercise. The same goes for patients with arthritis or fractures or ligamentous lesions in the area of the knee. In such patients, training of the quadriceps will have to be carried out under conditions of reduced lift.

5.6.4 Short and Sharp

"Short and Sharp" is a name we invented to characterize the small, precisely defined hand movements this exercise requires.

■ Goal of the Exercise

The goal is for the patient to be able to activate strongly the abdominal, back and neck muscles reactively and selectively, lift-free and with reduced lift, using small accelerating and braking arm movements.

▶ Functional Analysis in Therapist Language

● Conception of the Exercise

This exercise represents a treatment technique that can be employed often. The following selected examples show how it is used to selectively utilize the multitudinous functional possibilities of the abdominal, back and neck muscles.

Path Through Space of the Critical Distance Points
The critical distance points must be on the hand, because it is at its outermost point that the inherently mobile system of the arm, with its more than 30 articulating skeletal parts, is best able to follow a precise, specific path through space in any one of many directions.
The path traced by critical distance points through space should be about 20 cm long. To ensure that it is a straight path, none of the joints must be allowed to reach end-stop, because that can very quickly deflect the movement out of its prescribed direction.

Accelerating and Halting the Movements
The acceleration and halting of the movements trigger reactive activation of the abdominal, back and neck muscles. Without stabilization in the spinal column, the arm cannot perform swift straight movements at all, because the shoulder girdle needs a stabilized thorax in order to gain the necessary purchase and avoid a whiplash effect. The abdominal, back and neck muscles are activated in continuing movement and active buttressing. The arm movement is halted because the stipulated straight path is checked. Since end-stop movements are not allowed, the movements are halted by active buttressing. Because this has to happen suddenly, there is often a rebound movement, an avoidance mechanism which can destroy the entire stabilizing effect. The patient will need careful instruction if he is to learn these short accelerating and halting movements.

Vigorous Reduced-Lift Activation of the Abdominal, Back and Neck Muscles
In the starting position the spinal column is roughly in neutral. Activation of all the spinal muscles takes place without any movement excursions in the joints. This protects the passive structures. The not-moving, or rather the stabilization, which affects agonists and antagonists, is automatic only because the movement of the arm is swift and therefore the activation of the muscles powerful.

Direction of the Arm Movements

Because the movements are accelerating, gravity is of no particular significance to the direction of movement. This direction is roughly perpendicular to the movement axes of the spinal column and is determined by the lie of the fibres in the targeted muscles. For preference, the movement should take place within the patient's field of vision and the critical distance points should be a comfortable distance from BSs pelvis, thorax and head. The targeted group of abdominal, back and neck muscles to be activated are assigned the task of providing active buttressing.

● Position and Activation in the Starting Position

Short and Sharp can performed in any starting position desired. However, it is advisable to have the spinal column in neutral position, i.e. to constitute the virtual long axis of the body in the optimum way. It is also a good idea to first practice the exercise with the long axis of the body vertical. Figures 109a and 90a show good starting positions.

● Actio – Reactio of the Movement Sequence

Actio: The Primary Movement

Since the movement is small and the weight of the arms very light in relation to the total weight of the body, and since the acceleration means that the effect of gravity is only of relevance in the starting position, activated passive buttressing and changes in the support area are for the purposes of our analysis unimportant.

● Conditio – Limitatio of the Movement Sequence

Conditio: Constant Distances Between Body Distance Points
Limitatio: Active Buttressing and Stabilization

In Short and Sharp, the conditio of keeping constant distances between body distance points and the limitatio in the form of active buttressing are fulfilled reactively because of the acceleration of the primary movements.
The following is a list of frequently used exercises.

Exercise 1

Targeted actively buttressing muscles: Ventral tract of the straight rectus abdominis muscle.
Accelerated and halted primary movement: DPs right and left hands accelerate symmetrically upwards, about 20 cm in front of the ventral aspects of BSs pelvis and thorax, starting a little below the horizontal transverse plane through the navel. The thumbs touch the tip of the third fingers as if forming a tube. The wrists are in extension and the flexion/extension axes are vertical.
Muscles activated by the continuing effect: Back extensors.

Exercise 2

Targeted actively buttressing muscles: Back extensors
Accelerated and halted primary movement: DPs right and left hands accelerate symmetrically downwards, about 20 cm in front of the ventral aspects of BSs pelvis

and thorax, starting roughly in the horizontal transverse plane through the fronto-transverse diameter of the thorax.

Muscles activated by the continuing effect: Ventral tract of the straight rectus abdominis muscle.

Exercise 3

Targeted actively buttressing muscles: Oblique tracts of the abdominal muscles.

Accelerated and halted primary movement: For the muscles running from right/below/in front to left/above/in front, we take DP left palm as critical distance point. This distance point starts at an angle of about 45° to the horizontal midtransverse plane, facing to the right/backwards/upwards. At a comfortable distance to the ventral aspects of BSs pelvis and thorax, it moves from right/below to left/above, crossing the plane of symmetry.

Muscles activated by the continuing effect: Oblique tracts of the back muscles from left/above/behind to right/below/behind.

For the muscles running diagonally from left/below to right/above, the opposite holds. Here the critical distance point will be DP right palm, facing left/backwards/upwards.

Exercise 4

Targeted actively buttressing muscles: Oblique tracts of the back muscles.

Accelerated and halted primary movement: For the muscles running from left/above/behind to right/below/behind, we take DP left palm as critical distance point. This distance point starts at an angle of 45° to the horizontal midtransverse plane, facing right/backwards/upwards. At a comfortable distance to the ventral aspects of BSs pelvis and thorax, it moves in a frontal plane from left/above to right/below, crossing the plane of symmetry.

Muscles activated by the continuing effect: Oblique tracts of the abdominal muscles from left/above/in front to right/below/in front forwards.

For the oblique tracts of the back muscles from the right/above/behind to left/below/behind, the opposite holds. Here the critical distance point will be DP right palm, facing left/backwards/upwards.

Exercise 5

Targeted actively buttressing muscles: Lateral muscle tracts that lateroflex the spinal column.

Accelerated and halted primary movement: For the muscle tracts on the left side that effect left-concave lateroflexion in the lumbar and thoracic spine, we take DP left hand as critical distance point. At the start this is positioned in a grasp, with the thumb touching the third finger. The wrist is in extension with its flexion/extension axis vertical. The hand is in the vertically positioned sagittal plane of the left shoulder joint, at about the level of the midtransverse plane, which is horizontal. The accelerated and halted primary movement of DP left hand is directed upwards. For the muscle tracts on the right side that effect right-concave lateroflexion in the lumbar spine and thoracic spine, the primary movement of the left hand is downwards.

Muscles activated by the continuing effect: When DP left hand moves upwards, these are the lateroflexors on the right side. When it moves downwards, they are the ipsilateral lateroflexors.

NB: For rhythmic stabilization of the flexor/extensor muscle tracts, the respective primary movements can be performed as a to-and-fro movement.
For rhythmic stabilization of the oblique ventral and dorsal muscle tracts, the primary movements of the left and right hand can be performed simultaneously and symmetrically.
For rhythmic stabilization of the lateroflexional muscle tracts, the primary movements of the left or right hand can be performed as a to-and-fro movement; or, to increase the active buttressing and the continuing effect, the left and right hands can perform their movements simultaneously and counter-rotationally.

Conditio of Movement Speed
Limitatio of Economical Activity by Finding the Optimal Speed
In the early learning stages the patient has to learn the extent of the movement by conscious perception before speeding it up. Even during this slow learning phase, enough time should be allowed to carry out the halt properly. The acceleration is at its best when powerful reactive muscle activation can be seen. If the movement is being repeated, each movement – including the halt – should take 1 second, of which the movement itself should take about 10% and the halt about 90%.

5.6.5 Hocus-Pocus (Figs. 110 and 111)

Hocus-Pocus is an invented name, indicating that by accelerating some parts of the body we can make others appear lighter than they are.

■ Goal of the Exercise

The goal is for the patient, using small accelerated and halted movements of some parts of his body, to learn to reduce lifting stress in other parts, increase his lifting strength, or to compensate for weakness in lifting.

▶ Functional Analysis in Therapist Language

● Conception of the Exercise

The technique in Hocus-Pocus is used all the time in normal motor behaviour. In physiotherapy patients, however, it often appears in the form of a harmful avoidance mechanism that can considerably aggravate already existing deficits.

In movement sequences with predominantly vertical direction components, the entire weight of the body or of parts of the body has to be lifted or lowered with braking activity. Depending on the movement sequence, positive or negative lift is demanded of different joints. If the strain is too much for a given joint, the familiar injuries due to overstressing occur. However, it is possible to utilize the weight of an arm or leg by carefully planned acceleration in order to relieve stress on the affected joint or weak muscles. This "technique" can have a harmful effect if the accelerated weight is too small or too large, i. e. if the goal is under- or over-shot. The therapist using this technique must plan the movement analytically and practise it without risk to the patient. The following points should be remembered:

- To lift one part-weight of the body with the help of another, we can accelerate the latter – the auxiliary weight – upwards. However, we can also think in terms of a set of beam scales in the body, and lift one part by lowering and possibly accelerating another downwards as a counterweight.
   In the lifting itself, the horizontal direction component should be kept as small as possible. This component depends on the type of joint being relieved and on the length of the lever being mobilized.
   If we work with the scales system, it is helpful if the auxiliary weight is horizontal.
- The smaller the available auxiliary weight, the faster the acceleration must be.
- If we want to compensate for poor or absent lifting strength in a muscle, the direction of movement of the accelerating weight is determined by the optimal form of the movement sequence; for example, to make the bottom move upwards/forwards in rising from a chair, the arms should similarly be moved upwards/forwards. In this way, avoidance mechanisms are prevented before they start.

Example 1
Getting up from a chair with relief of stress on the knee or on a compromised quadriceps by accelerating the arms upwards (see *Functional Kinetics*, p. 132).

Example 2 (Fig. 110)
Sitting up from sidelying using the scales system keeping the spinal column in roughly neutral position, to relieve stress on insufficient abdominal and back muscles and protect the passive structures of the spinal column.

Starting position: Left sidelying. BSs pelvis, thorax and head are aligned in the horizontal long axis of the body. The thighs are flexed to 90° in the hip joints, the lower legs flexed slightly more than 90° in the knee joints. The knee joints project somewhat over the long edge of the treatment bench.

Body part of be lifted: BSs pelvis, thorax and head, constituting the long axis of the body, are to be brought vertical.

Auxiliary weight to be accelerated horizontally and downwards: Right (upper) leg.

Pivot support of the scale beam: Long axis of the left thigh.

Bolster of the movement sequence: Arms, which coordinate their pushing off with the caudal/downward acceleration of the weight of the right leg to bring the weight of BSs pelvis, thorax and head to shoulder height.

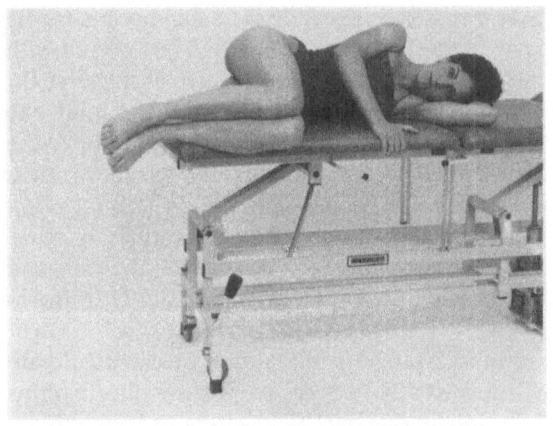

a

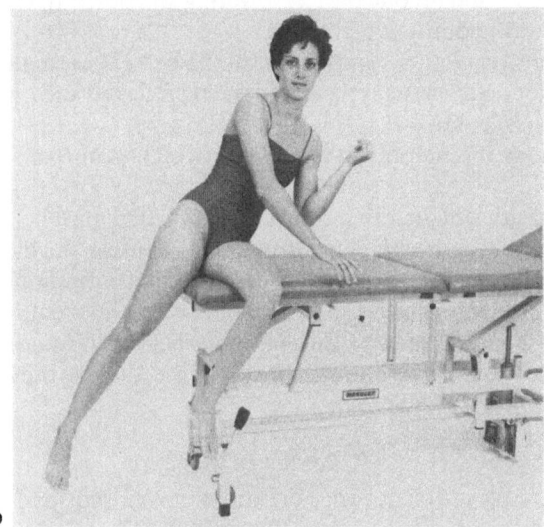

b

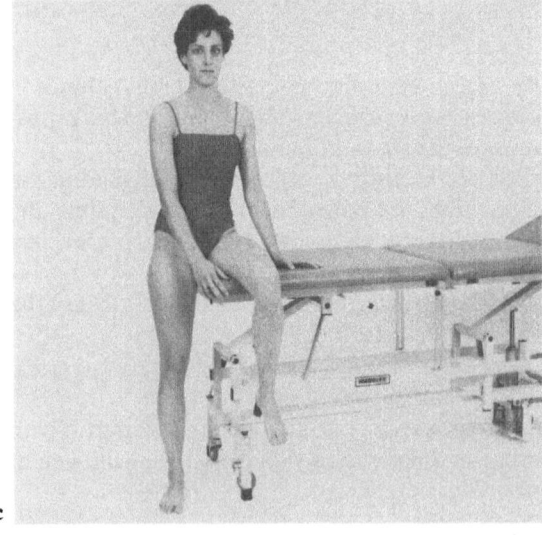

c

Fig. 110 a–c. Hocus-Pocus. Sitting up from sidelying, beam-scale system. **a** Starting position, **b** middle of the movement, **c** end position

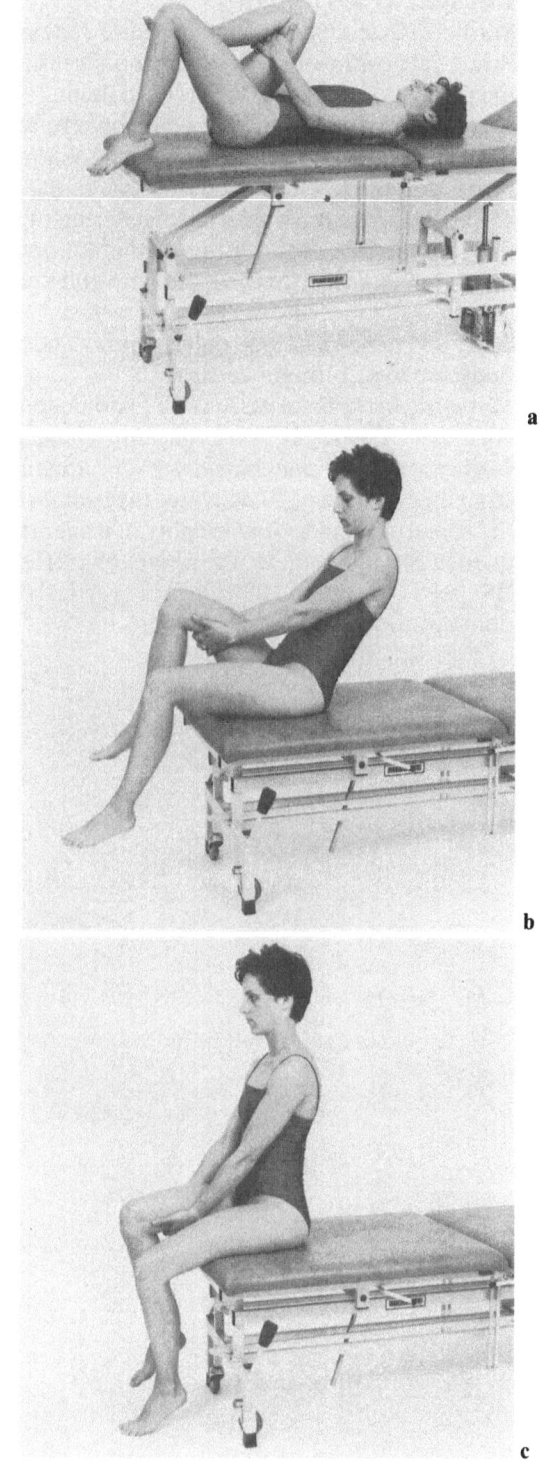

Fig. 111 a–c. Hocus-Pocus. Sitting up from supine, beam-scale system. **a** Starting position, **b** middle of the movement, **c** end position

Example 3 (Fig. 111)

Sitting up from supine using the scales system keeping the spinal column in roughly neutral position, to relieve stress on insufficient abdominal muscles and protect the passive structures of the spinal column.

Starting position: Supine in bed or on a treatment bench. BSs pelvis, thorax and head are aligned in the horizontal long axis of the body.

In BS legs, the left heel is on the edge of the bed. The left thigh is flexed to about 45° in the hip joint. By fulcrum displacement the knee is in about 125° flexion. The forefoot projects out over the edge of the bed. In BS arms, the folded hands clasp the right thigh close to the knee. Hip and knee joints are in extreme but comfortable flexion.

Body part to be lifted: BSs pelvis, thorax and head, constituting the long axis of the body, are to be brought vertical.

Pivot support of the scale beam: Flexion/extension axis of the hip joints.

Auxiliary weight to be accelerated horizontal and downwards: Left leg.

Bolster of the movement sequence: The arms and the weight of the right leg hanging from them. This weight activates the back extensors and thus makes it possible for the spinal column to stay roughly in its neutral position during the movement sequence. Simultaneously, the weight of the flexed leg pulls the inherently stabilized BSs pelvis, thorax and head into the vertical position with reduced stress on the abdominal muscles.

6 Tips, Insights, Hypotheses

Pain is a necessary signal to the patient. It is the body's way of saying, "Understand me, learn how to deal with me." There is no virtue in putting up with pain, and no reward. To learn to understand it, to try to reduce it or avoid it altogether is absolutely normal. If pain persists even during truly lift-free mobilization of the spinal column, movement is contraindicated.

Teaching a patient a carefully and precisely planned movement sequence can only succeed if the patient is able to consciously perceive the changes in position of the distance points in relation to space and to his own body and can translate these directly into movement.

It is the fine differentiations (conditio) and restrictions (limitatio) that make movement economical.

Whenever possible, the therapist should always try to have the critical distance point of any movement sequence move in a straight line. This makes it considerably easier for the patient to learn. To achieve this straight path, the distance points of the joints participating in the movement must move in effortlessly curving paths to ensure optimum coordination.

The fine differentiations in a movement sequence ensure that all the stress is never concentrated on one spot.

The more the differentiating conditios in a movement sequence, the clearer the dominant direction of movement becomes, until, ultimately, the various partial buttressings are integrated into one continuing flow of movement. The more a movement sequence becomes integrated into the normal movement pattern, the more natural the conditio-imposed differentiation appears – indeed, this differentiation is the very cause of ease of movement. This is why economical activity is easy for any patient once it is learnt, while for the therapist using the functional analytical approach it always remains complex.

To analyse movement always means to differentiate, to break down. To instruct always means to reassemble, to summarize, to discover signals that speak to the patient and call into action his natural capacity for coordination.

7 Glossary

Actio
In a movement sequence, the *actio* is the primary movement; it leads to the movement goal and dominates the patient's awareness. The *actio* displaces weights in the direction of movement; if it includes horizontal components, it has an accelerating effect on the movement.

Active insufficiency
A muscle is actively insufficient if it is unable to contract sufficiently to actively fix, in the end-stopped position, the levers, pointers or gliding bodies of the switchpoint it bridges.

Activity state
The multiplicity of possible postures and movements and their position in space under the influence of gravity demands different states of activity of the musculature. When we have defined these various activity states, we are in a position when analysing posture and movement to identify them, relate them to particular body segments, name them, and bring them about.

Angle of the body diagonals
The caudal or cranial angle formed where the body diagonals cross.

Antetorsion, angle of
If you lay a femur on a table, its neck points inwards/upwards. The angle formed between the axis of the femoral neck and the axis of the femoral condyles is the angle of antetorsion.

Avoidance mechanisms, avoidance movements
Uneconomical, unwanted continuing movements deviating out of the direction of movement, changes in the support area, or buttressing of continuing movements.

Axis of movement
The place at which levers and pointers rotate, i.e. the place at which movements of the joints take place.

Base plane
Transverse plane tangential to the soles of the feet.

Basic gait test
Test which may be carried out during the assessment of the functional status in order to analyse limping mechanisms.

Bridging activity
When, in any body posture or movement, the support area is determined by more than one point of

	contact between body and base support, the body segments or parts of them which provide the contact with the base supports form bridges with their neighbouring body segments. The muscle activity which braces the arch of this bridge is called bridging activity.
Body diagonal	Line connecting the midpoint of one hip with the midpoint of the contralateral shoulder.
Body segment	Each functional body segment has several levels of movement, whose motor behaviour may be regarded as a functional unit.
Buttressing mobilization	Buttressing mobilization of a joint always concentrates on a single fulcrum. The buttressing must take place in the fulcrum itself. In this way it becomes possible to exhaust the movement tolerance up to end-stop. This mobilization should if possible be performed lift-free, or at least with reduced lift.
Buttressing of continuing movement	Limitation of a continuing movement by counterweighting, counteractivity or countermovement.
Buttressing of continuing movement, activated passive	Automatic engagement of muscle activity to adjust the lever arm(s) of the counterweight of a primary movement to the length needed. Buttressing a continuing movement with a counterweight is an automatic equilibrium reaction. The counterweight works against the horizontal component of the primary movement and has a braking effect upon it.
Buttressing of continuing movement, active	Buttressing of continuing movement by antagonistic muscle activity.
Buttressing of continuing movement, passive	Purely passive buttressing rarely occurs, because the parts of the body used for the buttressing are inherently mobile.
Caudal/caudally	'Caudal' indicates position and means 'on the feet or the part containing the feet'; 'caudally' indicates direction and means 'towards the feet or in the direction in which the feet point'.
Cervical kyphosis	Kyphosis in the area of the upper thoracic and lower cervical spine, which involves stiffness of these parts of the vertebral column and has an unfavourable effect on the postural statics of the head. Also called 'neck kyphosis'.
Concentric isotonic	Describes active contraction of a muscle.
Conditio	In a movement sequence, the *conditio* is the sum of the conditions which make define the movement finely and precisely. The patient must be conscious of the *conditio* and this will make it easier for him to perform movements with precision.

Condition	The influence which a patient's social position and psychic and somatic state have upon his motor behaviour.
Constant-location movement	Describes movement sequences in which either the support area does not change at all or changes take place only within the support area.
Constitution	The influence which the lengths, widths, depths and weights of a patient's body segments have upon his motor behaviour.
Continuing movement	When any given point on the body is moved by a movement impulse in a particular direction and movement excursions occur at neighbouring joints which help to bring about this movement, a continuing movement has taken place.
Cranial/cranially	'Cranial' indicates position and means 'on the head or the part containing the head'; 'cranially' indicates direction and means 'towards the head or in the direction in which the head points'.
Degree of freedom	One way in which a lever, pointer or gliding body can move to and fro at its joint connection. Each degree of freedom has two components of movement.
Detorsion	The normal process of reduction of the natal angle of antetorsion during development to adulthood.
Distal/proximal	These terms relate to the functional centrepoint of the body. 'Distal' means 'further from the body's centrepoint', proximal means 'closer to the body's centrepoint'.
Distance points	The distance points of a joint movement are the furthest points on levers and pointers from the axis of movement.
Eccentric isotonic	Describes active extension of a muscle.
Effectors	From the functional point of view, muscles are effectors of posture and movement. They can act as lifters and movers of weights, as brakes on falling weights, and as preventers of weights from falling.
End-stop, end-stopping	Limitation of joint mobility by the passive structures of the movement apparatus.
Equilibrium reaction	When displacement of the centre of gravity threatens a person's equilibrium, reactions using counter-weighting, counteractivity, countermovement and/or a change in the support area ensure that the equilibrium is maintained.
Extensional activity	Activity of the muscles normally involved in extension at a joint.
Flexional activity	Activity of the muscles normally involved in flexion at a joint.

366

Free play function	Activity state which arises when an extremity is proximally suspended from the body and can move its distal end freely.
Frontal plane	Any number of parallel planes can be positioned between the front and back sides of the homunculus' cube. Where they cut the homunculus they divide him into a ventral and a dorsal part. All these planes are frontal. They relate to the body and not to space.
Frontosagittal axes	Lines of intersection of the frontal and sagittal planes of the body which pass through the centre of the joints of the vertebral column and proximal extremities.
Frontotransverse axes	Lines of intersection of the frontal and transverse planes of the body which pass through the centre of the joints of the vertebral column and proximal extremities.
Functional centrepoint of the body	Point of intersection of the two body diagonals.
Functional kinetics	Technique of direct observation and analysis of human posture and movement.
Hanging activity	Activity state which arises when the whole body or particular body segments or parts of segments hang from a suspension device; traction occurs at the joints involved.
Horizontal plane	A plane relating to space. When a person stands upright, his transverse planes are horizontal; on his back or his stomach, his frontal planes are horizontal; on his side, his sagittal planes are horizontal.
Isometric	Describes muscle activity which prevents possible movements: the length of the active muscle does not change.
Lift-free movement	Movement which does not require the parts of the body involved to be lifted against gravity.
Limitatio	In a movement sequence, the *limitatio* is the effect of the *conditio*.
Location-changing movement	Describes movement sequences in which the whole movement system of the inherently mobile human body moves to another place and has a new support area.
Long axis of the body	Line of intersection between the plane of symmetry and the midfrontal plane. It passes through the body's centrepoint and the vertex.
Lumbar kyphosis	Kyphotic alteration of the vertebral column at the lumbosacral junction. It may extend as far as the lower thoracic spine. A distinction is made between

structural and functional lumbar kyphoses; the latter disappear when the ischiocrural musculature is relaxed. A lumbar kyphosis has a bad influence on posture and is often the cause of loss of potential mobility of the pelvis at the hip and lumbar vertebral joints.

Midfrontal plane	Frontal plane which passes through the body's centrepoint.
Midtransverse plane	Transverse plane which passes through the body's centrepoint.
Mobile	Body segment which, in a given posture or movement, is predominantly potentially mobile.
Mobility	The extent of passive and active movement tolerance at the joints.
Neck kyphosis	*See* Cervical kyphosis.
Observation criterion	A feature which has been isolated by systematic observation and manipulation of the human body at rest and in motion, and which helps to differentiate the pathological from the normal.
Observer's bisecting plane	This is the vertical plane of symmetry of the eyes of the observer, projected until it meets the patient, bisecting him into a right and a left part. If the observer aligns her bisecting plane with the patient's centre of gravity, she can assess the potential accelerating and braking weights of the patient's body in movement in a direction at right angles to the bisecting plane.
Observer's horizontal plane	This is the horizontal transverse plane through the eyes of the observer, projected forwards until it meets the patient, dividing him into an upper and a lower part.
Observer's parallel plane	This is the vertical frontal plane through the eyes of the observer, displaced forwards in a parallel movement until it meets the patient. It enables one to judge actual distances on the patient's body and make comparisons between them.
Observer's planes	The observer's planes help the therapist to avoid being misled by perspective in her optical perception of the patient. The observer's eyes must be horizontal and their plane of symmetry vertical.
Parking function	Activity state present in a body segment or part of it which is in contact with a base support and exerts on this only the pressure of its own weight.
Passive insufficiency	A muscle is passively insufficient if it cannot be stretched far enough to allow levers, pointers or gliding bodies at the level of movement it bridges to move until end-stopped.

Plane of symmetry	Sagittal plane through the body's centrepoint, also called the median or midsagittal plane.
Plane of the vertex	Transverse plane tangential to the vertex.
PNF pattern fist	Closed fist as in the PNF pattern, with flexion of all joints of the fingers and palmar flexion of the wrist.
PNF open hand	Open hand as in the PNF pattern, with extension of all joints of the fingers and dorsiflexion of the wrist.
Potential mobility	Activity state: Readiness of muscles to respond to stimulation with movement, i. e. with changes in the position of the joints.
Pressure activity	Activity state: Muscle activity which increases the pressure exerted by a body at a point of contact with a base support. Pressure activity causes compression at the joints involved.
Primary movement	The initial movement towards the stated movement goal.
Proximal/distal	*See* Distal/proximal
Pushing off activity	Muscle activity which makes use of a point of contact between the body and a base support or supportive device to achieve a purposive thrust.
Reactio	In a movement sequence, the *reactio* is the name given to the automatic equilibrium reactions which arise in response to the primary movement or *actio*.
Reduced-lift movement	Movement in which as little as possible of the weights of the body is lifted against gravity.
Sagittal plane	Any number of parallel planes can be positioned between the left and right sides of the homunculus' cube. Where they cut the homunculus, they divide him into a right lateral and a left lateral part. All these planes are sagittal. They relate to the body and not to space.
Sagittotransverse axes	Lines of intersection of the sagittal and transverse planes of the body which pass through the centre of the joints of the vertebral column and proximal extremities.
Stabile	Body segment which, in a given posture or movement, is predominantly stabilized.
Stabilization	Activity state: Muscular fixation of one or more joints in a given position.
Statics, postural	The influence which a patient's posture has on his motor apparatus with regard to stress.
Support area	The smallest area which includes all the points of contact between activated body segments and their base support.
Supported leaning activity	Activity state which, when the body is leaning against a supportive device, arises in the braced muscles on the side of the body facing the support.

Supporting function	Activity state which arises when one of the extremities is in contact with a base support and exerts more pressure on it than is due to its own weight.
Switchpoint of movement	This term emphasizes how, in functional kinetics, the interest in the joint is that it is the place at which movements occur through changes in the position of levers, pointers and gliding bodies.
Transverse plane	Any number of parallel planes may be positioned between the base plane and the plane of the vertex of the homunculus' cube, each dividing him into a cranial and a caudal part. All these planes are transverse. They relate to the body and not to space.
Vertex	Point of intersection of the plane of symmetry, the midfrontal plane and the plane of the vertex.
Virtual body axes	These are axes which exist only in the imagination but which, within the inherently mobile system of the body, are brought into being by maintenance of a particular posture. Thus the long axis of the body is formed by a particular arrangement of the pelvis, thorax and head, or the long axis of the foot is that (imaginary) one about which the foot arcs when twisting from resting on the medial to resting on the lateral border. By contrast, for instance, the long axis of the thigh is a real and unchangeable axis.

8 Addendum: Selective Muscle Training in Klein-Vogelbach's Functional Kinetics

The following concerns the now widely discussed concepts of "selective muscle training" and "selective use of muscles" that come from Klein-Vogelbach's Functional Kinetics and deserve special attention in physiotherapy. The theory behind them is explained in the training courses "Selective Training of the Abdominal and Back Muscles" and "Selective Training of the Muscles of the Extremities", and they are employed in practical physiotherapy. These concepts are of great help in the analysis of movement.

There are many different kinds of selection:

1. Selection of whether a muscle is to lift weights (i.e. move them upwards), or lower weights with braking activity (i.e. move them downwards), or shift weights horizontally (i.e. right/left/forwards/backwards while remaining upright), or hold weights (i.e. prevent them from falling).

Example for the Quadriceps Muscle
Lifting weights: Standing up from kneeling (moving weight upwards).
Lowering weights with braking activity: Kneeling down (moving weight downwards).
Shifting weights horizontally: In sidelying with knee and hip joints in 90° flexion, moving the knees footwards/backwards or the feet abdomen-wards/headwards.
Holding weights: Standing on one leg with the knee not locked in extension (quadriceps activity works against the tendency of the knee joint to give way, i.e. it exerts fall-preventing activity).

2. Selection of whether particular muscles should be stressed with the weights of body parts or with outside weights.

Example for the Triceps Brachii
Stressing with body weights: The positive and negative lifting performed by the triceps during press-ups.
Stressing with outside weights: The positive and negative lifting performed by the triceps in raising a weight with the arms.

3. Selection of whether particular muscles should, by linking the weights of parts of the body appropriately, increase or reduce the force exerted by the weight of the body at its points of contact with the environment: the pressure exerted by the weight of the body at its points of contact with a base support, the pull exerted by

the weight of the body at its points of contact with a suspension device, or the body's tendency to slip at its points of contact with a supportive device against which it is leaning.

Example 1
Sitting upright. By supporting oneself on one's arms, BSs pelvis, thorax and head can be suspended from the shoulder girdle by the activity of the latissimus dorsi, pectoralis and trapezius muscles. This leads to an increase of pressure at contact points palms/seat and a reduction of pressure at contact points right and left ischial tuberosity/seat.

Example 2
Environment as a base support: When a patient is lying in as comfortable a position as possible on a treatment bench, all body segments are in parking function, the activity state at which the intensity of economical activity is at its lowest.
Environment as a supportive device: In leaning back against a wall at shoulder level, the extensors of the hip joints and lumbar and thoracic spine are activated in bridging activity.
Environment as a suspension device: In sitting on a high treatment bench and leaning backwards, BSs head, arms, thorax and pelvis become suspended via BS legs from the front edge of the bench, with activation of the flexors of the knee joints.

4. Selection of whether to activate particular muscles by imagining nonexistent weights, resistances or pulls.

Example
Starting position: Sitting upright on a chair with footsole/floor contact. Imagining the sole of one's right foot is firmly stuck to the floor, and trying "unsuccessfully" to tear it free, activates the extensors and flexors of the toes, the dorsiflexors and plantarflexors of the ankle, the flexors and extensors of the hip joint, and the flexors and extensors of the lumbar region. Imagining one wants to move this stuck right foot forwards but is unable to do so activates the extensors and flexors of the knee joint.
The co-contractive activation of the muscles takes place because, although it would in reality be possible to perform the imagined movement of the foot on the floor, the pretence that the foot is stuck to the floor forces the antagonistic muscles to prevent the movement.

5. Selection of whether particular muscles are needed or are to be brought into play to bring about or maintain a particular activity state, e.g. free play, bridging activity or dynamic stabilization.

Example for the Gluteus Maximus
Free play: In lifting one leg out of the all-fours position, extension at the knee and hip joints.
Bridging activity: In lifting the pelvis out of supine lying with the feet propped up with their soles on the base support.

Dynamic stabilization: In performing the horizontal balance position from one-legged standing upright, extension at the hip joint connecting the "tower" and the free-play leg.

6. Selection of whether polyarthric muscles should be contracted or stretched or maintain the same length at the switchpoints they cross.

Example
For correct physiologic contraction of the abdominal muscles with economical posture and respiration when the abdominal muscles are under stress, the caudal portion of the straight and oblique muscles must be contracted and the cranial portion increase tone without contracting. Only in this way can the transverse muscle together with the oblique muscles perform the contraction.

7. Selection of whether, in the case of muscles that can activate various components of movement at a joint with more than one degree of freedom, one wishes to stress the muscles differently in regard to conditions of lift, reduced lift, or freedom from lift.

Example
When, in upright standing with the long axis of the arm sagittotransverse, the arm is moved in transverse extension/flexion and rotation, the middle portion of the deltoid performs holding work under lifting stress while the anterior and posterior portions of the deltoid perform lift-free transverse flexion/extension and rotation.

8. Selection of whether antagonistic muscles on the vertebral column that move or stabilize many joints should be made to work in different activity states.

Example
If, in the end position of Ball Exercise "The Indian Fakir", one leg is raised, the extensors of the vertebral column work in bridging activity while the weight of the raised free-play leg activates both the straight and the oblique abdominal muscles by continuing movement.

9. Selection of whether one wishes to use a quickening of movement speed to stress certain muscles heavily in order to reduce the stress on others.

Example
Standing up from a chair using small accelerated and then halted arm movements to reduce the stress on the quadriceps muscles.

10. Selection of whether or not to override insufficiency of a muscle by altering the movement speed.

Example
Sitting up from supine with accelerated arm movement to aid insufficient abdominal muscles and avoid contraction of the straight abdominal muscle in the upper abdomen.

11. Selection of whether to emphasize the motive or the compressive components of a particular muscle.

Example 1
Tremor movements of an elbow stabilized in the neutral position bring about co-contraction of the flexors and extensors of the elbow, compressing the joint.

Example 2
Boxing with the punchball trains the motive components of the flexors and extensors of the elbow joints.

12. Selection of whether to train the holding or the motive function of particular muscles.

Examples
In Therapeutic Exercise "The Snake", the muscles designed for holding function are trained in motive function.
In ballet, a pirouette trains the muscles of the supporting leg for holding function, although they are really designed for motive function.

In Functional Kinetics, What Is Meant by "Disturbed Coordination"?

In Functional Kinetics, particularly in gait training, "disturbed coordination" means exactly what it says. "Coordination" means the mutual attuning of various factors and processes; in medical terms in relation to muscle activity it means the harmonious interplay of all the muscles involved in a movement. *Functionally disturbed coordination* consists in inharmonious and therefore uneconomical interplay of muscles without irreversible neurological damage. Disturbances of coordination are thus "limping mechanisms" in reaction to gravity that bring about uneconomical interplay of fall-preventing muscles, because the muscles, in themselves healthy enough, are being subjected to inappropriate demands.

9 References and Further Reading

Benninghoff and Goerttler (1971) Lehrbuch der Anatomie des Menschen. Urban and Schwarzenberg, Munich

Bobath B (1976) Abnormal postural reflex activity caused by brain lesions, 2nd edn. Heinman, New York

Braune W, Fischer O (1985) On the centre of gravity of the human body. Springer, Berlin Heidelberg New York

Braune W, Fischer O (1987) The human gait. Springer, Berlin Heidelberg New York

Brügger and Rhonheimer (1965) Pseudoradikuläre Syndrome des Stammes. Huber, Berne

Debrunner HU (1971) AO-Gelenkmessung (Neutral-O-Methode), Längenmessung, Umfangmessung. „Dokumentation der DGOT Tübingen", Berne

Kapandji IA (1974) Physiology of the joints, vol 3: The trunk and vertebral column, 2nd edn. Churchill Livingstone, Edinburgh

Kapandji IA (1982) Physiology of the joints, vol 1: Upper limb, 2nd edn. Churchill Livingstone, Edinburgh

Kapandji IA (1987) Physiology of the joints, vol 2: Lower limb, 5th edn. Churchill Livingstone, Edinburgh

Kendall HO et al (1971) Muscles: testing and function. Willians and Wilkins, Baltimore

Klein-Vogelbach S (1990) Functional kinetics. Springer, Berlin Heidelberg New York

Klein-Vogelbach S (1991) Gangschulung zur funktionellen Bewegungslehre. Springer, Berlin Heidelberg New York (in press)

Knott M (1969) Proprioceptive neuromuscular facilitation. Hoeber-Harper, New York

Manter and Gatz (1958) Clinical neuroanatomy and neurophysiology. Davis, Philadelphia

Menschik A (1987) Biometry. Das Konstruktionsprinzip des Kniegelenks, des Hüftgelenks, der Beinlänge und der Körpergröße. Springer, Berlin Heidelberg New York

Sinclair DC (1975) An introduction to functional anatomy, 5th edn. Blackwell, Oxford

Tittel K (1974) Beschreibende und funktionelle Anatomie. Fischer, Jena

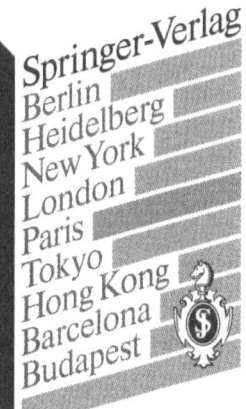

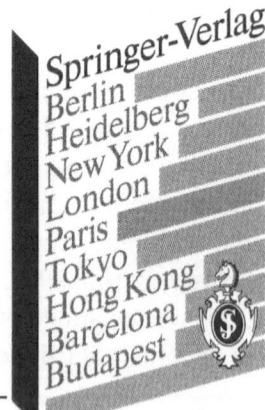